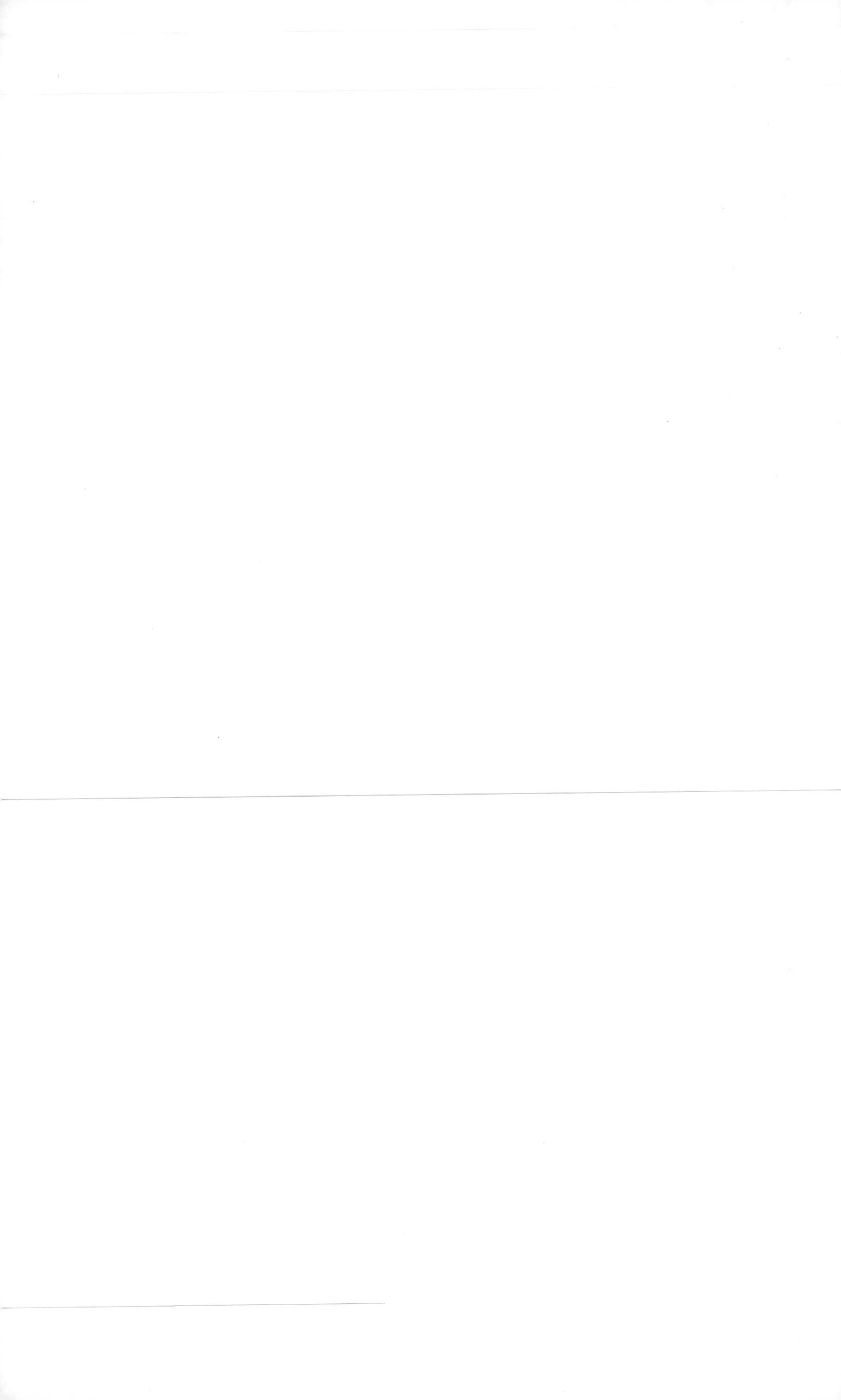

Health Informatics

(formerly Computers in Health Care)

Kathryn J. Hannah Marion J. Ball
Series Editors

Springer
New York
Berlin
Heidelberg
Barcelona
Hong Kong
London
Milan
Paris
Singapore
Tokyo

Health Informatics Series

(formerly Computers in Health Care)

Series Editors
Kathryn J. Hannah Marion J. Ball

Dental Informatics
Integrating Technology into the Dental Environment
L.M. Abbey and J. Zimmerman

Aspects of the Computer-based Patient Record
M.J. Ball and M.F. Collen

Performance Improvement Through Information Management
Health Care's Bridge to Success
M.J. Ball and J.V. Douglas

Strategies and Technologies for Healthcare Information
Theory into Practice
M.J. Ball, J.V. Douglas, and D.E. Garets

Nursing Informatics
Where Caring and Technology Meet, Third Edition
M.J. Ball, K.J. Hannah, S.K. Newbold, and J.V. Douglas

Healthcare Information Management Systems
A Practical Guide, Second Edition
M.J. Ball, D.W. Simborg, J.W. Albright, and J.V. Douglas

Clinical Decision Support Systems
Theory and Practice
E.S. Berner

Strategy and Architecture of Health Care Information Systems
M.K. Bourke

Information Networks for Community Health
P.F. Brennan, S.J. Schneider, and E. Tornquist

Introduction to Clinical Informatics
P. Degoulet and M. Fieschi

Patient Care Information Systems
Successful Design and Implementation
E.L. Drazen, J.B. Metzger, J.L. Ritter, and M.K. Schneider

Introduction to Nursing Informatics, Second Edition
K.J. Hannah, M.J. Ball, and M.J.A. Edwards

Information Technology for the Practicing Physician
J.M. Kiel

(continued after Index)

John S. Silva Marion J. Ball
Christopher G. Chute Judith V. Douglas
Curtis P. Langlotz Joyce C. Niland
William L. Scherlis
Editors

Cancer Informatics

Essential Technologies for Clinical Trials

With a Foreword by Richard D. Klausner

With 62 Illustrations

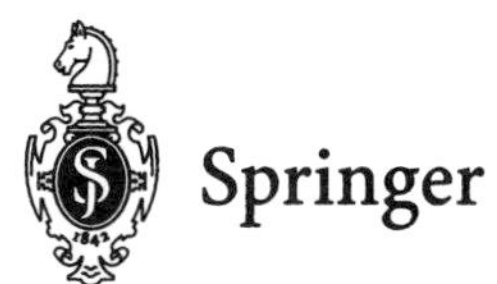

Springer

John S. Silva, MD
Center for Bioinformatics
National Cancer Institute
Eldersburg, MD 21784, USA
jc-silva-md@worldnet.att.net

Judith V. Douglas, MA, MHS
Adjunct Faculty
Johns Hopkins University
School of Nursing
Reisterstown, MD 21136, USA
judydouglas@home.com
Formerly Associate,
First Consulting Group
Faculty of Medicine
Baltimore, MD 21210, USA

William L. Scherlis, PhD
Principal Research Scientist
School of Computer Science
Carnegie Mellon University
Pittsburgh, PA 15213, USA
scherlis@cs.cmu.edu

Marion J. Ball, EdD
Vice President, Clinical Solutions
Healthlink, Inc.
Adjunct Professor
Johns Hopkins University School
of Nursing
Baltimore, MD 21210, USA
marionball@earthlink.net

Curtis P. Langlotz, MD, PhD
Assistant Professor of Radiology, Epidemiology, and Computer and Information Science
University of Pennsylvania
Moorestown, NJ 08057, USA
langlotz@rad.upenn.edu

Series Editors:
Kathryn J. Hannah, PhD, RN
Professor, Department of
Community Health Science
The University of Calgary
Calgary, Alberta, Canada
khannah@ucalgary.ca

Christopher G. Chute, MD, DrPH
Professor of Medical Informatics
Head, Section of Medical
Information Resources
Mayo Clinic
Rochester, MN 55905, USA
chute@mayo.edu

Joyce C. Niland, PhD
Chair, Division of Information
Sciences
Director, Department of Biostatistics
City of Hope National Medical Center
Duarte, CA 91010, USA
jniland@coh.org

Marion J. Ball, EdD
Vice President, Clinical Solutions
Healthlink, Inc.
Adjunct Professor
Johns Hopkins University School
of Nursing
Baltimore, MD 21210, USA
marionball@earthlink.net

Library of Congress Cataloging-in-Publication Data
Cancer informatics: essential technologies for clinical trials/editors, John S. Silva [et al.].
p.; cm. — (Health informatics)
Includes bibliographical references and index.
ISBN 0-387-95328-0 (alk. paper)
1. Cancer—Research. 2. Clinical trials. 3. Medical informatics. I. Silva, John S. II. Series.
[DNLM: 1. Neoplasms. 2. Clinical Trials—methods. 3. Medical Informatics. QZ 26.5 C215 2002]
RC267 .C363 2002
616.99'4—dc21

Printed on acid-free paper. 2001040097

Production coordinated by Chernow Editorial Services, Inc., and managed by Tim Taylor; manufacturing supervised by Joe Quatela.
Typeset by SPS Publishing Service (P) Ltd., Madras, India.
Printed and bound by Maple-Vail Book Manufacturing Group, York, PA.
Printed in the United States of America.

9 8 7 6 5 4 3 2 1

ISBN 0-387-95328-0 SPIN 10842666

Springer-Verlag New York Berlin Heidelberg
A member of BertelsmannSpringer Science+Business Media GmbH

Dedication

Here is a book dedicated to people who have experience with cancer, those who will benefit from the creation of a Cancer Informatics Infrastructure.

This book is the first to set forth this vision. To do so, it brings together a constellation of contributors who describe how information technology can improve clinical trials. It culls information from top institutions, associations, journals, and projects to explain how this informatics infrastructure can help translate cancer research into cancer care and control.

As this vision becomes real, it will accelerate knowledge about cancer, its causes, and its treatment, paralleling the creation by the National Library of Medicine, NIH, of the Clinical Trials Database, www.clinicaltrials.gov. Like that database, the Cancer Informatics Infrastructure reaches beyond basic science and its investigators to physicians and to patients, offering them resources that apply to each individual situation with its specific personal challenges.

Today, *clinicaltrials.gov* is an answer to the dilemma of what is the newest, most hopeful, available clinical trial and how to get into it. Tomorrow, the Cancer Informatics Infrastructure will join it in applying information technology to science and clinical medicine and making knowledge available to all.

Tenley E. Albright, MD
Harvard Medical School
Whitehead Biomedical Research Institute
Former Chairman, Board of Regents, National Library of Medicine

Foreword

It has become *de rigueur* to pronounce this the age of informatics in medicine and biology. Of course, at some level, this is a reflection of the larger information age that pervades so much of modern society. Despite the new automaticity of this claim, the pronouncement speaks the truth. Yet, in medicine and biology, the age of informatics is not a statement about the current reality but rather a vision of where we must go.

The transformation of biology, or rather of biologic research, from an experimental to an experimental plus information science is deep and profound. It reflects not just a new approach to doing research (although that too is happening) but a fundamental evolution in how biologic questions are asked, how data are acquired and analyzed, and how we begin to grapple with both the daunting complexity of biology and its enormous and essential variability. Biologic research is asking and answering questions about living systems and life processes. That information lay at the core of biology is not new but rather directly reflects the great biologic revolution of the mid-twentieth century with the discovery of the structure of DNA, the genetic code, and the emergence of molecular genetics/molecular biology. With these developments, biology fundamentally became the study of the storage, transmission, and decoding of information, on the one hand, and the function and structures of the decoded information products, on the other hand. It is interesting, and not coincidental, that a qualitative change in the approach to biology as an information intense science comes at the same time that the rest of society is entering the information age. The capacity to cope with, analyze, exchange, and communicate large amounts of information and the wide dissemination of that capacity in biology is a reflection of the same microprocessor revolution that has enabled the broader information age. The human genome project, genomics, and the proliferation of other "-omics" are all possible because of high capacity computing. Equally important, the dissemination of these changes to the broad scientific community was made possible by the distribution of computers, networking and a sociology of computer literacy/familiarity within the biologic research community. High-throughput analyses of biologic systems are producing data sets of extremely high dimensionality. A growing collection of measurement tools, more extensive laboratory and imaging data acquisition, and an emerging domain of inquiry (including organ and organismal biology, genetic variation, polygenic traits, structural biology, population science), and a growing acceptance of the possible role of computational modeling as of real value to biology are all ushering in the need to marry biology with computational and information sciences.

On the other end of the biology–medicine spectrum is the recognition of the role of information sciences in clinical medicine. This is driven by three factors. First are the administrative demands for more efficient and accurate "business" systems for medical records, pharmacy, laboratory, and special studies, as well as billing, quality control, and, when applicable, reporting requirements. Second is the need to access a growing amount of information in all aspects of medicine. Third is the need to provide that information to multiple users and to couple its accessibility with the ability to communicate.

About four years ago in a speech to the American Society of Clinical Oncology, I proposed the need for a Cancer Informatics Infrastructure (CII) to enable the cancer research enterprise and to link it to the delivery of cancer care. I envisioned this as a difficult but essential undertaking for the National Cancer Institute (NCI). The goal was to develop a process and commit the resources for the creation of an enabling architecture, a set of standards, a means of dissemination and training, and, when appropriate, the development, adoption, and modification of tools and applications. Although these issues needed to be addressed for all aspects of the National Cancer Research Program, we felt we should turn to clinical trials as the centerpiece and starting point for the CII.

Why Clinical Trials?

First, clinical trials represent the crucible through which the insights, ideas, and tools of basic science and technology meet clinical practice through the testing of hypotheses in human beings and the garnering of evidence that will drive the changing behavior of the medical and public health systems. If we were to begin to meaningfully ask precise, detailed, and intelligent questions about biology, pharmacology, physiology and pathology in human beings, the crucible of the clinical trial needs to be up to the task; this would require the capacity to ask and answer these increasingly complex questions and to monitor states that would be rich and complex in information content. Furthermore, if we were going to be able to develop meaningfully the interfaces between the description of clinical states, molecular pathology, complex imaging data, genetics, and chemistry to create scientifically intense clinical trials, common language and compatible data sets would be essential.

Second, clinical trials, especially multi-site clinical trials, have always been enterprises that could only work if standards were established and applied and if data from disparate sites could be reliably merged.

Third, we recognized the need to re-evaluate the actual functioning of the clinical trials system to achieve a number of goals:

1. The design, implementation, monitoring, and reporting of clinical trials had to become more efficient and less administratively burdensome.
2. We needed to move towards a truly national system, in which access to available clinical trials was made broader and more facile for physicians and patients.
3. We needed to smoothly link the clinical trials system to an open, accessible information and communication system available to physicians, patients, healthcare organizations, sponsors, and funders.

Clearly, none of these goals could be achieved without an information system through which clinical trials could be designed, executed, analyzed, and reported.

With these considerations, we embarked on a program to begin to create a CII for cancer clinical trials. We recognized multiple challenges:

1. *Strategic Vision.* We needed to articulate an overall set of concepts about the models upon which the CII would be built, the principles underlying those models, the nature of the system architecture, and the scope and definition of standards.
2. *Tactical Approach.* We needed next to define the planning, oversight, and implementation processes. These included critical technical decisions and establishing affordable budgets. Decisions had to be made about the order of development, how to deal with legacy systems, what to specify and what not to specify, what to develop or adopt, and what to adapt, purchase, or leave to users to solve. We needed to establish how the CII would integrate with other standard developers, both conceptually and technically.
3. *Sociologic Issues.* The success or failure of the CII will rest not only with these strategic and tactical decisions or even with the products per se. Rather it will succeed or fail with the users. Only an approach that would satisfy their needs and be perceived and experienced as satisfying these needs and as being of benefit could be adopted. This would require buy-in from the beginning, ongoing input, usability-based development, and a realistic plan for dissemination, distribution, and adoption.

There is no question that the only way we will fully realize the potential of cancer research is to develop better tools for acquiring, analyzing, sharing, and communicating data and for being sure that we optimize how data are turned into meaningful information. This volume, many of whose contributors are actively engaged in the realization of the concept of a Cancer Informatics Infrastructure, describes current thinking about how such an infrastructure might be constructed. It is hard to produce a book in areas such as informatics and clinical trials that will remain relevant in the face of rapidly changing technologies, evolving policy issues, and ever-expanding expectations. Despite that challenge, this volume lays out principles and processes that are of interest and value and will remain relevant for some time to come.

Richard D. Klausner, MD
Director, National Cancer Institute

Series Preface

This series is directed to healthcare professionals who are leading the transformation of health care by using information and knowledge. Launched in 1988 as Computers in Health Care, the series offers a broad range of titles: some addressed to specific professions such as nursing, medicine, and health administration; others to special areas of practice such as trauma and radiology. Still other books in the series focus on interdisciplinary issues, such as the computer-based patient record, electronic health records, and networked healthcare systems.

Renamed Health Informatics in 1998 to reflect the rapid evolution in the discipline now known as health informatics, the series will continue to add titles that contribute to the evolution of the field. In the series, eminent experts, serving as editors or authors, offer their accounts of innovations in health informatics. Increasingly, these accounts go beyond hardware and software to address the role of information in influencing the transformation of healthcare delivery systems around the world. The series also will increasingly focus on "peopleware" and the organizational, behavioral, and societal changes that accompany the diffusion of information technology in health services environments.

These changes will shape health services in the new millennium. By making full and creative use of the technology to tame data and to transform information, health informatics will foster the development of the knowledge age in health care. As coeditors, we pledge to support our professional colleagues and the series readers as they share advances in the emerging and exciting field of health informatics.

Kathryn J. Hannah, PhD, RN
Marion J. Ball, EdD

Editors' Preface

A digital revolution has raced across the heart of the world's digital community; today, advances in information technology (IT) have totally transformed the way businesses do business. Now, interconnected networks of suppliers, producers, resellers, and distributors are working together with substantially lower administrative costs and clearly improved efficiencies. These "frictionless transactions" have contributed to a dramatic improvement in productivity in nearly all business sectors. Similar advances in IT and gene sequencing technologies have produced the first complete map of the human genome. As a result, cancer cells are yielding their secrets to researchers who are finding the errors in genes, the gene protein products, and the pathways that regulate all cell functions. These discoveries are generating a profound increase in cancer-specific target compounds—the cancer equivalents of laser-guided bombs—that hold the promise to cure or prevent cancer as we know it.

Moving research discoveries into practice requires an essential step: the clinical trial. Clinical trials establish that the new drug is safe for humans, that the drug is effective, and that the drug is in some way better than current treatments. Despite the IT transformations in other industries, many of today's clinical trials are bound to paper. The clinical trial protocol is created on paper by an investigator. The myriad protocol approval and tracking processes are managed on paper. This process is so cumbersome that it often takes in excess of two years from the time an investigator begins working on a clinical trial until the first patient is enrolled. Patient data are collected on paper case report forms and in such a manner that performing the clinical trial is very different from taking care of the patient. These paper case report forms are mailed to the clinical trials study centers and manually entered into databases for analyses of the clinical trial. Any errors in the forms require mailing them back to the investigator, who corrects the errors and returns the forms by mail. The final reports of the clinical trials are published on paper.

The foregoing inefficiencies are compounded by the critical need for patients. It is estimated that ten times more patients are needed on clinical trials than are currently available, just to test currently available drugs. The explosion of promising target compounds will overstress today's clinical trials systems and result in many promising drugs lying fallow until we can get around to them. The pharmaceutical industry, clinical research organizations, and the Federal Drug Administration (FDA) have efforts underway to improve this situation. Most of these are focused on reducing the paper logjam. Leading pharmaceutical and biotechnology companies are sponsoring remote data entry of case report forms directly into their study centers. The FDA is promoting electronic submissions of all drug information. A nonprofit Clinical Data Interchange Standards Consortium (CDISC) is working to coordinate 150 industry, academic, and government organizations that are implementing the FDA s Guidance for Industry. CaPCURE, a private foundation supporting prostate cancer research, and Oracle Corporation, which underwrote the effort, recently completed development of a clinical research information system to enhance data collection for prostate cancer trials in major cancer centers.

Recognizing the systemic nature of the problem, the National Cancer Institute (NCI) is planning a Cancer Informatics Infrastructure (CII) that will speed discovery and clinical trials processes. The CII will exploit the best components of the existing national information infrastructure to increase the efficiency and ease of doing clinical trials. A Long Range Planning Committee helped develop a vision for the CII and recommended a series of steps to hasten its development. Already, NCI has developed standard data and criteria for reporting all data collected during a clinical trial. These common data elements, common forms, and terminology have significantly reduced the hassle factors associated with clinical trials. An NCI enterprise system for clinical trials is well underway to create an information architecture for clinical trials and to realize improved efficiencies by managing data more effectively. This book extends the committee s report by focusing on bridging the chasm between discoveries and best clinical practices. Its thesis is that advanced information technologies and concurrent process enhancements will transform clinical trials, just as they have businesses. The result will dramatically accelerate the introduction of safer and more effective treatments into practice.

The book s section editors were part of a team that met to assist the early formulation and implementation of the principles of the CII. As we discussed many of the issues, it became clear that the committee s report would be insufficient to describe the myriad interconnections among the people, the organizations, and the technologies. Each section leader assembled a diverse group of experts to describe major contributions from the technology sector (Section 2), from standards and vocabularies activities (Section 3), and from actual implementation examples of visionary systems (Section 4). These chapters portray how activities from other sectors, such as e-commerce, can be exploited for the CII or how activities within health care make possible our vision of clinical research. They are designed as an initial point of exploration into the CII and the transformed clinical research it could foster. We hope our messages will motivate our readers to become actively involved in building this vision. Only then can we fundamentally improve our clinical trials system and realize the potential the information revolution holds.

The recent Institute of Medicine (IOM) report, *Crossing the Quality Chasm*, is a harsh call for reengineering the healthcare system at the national and local levels. The report specifically highlights that the information revolution has not transformed health care despite its obvious effect on other sectors. The IOM report s Recommendation 9 calls for building an information infrastructure that pervades all healthcare services in such a manner that handwritten clinical data would be eliminated by the end of the decade. Further, it states that information technologies must play a central role in the transformation.

In this context, the National Information Infrastructure (NII) supplies essential materials that we must use to construct our bridge over the quality and clinical trials chasm. For example, e-commerce has robust security services. Could we not re-use those services to meet (or exceed) the privacy, confidentiality, and security requirements of the Health Information Portability and Accountability Act (HIPAA)? We believe the answer is an emphatic *yes*! Could we not re-use the frictionless transactions of IT-transformed businesses for our own information exchanges? We believe the answer is an emphatic *yes*, but it will take *lots* of work. Indeed, we would suggest that clinical trials and protocol-based care delivery (clinical trials without a research arm) are the process infrastructure tools that will enable our taking the NII girders and constructing early versions of bridges to span the chasm. We believe that this book describes a vision for information creation, delivery, and use that is consistent with the IOM report recommendations. The principles and practices enunciated in the CII vision and this volume could catalyze the rapid implementation of those recommendations in the cancer research community.

As authors and editors, we have put more than a bit of ourselves into this volume. We hope our efforts will foster a speedy embracing of the information revolution by clinical research communities initially, followed by widespread adoption throughout the healthcare system.

John S. Silva, MD
Marion J. Ball, EdD
Judith V. Douglas, MA, MHS

Acknowledgments

As editors, we join in thanking all the colleagues who contributed to the concept of cancer informatics that is the heart of this book. In addition to the chapter authors, whose role is clear, there are many more who gave of their time, their intellect, and their energy to translate their thoughts, and the thoughts of others, into the pages that follow. Their support and the support of our families were invaluable to us. Our thanks also go to Nhora Cortes-Comerer, for shepherding us through the proposal development process; to David Beaulieu, for helping us complete this project; and to Jennifer Lillis, for lending her editorial hand.

John S. Silva, MD
Marion J. Ball, EdD
Christopher G. Chute, MD, DrPH
Curtis P. Langlotz, MD, PhD
Joyce C. Niland, PhD
William L. Scherlis, PhD
Judith V. Douglas, MA, MHS

Contents

SECTION 2 THE INFRASTRUCTURE

William L. Scherlis
Section Editor

SECTION 3 STANDARDS AND VOCABULARY

Christopher G. Chute and Curtis P. Langlotz
Section Editors

Contributors

Marion J. Ball, EdD
Vice President, Clinical Solutions Healthlink, Inc.; Adjunct Professor, Johns Hopkins University School of Nursing; Formerly, Vice President, First Consulting Group, Baltimore, MD 21210, USA (marionball@earthlink.net)

Aziz A. Boxwala, MBBS, PhD
Instructor, Decisions Systems Group, Brigham & Women's Hospital, Boston, MA) 02115, USA (aziz@dsg.harvard.edu)

William R. Braithwaite, MD, PhD, FACMI
Senior Adviser on Health Information Policy, U.S. Department of Health and Human Services, Washington, DC 20201, USA (BBraithw@osaspe.dhhs.gov)

Keith E. Campbell, MD, PhD, FACMI
Chief Technology Officer, Inoveon, Inc., Oklahoma City, OK 73104, USA; and Assistant Adjunct Professor of Medical Informatics, University of California, San Francisco, San Francisco, CA 94143, USA (campbell@informatics.com)

John S. Carter, MBA
Doctoral Fellow, Medical Informatics, University of Utah, Salt Lake City, UT 84108, USA

Christopher G. Chute, MD, PhD
Professor of Medical Informatics, Head, Section of Medical Information Resources, Mayo Clinic, Rochester, MN 55905, USA (chute@mayo.edu)

Sherri de Coronado, MS, MBA
Senior Program Analyst, Center for Bioinformatics, National Cancer Institute, Rockville, MD 30852, USA (sc61s@nih.gov)

Judith V. Douglas, MA, MHS
Adjunct Faculty, Johns Hopkins University School of Nursing; Formerly, Associate, First Consulting Group; Reisterstown, MD 21136, USA (judydouglas@home.com)

John H. Gennari, PhD
Assistant Professor, Department of Information and Computer Science, University of California, Irvine, Irvine, CA 92697, USA (Gennari@ics.uci.edu)

L. Michael Glodé, MD
Robert Rifkin Professor of Medicine, University of Colorado Health Sciences Center, Denver, CO 80262, USA (Mike.Glode@uchsc.edu)

Howard S. Goldberg, MD
Director of Clinical Research and Development, Clinician Support Technology, Inc., Framingham, MA 01701, USA (hgoldberg@cstlink.com)

Robert A. Greenes, MD, PhD
Director, Decision Systems Group, Brigham & Women's Hospital, Harvard Medical School, Boston, MA 02115, USA (Greenes@harvard.edu)

Douglas Hageman, MPA
Director, Office of Clinical Informatics, National Cancer Institute, Bethesda, MD 20892, USA (Hagemand@exchange.nih.gov)

M. Elizabeth Hammond, MD
Chairman, Department of Pathology, Urban Central Regional Hospitals, Intermountain Health Care; and Professor of Pathology and Internal Medicine, University of Utah School of Medicine, Salt Lake City, UT 84143, USA (ehammon@ihc.com)

W. Ed Hammond, PhD
Professor, Community and Family Medicine, Duke University, Durham, NC 27710 USA (hammon001@mc.duke edu)

Francis W. Hartel, PhD
Project Officer, Center for Bioinformatics, National Cancer Institute, Rockville, MD 20852, USA (Hartel@exchange.nih.gov)

Robert A. Hiatt, MD, PhD
Deputy Director, Division of Cancer Control and Population Sciences, National Cancer Institute, Bethesda, MD 20892, USA (robert.hiatt@nih.gov)

Stanley M. Huff, MD
Medical Informatics, Intermountain Health Care, Salt Lake City, UT 84120, USA (coshuff@ihc.com)

Susan M. Hubbard, BS, RN, MPA
Special Assistant for Communications, Office of the Director, National Cancer Institute, Bethesda, MD 20892, USA (shubbard@mail.hih.gov)

Kevin D. Keck, BS
Keck Labs, Alameda, CA 94501, USA (Keck@kecklabs.com)

Curtis P. Langlotz, MD, PhD
Assistant Professor of Radiology, Epidemiology, and Computer and Information Science, University of Pennsylvania, Moorestown, NJ 08057, USA (langlotz@rad.upenn.edu)

Ronald L. Larsen, PhD
Executive Director, Maryland Applied Information Technology Initiative, University of Maryland, College Park, MD 20742, USA (rlarsen@deans.umd.edu)

Deborah K. Mayer, RN, MSN, AOCN, FAAN
Chief Medical Officer, CancerSource.com South Easton, MA 92375, USA (Dmayer@cancersource.com)

Alexa T. McCray, PhD
Director, Lister Hill National Center for Biomedical Communications, National Library of Medicine, Bethesda, MD 20894, USA (Am97t@nih.gov)

Mitchell Morris, MD
Vice President, First Consulting Group; and Adjunct Professor of Health Informatics, University of Texas Health Science Center, Houston, TX 77046, USA (Mmorris@fcg.com)

Clifford Neuman, PhD
Senior Research Scientist, University of Southern California, Marina del Rey, CA 90292, USA (bcn@isi.edu)

Joyce C. Niland, PhD
Chair, Division of Information Sciences; and Director, Department of Biostatistics, City of Hope National Medical Center, Duarte, CA 91010, USA (jhiland@coh.org)

Mor Peleg, PhD
Medical Informatics, Stanford University, Stanford, CA 94305, USA (Peleg@smi.stanford.edu)

Dianne M. Reeves, RN
Senior Research Nurse Specialist, Center for Cancer Research, National Cancer Institute, Bethesda, MD 20892, USA (Reevesd@mail.nih.gov)

Charles Safran, MD
Chief Executive Officer, Clinician Support Technology, Inc.; and Associate Clinical Professor of Medicine, Harvard Medical School, Framingham, MA 01701, USA (Csafran@cstlink.com)

William L. Scherlis, PhD
Principal Research Scientist, School of Computer Science, Carnegie Mellon University, Pittsburgh, PA 15213, USA (scherlis@cs.cmu.edu)

Jean Scholtz, PhD
Program Manager, Defense Advanced Research Projects Agency, Arlington, VA 22203, USA (Jscholtz@darpa.mil)

Abdul-Malik Shakir
Senior Advisor, e-Intelligence Solutions Group, IDX Systems Corporation, Alameda, CA 94502 (Abdul-malik_shakir@idx.com)

Edward H. Shortliffe, MD, PhD
Professor and Chair, Department of Medical Informatics, College of Physicians and Surgeons, Columbia University, New York, NY 10032, USA (shortliffe@dmi.columbia.edu)

John S. Silva, MD
Center for Bioinformatics, National Cancer Institute, Eldersberg, MD 21784, USA (jc-silva-md@worldnet.att.net)

Donald W. Simborg, MD
Chief Executive Officer, iKnowMed, Berkeley, CA 94710, USA (Dsimborg@iknowmed.com)

Kent A. Spackman, MD, PhD
Associate Professor, Department of Pathology, Oregon Health Sciences Unversity, Portland, OR 97201, USA (spackman@ohsu.edu)

Douglas C. Stahl, PhD
Director, Biomedical Informatics, City of Hope National Medical Center, Duarte, CA 91010, USA (dstahl@coh.org)

Walter Sujansky, MD, PhD
Director, Product Development, ePocrates, Inc., San Carlos, CA 94070, USA (wsujansky@epocrates.com)

Jay M. Tenenbaum, PhD
Chief Scientist, Commerce One, Pleasanton, CA 94025, USA (Marty.tenenbaum@commerceone.com)

Samson Tu, MSc
Senior Research Scientist, Section on Medical Informatics, Stanford University, Stanford, CA 94305, USA (Tu@stanford.edu)

Mark S. Tuttle, FACMI
Vice President, Business Development, Apelon Federal Systems, Apelon, Inc., Alameda, CA 94501, USA (Mtuttle@apelon.com)

Warren G. Williams, MPH
Centers for Disease Control and Prevention, Atlanta, GA 30341, USA (wxw4@cdc.gov)

Section 1
The Vision

John S. Silva, Marion J. Ball, and Judith V. Douglas
Section Editors

Introduction
Envisioning a National Cancer Information and Knowledge Environment

JOHN S. SILVA

Section 1 of this book sets forth a vision of a national cancer information and knowledge environment that will greatly accelerate moving cancer discoveries into cancer practice. This environment supports the next generation of clinical trials from the dawn of a new idea to the design, activation, and conduct of a trial, on through the use and creative re-use of all the outcomes of studies to influence subsequent clinical research. The National Cancer Institute has described a Cancer Informatics Infrastructure (CII) that exploits the National Information Infrastructure to make the clinical trial processes truly frictionless—a CII that builds on existing tools and initiatives to serve the needs of the cancer community.

As an enabler and catalyst, the CII will adopt proven models and existing information technologies to expedite information exchange, both within the National Cancer Institute and across the national cancer community. A group of national experts in cancer care and research helped define the CII vision; their findings and recommendations are reported in Chapter 1, the CII is designed to serve the needs of the full spectrum of its users. The visionary scenarios of how the CII may transform cancer care are described in Chapter 2. Author Mike Glodé presents a crisp summary of today's resources for the cancer patient and health professional in Chapter 3.

The CII's overarching principles are simple yet profound:

- User focused—meet the needs of multiple stakeholders, including clinicians, consumers, regulators, insurers, NCI, and other sponsors.
- Private—ensure confidentiality, patients' right to privacy; limit access to authorized users only.
- Shareable—make it interoperable with standards in the clinical environment, meaningful, analyzable, and "entered once, used many times."
- Integrative—design a seamless system to meet the users' needs; integrate research resources and clinical practice; make it transparent.
- Valuable—provide immediate, tangible value for clinicians, patients, and other stakeholder groups; ultimately improve cancer care by defining the efficacy of formal clinical trials and standard-of-care treatments.

- Evolvable and innovative—provide a basis for state-of-the-art systems that exploit the existing technology base.

Further, our analyses identified the clear need to employ a "macro ergonomic model" that brings together the mission, processes, and work culture of cancer research and care; the stakeholders and "consumers" of research and care; and the tools and technologies that people use to do the work.

In a broader sense, this volume may address many of the fundamental challenges facing the US healthcare system identified in the recent Institute of Medicine (IOM) report, *Crossing the Quality Chasm: A New Health System for the 21st Century* (2001). This report is candid in its assessment: "The current care systems cannot do the job. Trying harder will not work. Changing systems of care will (p. 4)." The IOM calls for redesigned systems of care built upon integrative information technologies and a set of rules for the new systems of care that include shared knowledge and free flow of information, evidence-based decision making, safety as a system property, and transparency (p. 8). It calls for the public and private sectors to create "an infrastructure to support evidence-based practice."

The Cancer Informatics Infrastructure may well be an early exemplar of the IOM's vision for a 21st century healthcare system. This and subsequent sections describe a vibrant vision for cancer care. They describe the initial steps in a shared quest for achieving the best health by efficient access to ubiquitous information at the point of decision making.

References

Institute of Medicine. 2001. Crossing the Quality Chasm: A New Health System for the 21st Century. Washington, DC: National Academy Press.

1
Translating Cancer Research into Cancer Care: Final Report of the Long Range Planning Committee

Long Range Planning Committee*

Background

First convened in July 1998, the Long Range Planning Committee (LRPC) met again in January and July of 1999 and concluded its deliberations in February 2000. With membership from across the nation and expertise in clinical trials, informatics, statistics, computer science, and medicine, the LRPC worked with the senior editor of this volume in his role as Director of the Office of Informatics (OI) at the National Cancer Institute (NCI). Charged with developing a vision for a new Cancer Informatics Infrastructure (CII), the LRPC prepared a report at the director's request, advising him on what he should do in the near future to move the CII initiative forward. This report, which provides the conceptual underpinnings for this volume, follows.

Executive Summary

The Long Range Planning Committee envisions a national cancer information and knowledge environment that will translate cancer research into cancer care. To this end, the Committee recommends the creation of a Cancer Informatics Infrastructure (CII) that exploits the National Information Infrastructure to speed the clinical trial process. As an "enabler," the CII will expedite information exchange, both within the National Cancer Institute and across the national cancer community.

To move the CII from theory into practice, the Committee recommends that the Office of Informatics:

- Formulate the role of the National Cancer Institute in the national standards development process.

*A list of members appears at the end of this chapter.

- Convene a national advisory meeting on oncology-related terminology and standards, focusing on the development of common data elements.
- Focus on demonstration and evaluation projects that enhance the Institute's mission, by building on ongoing mainstream informatics initiatives and Internet technologies.
- Develop a process to strategically and tactically diffuse the products and concepts of recommendations 1, 2, and 3 throughout the cancer community.

In 2004, the CII will support all stakeholders—patients and physicians, investigators, trial managers, and payers—as they make vital decisions affecting the course of cancer treatment and research. Clinical trial results will drive cancer care, and care results will drive future research.

Introduction

The goal of the Cancer Informatics Infrastructure (CII), as we envision it, is to create a national cancer information and knowledge environment that speeds the discovery process and the translation of best discoveries into clinical trials. The CII will be the "enabler" that integrates the efforts of individual researchers, clinicians and patients in ways previously impossible, given the myriad of incompatible information systems within NCI and across the national cancer community. By fostering collaboration within and beyond NCI and by exploiting the potential of the Web, the CII will dramatically improve all aspects of cancer research and clinical care. It will expedite the process of converting the growing knowledge of genes, proteins, and pathways into the most appropriate preventative, diagnostic, and therapeutic measures.

Picturing the CII and Its New Model of the Clinical Trial Process

Our schema for the CII sets forth an architectural base for moving information across the continuum of cancer research: basic, clinical, translational, and population-based research. It is a model that brings together:

- The mission, processes, and work culture of cancer research, care, and policy
- The stakeholders and "consumers" of research and care
- The tools and technologies (including hardware and software) that people use to do the work.

With the National Information Infrastructure (NII) at its core, the CII will make maximum use of existing commercial capabilities and be poised to harvest the new technologies of the twenty-first century (the inner circle

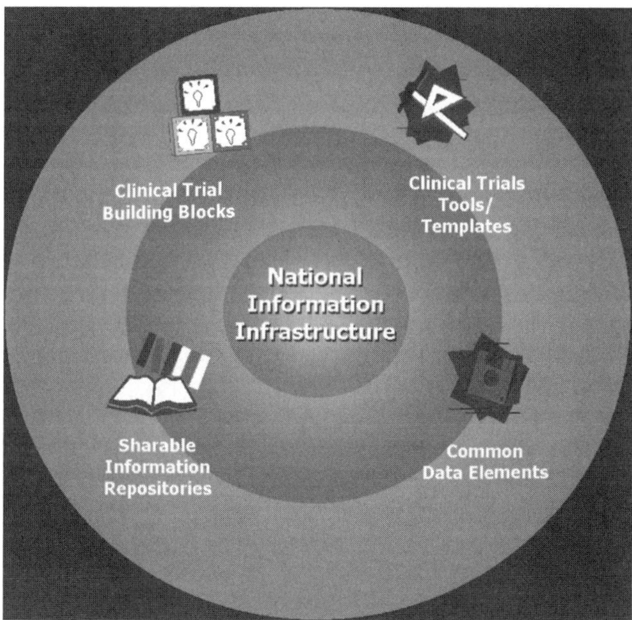

Figure 1.1. Model for cancer informatics infrastructure.

shown in Figure 1.1). Today's Web is an essential element of the NII. It provides people with unprecedented access to online information and services. However, because the information is unstructured, computers cannot readily "understand" it. This limitation helps explain why information on the Web is hard to find, integrate, and automate. The enabling technology for the next generation Web is a new standard called XML (eXtensible Markup Language). Developed by the World Wide Web Consortium, XML makes it easy to create specialized markup languages—sets of tags that tell a computer what data mean, rather than merely how to display them, as is the case with the current Web standard called HTML (HyperText Markup Language). Using XML, a number can be "understood" by the computer to be a specific laboratory result, patient history, physical finding, or patient identifier, etc. With HTML, these numbers are unstructured text that the computer does not understand.

The CII will overcome these limitations by using core technologies, such as XML, to provide information and services in a structured form readily accessible to both people and computers. Sites will publish patient records, trial results, eligibility requirements, treatment schedules, and the like, so that they are available to anyone—or any Web-enabled application—with the proper authorizations. They will also publish services that enable members of the cancer community to analyze data, run disease and diagnostic models, book appointments, and so forth. Thousands of sites will build on each other's information and services, creating innovative networked medical centers and hybrid treatment protocols that accelerate the path from research to cure.

The NCI should build only those capabilities that are specific to its needs: common data elements, research building blocks, and tools to support the conduct of cancer related research. This report addresses the specific case example of how this might be implemented within the context of NCI clinical treatment and diagnostic trials. This methodology is expected to have broad application to NCI's extensive research mission from basic to applied observational, population-based research.

Although the specifics of how it might be applied to those diverse settings will need to be addressed with specific efforts, the model proposed here stresses interoperability among technologies and collaboration among communities to develop and share relevant knowledge about cancer. For NCI, this means that the CII can provide totally new ways to collaborate, such as the linkages among basic biologists, mouse researchers, genomics researchers, and clinicians studying human cancers in the Mouse Models of Human Cancer Consortium. For organizations outside NCI, this means that the CII can provide links among local systems that were heretofore incompatible.

To make our vision of the CII more "real," we developed a model of what clinical research will look like in 2004. This model is presented in Chapter 2. Using the CII, ideas are generated, funding and protocol approvals are obtained, clinical trials are conducted, findings are analyzed, and more new ideas are generated, as shown in Figure 1.2. The entire drug development process is greatly enhanced by eliminating redundancy and most of the

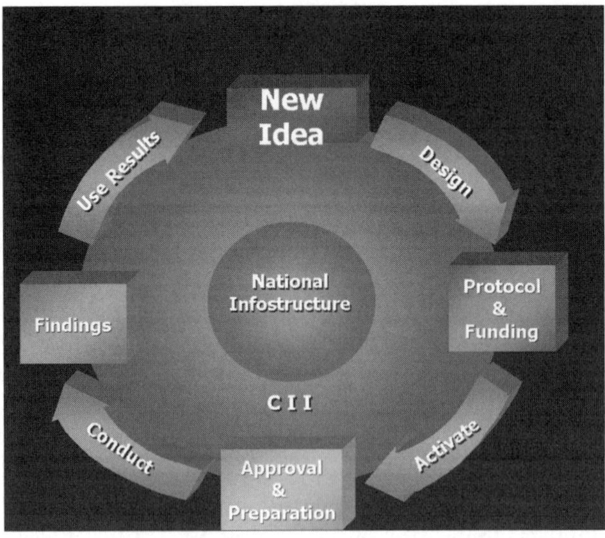

Figure 1.2. Clinical trial life cycle.

paper and expediting each step. Trials are authored that focus on the science of the trial, not the text of the protocol document. They are authored collaboratively by appropriate members of the community and approved within 60 days. Patients are accrued more rapidly since clinical trials are integrated in the standard of care. Chapter 2 contains detailed scenarios of use of our model system from the perspective of patients, physicians, investigators, trials managers, and payers.

Recommendations

Recommendation 1. Formulate the role of the National Cancer Institute in the national standards development process.

- **Create a standing review panel for NCI information standards.** This body will peer review and seek consensus from relevant stakeholders on proposed information standards unique to the CII enterprise. Operating under one of NCI's existing advisory committees, it will liaison with other appropriate federal agencies and organizations.
- **Ensure that NCI efforts to develop or promote oncology-specific information standards are tightly coordinated with the broader health information standards community.** Coordination needs to extend to include standards development organizations (SDOs), such as HL7 and SNOMED, umbrella organizations such as ANSI HISB and ISO TC 215, and larger communities of interest such as FDA and the pharmaceutical industry, NLM's UMLS, and most importantly, practicing scientists and clinicians.
- **Include in the approach dynamic processes for content management and configuration control for the entire lifecycle of standards.** Content management is critical given the need to continuously revise common data elements to reflect changes in the science. Configuration management—for example, appropriate content maintenance, version control, and seamless integration of updates—is also essential to make the implementation of standards "transparent" and as effortless as possible for cancer centers, the pharmaceutical industry, the Food and Drug Administration, and the National Cancer Institute itself.

Recommendation 2. Convene a national advisory meeting on oncology-related terminology and standards.

The LRPC commends the National Cancer Institute for its terminological development efforts. The implementation of the Cancer Informatics Infrastructure (CII) requires commonality, such as is provided by common toxicity criteria (CTCs). The development of common data elements (CDEs) is unique to the National Cancer Institute and critical to the CII.

We recommend that a working group be convened to consider oncology-related terminology and standards (ORTS), led by Curtis Langlotz, MD,

PhD. Details of his work to date are included in the appendix on the CDE development model for spiral computed tomography in lung cancer. Assisted by Christopher Chute, MD, DrPH, other experts, and NCI staff, this working group will advise the Office of Informatics on how best to do the following:

- **Identify oncology-related terminology and standards that should be supported throughout their lifecycle by NCI.** It is critical to distinguish between oncology-relevant standards, such as SNOMED, UMLS, HL7, XML, and DICOM, and cancer-specific standards, such as CDEs and common toxicity criteria (CTCs). The ORTS working group will define the responsibility of NCI for the lifecycle of cancer-specific standards and clarify the role of NCI in the area of oncology-related standards, including appropriate linkages and participation.

- **Institute formal change management processes for CDEs and other oncology-related terminology.** As CDEs are developed and adopted, NCI will need to re-focus on monitoring adherence and providing technical assistance to support adoption and implementation for all stakeholders. Processes must ensure that terminological standards evolve in parallel with and support of clinical and research needs, including those of the pharmaceutical industry and the FDA. The ORTS working group will identify activities to:

- develop guidelines and resource materials formalizing best practices to assist participants in CDE development
- elicit clinical input from designated "champions" early in each round of terminological development.

- **Propose initiatives to augment the CDE information model.** To succeed, terminologies must develop associated meta-knowledge and meta-data about each term to provide linkages between terms, logical contexts for terms, and specifications on instantiating and using terms to clarify interrelationships. The ORTS working group will propose initiatives to:

- describe the CDE database schema and information model in detail, for public review and comparison to other models and terminologies based on meta-data standards and in collaboration with ongoing efforts to harmonize medical standard repositories (HFCA's meta-data repository)
- establish a rich, consistent information model for CDEs, by building on existing CDE "Categories" and ultimately employing knowledge representation techniques like semantic networks and description logic
- create detailed data dictionary entries for new data elements, including nontextual data (e.g., imaging), to minimize variations.

- **Recommend methods to encourage the dissemination and use of CDEs.** In the effort to establish CDEs as a *de facto* standard for oncology data collection, NCI now makes them available for free on its Web site. More work is needed to increase the use of CDEs inside and outside of the cooperative groups. New functionalities are key to attracting additional researchers to use the CDEs and other CII technology. The ORTS working group meeting will identify approaches to:

- enhance the Web-enabled interface to CDEs, making it easier for new users and users outside the cooperative groups
- automate the connection between the CDE Web site and research systems using CDEs by encouraging projects at different phases of the cancer lifecycle to download and incorporate CDEs into data collection systems for clinical trials, possibly through funding supplements to existing trials
- enhance download formats, including case report form (CRF) templates, draft database designs, and XML, enabling users to search for and download relevant CDEs and evolving the CDE resource into a meta-data repository.

Recommendation 3. Focus informatics efforts on demonstration and evaluation projects that enhance NCI's ability to carry out its mission, by building on ongoing mainstream informatics initiatives and Internet technologies.

Implementing the CII is a complex and long-term task, but most of the technologies and applications required to support it are available now. Creation of the CII requires a set of common infrastructure services, such as medical informatics standards and tools, digital libraries, collaboration tools, security services, and electronic transaction support.

In order to maximize impact in the NCI community, we recommend that the Director of the Office of Informatics exploit existing and emerging technologies and capitalize on initiatives underway outside the National Cancer Institute. The NCI operates in an environment of diverse stakeholders, rapidly evolving policy and technology, extensive interdependency with externally developed informatics and Internet infrastructure, and long-lived data and processes associated with trials. In the overall process of developing the CII, we therefore recommend that the NCI fulfill three specific roles.

First, NCI is the principal stakeholder for the long-term interests of the cancer-trials community. NCI should therefore emphasize investments that address issues of future concern, such as support for the evolution of standards, or consideration of issues relating to the scaling-up of the extent of CII deployment among the diverse participants in NCI activities. For example, when new standards are proposed (such as CDEs), the NCI should, from the outset, assure that the designs do not preclude smooth transitions to exploit anticipated future developments in health care and in information technology. In special cases, these investments can include generic information technologies that play a critical role in NCI infrastructure development. (It may be appropriate to co-manage these investments with other agencies that serve in a more primary role in technology development.)

Second, NCI has a principal role in buying down the risks of creating and adopting new technologies. For example, NCI should make targeted investments to assist early adopters in evaluating CII technologies. NCI can also undertake targeted experiments to assess how new standards and processes may introduce or eliminate barriers to efficient trials management and broad participation.

Third, the NCI needs to make specific investments that address compelling nearer-term needs. This includes "bootstrapping" new efforts in the development of standards and technology. It is essential that these investments be made in a manner that is consistent with the long-term CII vision. This keeps the CII vision grounded in the baseline of present practice (and it may entail adapting the CII vision). By getting involved at very early stages, NCI can exert greater leverage with its investment. This approach assures that NCI informatics investment is consistent with overall strategy. Within the overall strategy, of course, there may be a need to explore diverse approaches to particular problems.

In carrying out these roles, the NCI Office of Informatics can maximize the return on its investment by leveraging ongoing informatics and Internet technology efforts to address NCI-specific needs. For example, CDE standards developed under NCI sponsorship should be integrated into mainstream framework efforts such as HL7.

As an example of successful mediation of community standards development efforts, we note the work of the Internet Engineering Task Force (IETF), which has been the governing body for Internet standards since the early 1970s. The IETF has succeeded in building a national-scale community process to support an evolving collection of standards and capabilities. We recommend the IETF model because, in the rapidly evolving environment of cancer research and treatment, the only constant can be the principles that make up the process model:

- Provide mechanisms to facilitate stakeholder participation
- Leverage sponsorship rather than subsidize the entire CII
- Provide both a test bed and an infrastructure.

NCI should identify critical areas of standards and technology development in which it needs to participate in order to address the needs identified above. Standards development, in the IETF process, involves not only community consensus efforts, but also development of technology prototypes that can enable direct evaluation of candidate approaches to be undertaken.

With respect to standards, we advise Office of Informatics to undertake the following efforts:

- **Collaborate with radiologists and pathologists to ensure that their efforts to create digital libraries for large-scale multimedia records are compatible with the CII.** Building on its success in persuading vendors to adopt the DICOM standard, the Radiological Society of North America is actively pursuing the multimedia record and the integration of imaging information into the clinical record. Pathologists are pursuing similar efforts with tissue banks, with funding from NCI forthcoming for three to five institutions to develop shared tissue resources.

- **Participate in the Guidelines Interchange Format (GLIF) Workshop in March 2000 to draw upon and impact ongoing efforts to develop suites of building blocks.** This workshop includes multiple governmental sponsors along with the American College of Physicians–American Society of Internal Medicine. As such, it provides an opportunity to begin to consolidate the national cancer community and its diverse stakeholder groups in assessing current efforts (both intramural and extramural) and defining next steps.
- **Exploit e-commerce and emerging business models to support electronic transactions between parties.** Standard practices in e-commerce, notably business-to-business applications, have brought multiple legacy systems together. Similar mechanisms will enable basic researchers to collaborate with clinical researchers and result in the more effective use and reuse of knowledge in their own legacy systems. They will also allow for linkages with individuals and entities outside NCI, from patients to ancillary care providers.

With respect to technology development, we advise the Office of Informatics to undertake efforts such as:

- **Capitalize on work developing collaborative tools done by other federal agencies.** Issues surrounding scientific collaboration and research were recently explored at a workshop on Collaborative Problem Solving Environments, sponsored by the Department of Energy and attended by the NCI Office of Informatics. Their findings and work ongoing in the National Science Foundation and the Defense Applied Research Projects Agency should be analyzed for insight into issues central to the CII.
- **Exploit national initiatives to create security services needed to protect patient privacy and confidentiality.** Work by the Computer-Based Patient Record Institute (CPRI) and in conjunction with the Health Insurance Portability and Accountability Act (HIPAA) addresses the policy and technology issues critical to the CII and the patient-centric data it will include. The Office of Informatics should leverage this work rather than develop services independently.

Recommendation 4. Develop a process to strategically and tactically diffuse the products and concepts of recommendations 1, 2, and 3 throughout the cancer community.

In the cancer community there are a number of early adopters or visionaries of a comprehensive cancer informatics infrastructure and its potential impact on the clinical trials process. There is sometimes a "gap" between these early adopters/visionaries and the majority of others who are working in the cancer area. The goal of this recommendation is to develop systematic

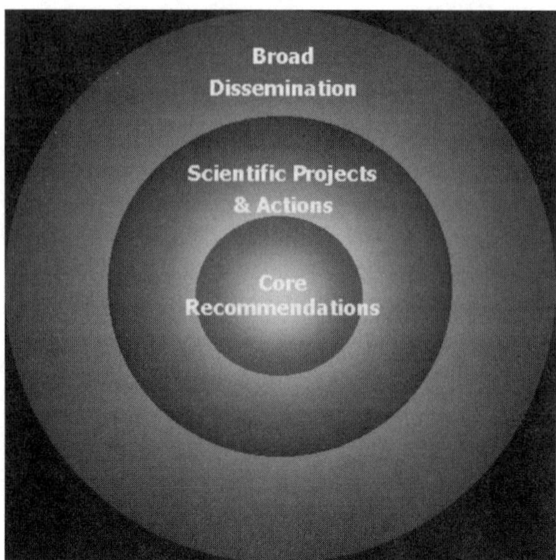

FIGURE 1.3. Dissemination model.

demonstration and evaluation efforts that will illustrate the impact to the people in the cancer community who can be called "early majority pragmatists."

We recommend a concentric circle model to demonstrate this change oriented diffusion process (Figure 1.3). The center circle within this model contains the three core product recommendations. The circle immediately touching the recommendations contains a number of specific projects and actions that are highly relevant to the current user community, e.g., centers, groups, NCI, and so on. To fulfill the demonstration effect of the items listed in this circle, people who are "early adopters" could be asked to complete demonstration projects. The types of items listed in the next concentric circle will be dissemination items to the people who are more conservative in their approach.

- **Convene a planning meeting/working group with representation from the recommendation developers and early adopters/visionaries who are respected within NCI and within the cancer community.** This meeting would plot needed efforts along a timeline and the concentric model, demonstrating the impact of each of the recommendations in a CII enabled process, that would be implemented by people highly respected by NCI and the cancer community.
- **Develop the processes, identify and remove the barriers, and request the completion of the targeted diffusion efforts.** The planning/working group will be responsible for the components in this portion of the diffusion plan. We strongly suggest that the planning group consider tactics for disseminating information on the CII in NCI announcements, including Requests for Applications (RFAs).

From Theory to Practice: Clinical Trials in 2004

In 2004, the Cancer Informatics Infrastructure (CII) will translate clinical trials results into clinical care, and care results will drive future research. With common processes and tools in place, the CII will expedite information exchange. Access to information will support all stakeholders—patients and physicians, investigators, trial managers, and payers—as they make vital decisions affecting the course of cancer treatment and research. In the end, the benefits will accrue to the patient, and the NCI will realize its ultimate mission: to bring better care to the American public.

The information and knowledge depicted in Figure 1.4 will make it possible for:

- Patients and their physicians to:
  - access up-to-date medical information
  - maintain patient-centric records
  - be partners in shared decision making.
- Investigators to:
  - design and obtain approval for a trial in 60 days
  - rapidly accrue patients into trials
  - populate research databases using clinical data.

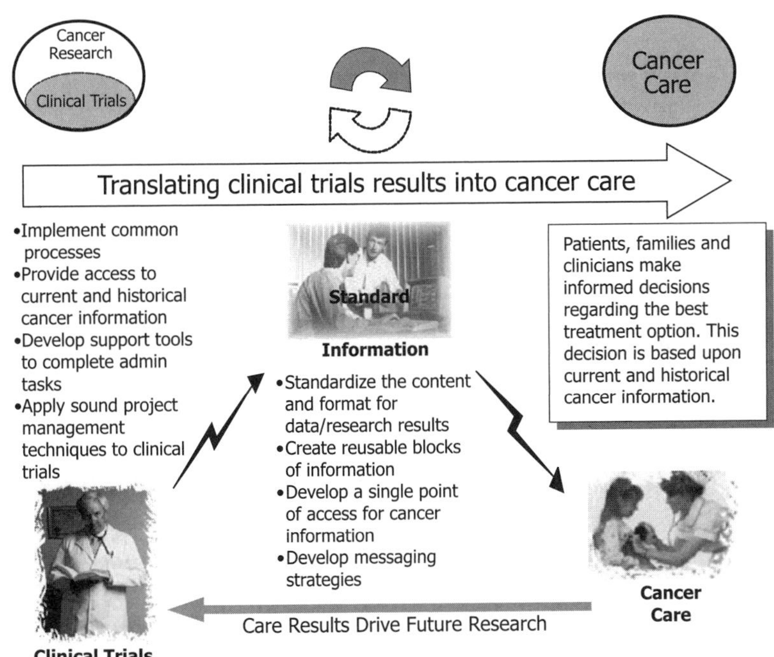

FIGURE 1.4. Cancer care and cancer research in 2004.

- Trial Managers to:
  - minimize time from scientific concept to first patient accrual
  - maximize patient participation in cancer clinical trials
  - exchange information to optimize effective studies
  - facilitate translation of clinical trial results into cancer care.
- Payers to:
  - provide high quality cancer treatment for their members
  - make a solid business case for participating in clinical trials.

We believe that moving the CII from theory into practice will help the National Cancer Institute achieve its mission of lessening the burden of cancer for all Americans, and we urge the Director of the Office of Informatics to continue working towards the vision we have presented in this report.

Acknowledgments. Throughout its deliberations, the Long Range Planning Committee drew upon expertise within the National Cancer Institute, including many NCI staffers in its meetings. In addition, the LRPC also consulted with experts from academia and the private sector. A small "tiger team," including Marion Ball, Michael Becich, Christopher Chute, Judith Douglas, Michael Glodé, Curtis Langlotz, and William Scherlis, assisted in developing the final report. The tiger team was briefed by representatives from Oracle and worked with a team from First Consulting Group led by C. David Hardison during phase 2 activities.

National Cancer Institute Long Range Planning Committee (LRPC) Members*. Marion J. Ball, First Consulting Group and Johns Hopkins University; Michael J. Becich, University of Pittsburgh School of Medicine; Douglas W. Blayney, Pomona Valley Hospital Medical Center; David N. Campbell; Christopher G. Chute, Mayo Foundation; Morris F. Collen, Kaiser Permanente; Don E. Detmer, University of Virginia; Alan Dowling, Ernst & Young; John P. Fanning, Department of Health and Human Services; L. Michael Glodé, University of Colorado Health Sciences Center; David Harrington, Dana-Farber Cancer Institute; Robert A. Hiatt, National Cancer Institute; Curtis P. Langlotz, University of Pennsylvania and EDICT Systems; Nancy M. Lorenzi, University of Cincinnati Medical Center; William L. Scherlis, Carnegie Mellon University; Eleanor McFadden, Frontier Science and Technology Research Association; Mitchell Morris, MD Anderson Cancer Center; Joyce Niland, City of Hope National Medical Center and Beckman Research Institute; Jane Reese-Coulbourne, National Cancer Institute; Howard R. Soule, CaPCURE; Juilian Smith, National Cancer Institute; Robert E. Wittes, National Cancer Institute; Jay M. Tenenbaum, Veo Systems; Yelena Yesha, University of Maryland Baltimore County.

---

*Affiliations are those held by members during the committee's deliberations.

2
Visions of the Future

Long Range Planning Committee*

Background

As the base for their recommendations, the Long Range Planning Committee developed scenarios of clinical trials enabled by the Cancer Informatics Infrastructure (CII). These scenarios, envisioned for the year 2004 and beyond, set forth the perspectives of patients, physicians, investigators, trial managers, and payers as they participate in clinical trials.

Patient/Physician Perspective on Clinical Trials

In 2004 and beyond, patients with cancer, their physicians, and anyone wanting to learn about cancer prevention and treatment will have access to up-to-date reliable medical information. Records will be patient-centric, making it possible to customize information and treatment choices to individual patient preferences. Software tools will search out and "translate" information, and support physicians and patients in shared decision making. By improving access to relevant information, the Cancer Informatics Infrastructure (CII) with its software tools will enable patients and physicians to partner in shared decision making, resulting in improved outcomes.

The goal is for the patient and physician to:

Access up-to-date medical information.

- Continuously updated, the CII will identify clinical trials appropriate to each patient's diagnosis.
- Information on the CII will carry the National Cancer Institute's "seal of approval" to assure its accuracy and timeliness.

*A list of members appears at the end of this chapter.

- Search engines—"intelligent" agents—will update physicians on developments in areas of interest.
- Identify and "translate" relevant information for patients.

Maintain patient-centric records.

- Patients will use "health partner" software to collect and contain their medical record, personal health journals and care preferences.
- Physicians will use a Web-based patient-centric record that holds all the information necessary for cancer treatment.
- Once a patient is in a trial, the CII will automatically:
  - transmit data from the patient's record into the clinical trial database
  - generate patient education materials relevant to the patient's care
  - provide clinical alerts and updates to physicians and caregivers
  - generate approvals for laboratory tests, imaging, etc.

Be partners in shared decision making.

- Patients and physicians will have the information they need as "partners in care."
- Patient "mediators" will help patients understand care options and determine how much and what kind of information they want to receive.
- Patient education materials relevant to their diagnosis and treatment will help patients understand and manage their care.
- Physicians will be better able to focus on the patient's needs and interpret (not simply download) information and clinical practice guidelines.
- NCI software tools for gathering, evaluating, and displaying relevant information will assist patients and physicians in making best informed decisions.
- While preserving the confidentiality of individual patients' records, more effective sharing of clinical information will empower patients, with their physicians, to make treatment decisions, tailored to patient preferences.

Scenario

Symptom-free since a right lumpectomy and radiation therapy three years ago, 55-year-old patient Judith Johnson has had some lower back pain for several weeks. When she discovers a lump below her right breast, she immediately telephones her primary care physician, Dr. Robert Simpson.

In the few days before her appointment, Judith Johnson uses her home computer to go to the Web. There she accesses her own patient record—her Personal Health Partner—which contains her medical history and her own entries, including her journal and her lists of her preferences on treatment and the level of information she wishes to receive. She uses her Personal Health Partner to focus her search on the Web for the latest information on recurring breast cancer. She receives the results of her search and confirms that she wants additional information as it becomes available.

On the Web, Judith Johnson visits her breast cancer survivor group with news of her possible recurrence. Words of support and advice from fellow survivors come quickly on the Web. She also leaves a message for Cathy Myers, who served as her "mediator" since she was first diagnosed, offering guidance and support during key decision points.

When patient Johnson arrives at Dr. Simpson's office, she has information from the Web in hand: questions on recurring breast cancer, a list of tests he is likely to recommend, and profiles of local surgeons who meet her preferences. Together they go through the information and agree on what will happen next. Patient Johnson will have lab work, a bone scan, a chest X-ray, and a biopsy of the lump. Dr. Smith, a surgeon, will perform the biopsy, and the test results will be sent directly to her Personal Health Partner at the same time they go to Dr. Simpson and the Cancer Knowledge Base.

The tests completed, Dr. Simpson receives the results. Patient Johnson's lab tests are normal, but her chest x-ray shows multiple nodules in both lungs, and her bone scan indicates that there are lesions in her spine and pelvis. The pathology report from her biopsy indicates that the lump is malignant. Dr. Simpson speaks with her about the results. His next step is to research her long-term outlook and treatment options, and he asks patient Johnson whether she wants to receive information when he does.

Although she indicates she herself is not ready to deal with more information now, she authorizes Dr. Simpson to use her data to find appropriate treatments on the Cancer Knowledge Base. Back home, patient Johnson calls Cathy Meyers, her mediator, to discuss her results before her next appointment with Dr. Simpson.

Dr. Simpson checks his Cancer Inbox for patient Johnson's results. (Responses to his queries regarding prognosis and treatment, specific to her clinical data, are done by an "intelligent agent.") He reviews the three treatment options appropriate for her. Had patient Johnson requested it, Dr. Simpson could have forwarded the same information to her. For each of the three treatment options identified, the details include:

- Clinical research results, including relevant publications
- Authorized oncologists, including contact information
- Outcomes for patients treated, including quality of life information
- Financial implications, including health plan coverage issues
- Patient education tools, including print and multimedia materials
- Web-based resources, including discussion groups.

One of the three options is the Phase III clinical trial of a new drug developed by PharmaCo. Named OncoDrug, it has been shown in preclinical studies to interfere with cell cycle progression, most notably in patients whose tumor markers predict high susceptibility to the drug. The principal investigator for the trial is John Carter, MD, PhD, chairman of Oncology at Gateway Medical Center, which is a member of the Mid-Central Oncology Cooperative Group (MCOG).

Plantation Medical Center, an MCOG member 25 minutes from Judith Johnson's home, is the closest facility offering the OncoDrug trial. Dr. Simpson sends the data used to identify treatment options to the authorized oncologist at the Center, Elizabeth Austin, MD; she will contact Dr. Simpson by phone about Judith Johnson's possible eligibility. He also queries the health plan about financial obligations associated with any of the treatment options.

The next day, Judith Johnson and her husband meet with Dr. Simpson to discuss the treatment options identified by the Cancer Knowledge Base. After reviewing the information, she and her husband decide to seek a second opinion and do some additional research. With Dr. Simpson, they look over the list of authorized breast cancer specialists who meet her preferences and select Dr. Maria Walton. Judith Johnson authorizes the release of her medical information to Dr. Walton and requests that the treatment option information be forwarded to her mediator, Cathy Meyers.

Once home, Judith Johnson accesses the Cancer Knowledge Base for more information on the OncoDrug trial. Information in hand, she calls her mediator and discusses her options. After talking matters through, patient Johnson decides that the OncoDrug clinical trial is her best option, if the second opinion concurs. Based on a review of her record and test results online, Dr. Walton confirms the diagnosis two days later.

When Judith Johnson and her husband meet with Dr. Simpson and indicate that the OncoDrug trial is her first choice, Dr. Simpson arranges to complete her eligibility assessment, including a special study of her genetic markers. He collects a specimen for analysis, and she authorizes release of her tissue to the research center. When the test shows the marker is positive, she is eligible for the OncoDrug trial.

Now Judith Johnson signs the electronic informed consent document. She authorizes the release of her patient record and clinical data for use in completing the trial study enrollment forms. She also authorizes the release of her subsequent clinical trial data to the study center, to Dr. Simpson, and her own Personal Health Partner. Confirmation of enrollment is sent to the patient, her physicians, her health plan, and the clinical facilities that will provide care, including the infusion center, clinical laboratory, and imaging center.

Upon confirmation, Beth Davis, the oncology nurse at the infusion center who works with Dr. Austin, sends patient Johnson educational materials about the trial, along with the date for her first infusion. At patient Johnson's request, nurse Davis forwards copies of the material to mediator Meyers. The educational materials include a review of possible side effects and a description of what occurs during a patient's first visit to the infusion center. A tentative schedule for patient Johnson lists dates for her medication infusions, laboratory tests, imaging procedures, and physical exams. Nurse Davis includes her telephone number and email address for patient Johnson's questions throughout the course of treatment. She also gives patient Johnson information on the secure Web chat room she can access to share experiences with other patients in the OncoDrug clinical trial.

At the first visit, nurse Davis and patient Johnson review the schedule. Once approved, it is routed online to the appropriate personnel, including Dr. Simpson, who is notified of the dates patient Johnson will need physical exams and laboratory tests to obtain her genetic data (to determine the medication dosage to order). Dr. Simpson's office schedules all procedures and confirms the times with Judith Johnson. Because her health plan has approved her participation in the trial, all the lab orders, imaging requests, and other services specified by the protocol are pre-authorized, and she will incur no added financial risk.

Shortly before each visit, Judith Johnson receives a reminder automatically from Dr. Simpson's office. Nurse Davis also receives a reminder the day Judith Johnson will be at the infusion center. After reviewing the lab values for patient Johnson and confirming they are acceptable, nurse Davis administers OncoDrug and enters in all the required data.

Before one visit, close to the end of the trial, Dr. Simpson and Dr. Austin are notified that patient Johnson's white blood cell count has dropped to a level indicative of an adverse response to the treatment. After reviewing the blood work and talking with Judith Johnson, they agree that she will stay in the trial. At this time, as throughout the trial, she visits the OncoDrug Web chat room and confers with her mediator, Cathy Meyers, for encouragement.

When Judith Johnson's course of treatment in the trial is over, Dr. Simpson continues to monitor her progress, arrange for the recommended follow-up exams/tests, and electronically approves transmission of reports from her medical record to the clinical trial database, while preserving confidentiality of the individual patient's data. When the trial is concluded, data analyzed, and results published and disseminated, copies are sent to Dr. Simpson and Judith Johnson. Patient Johnson also receives quality-of-life surveys on a periodic basis.

Investigator Perspective on Clinical Trials in 2004

In 2004 and beyond, investigators—the clinical researchers who develop and conduct clinical trials in cancer—will be able to design, obtain approval, and begin enrollment of their patients in less than 60 days. They will be able to gather research data at the same time they provide care to patients. Patients will be eager to enroll so that trials will be concluded quickly and results will be available widely. By easing their administrative burdens, the Cancer Informatics Infrastructure (CII) will free investigators to address more scientific questions and implement new advances into routine care more rapidly.

The goal is for investigators to:

Design and obtain approval for a trial in 60 days.

- Standard protocol templates and "starter toolkits," accessible on the researchers' desktop, will expedite the preparation of new protocols for trials.
- The NCI's Protocol Approval Tracking System (PATS) will enable parallel creation and review of components of the trial (e.g., drugs, statistics, and radiation therapy).
- Search engines—intelligent agents—will seek out required trial information, such as toxicities from multiple databases, including those not on MedLine.
- Researchers in other disciplines will receive notification of planned trials early in the creation phase, allowing co-development of important research questions to be answered during trials.
- A national Institutional Review Board (IRB) will approve clinical trials and facilitate review and approval by local IRBs.

Rapidly accrue patients into trials.

- Standard definitions—for example, common data elements (CDEs) and clinical states—will match patients with trials and assist in selecting the most appropriate treatment options.
- Clinicians, patients, and advocates will receive notification of trials under development and materials to promote approved trials.
- Collaboration among clinical researchers and local clinicians will remove geographical barriers to access and extend trials to all eligible patients.
- Pre-approvals for trials will eliminate financial barriers to patient enrollment.
- Simplified trials administration will eliminate patient and clinician "hassle" factors.
- Patients, if they request it, will receive information about appropriate resources for their diagnosis, including clinical trials, as a result of a positive pathology report.

Populate research databases using clinical data.

- Common data elements for both clinical encounters and research will allow trial information to be collected as a byproduct of clinical encounters.
- Standardized clinical trial data will enhance meta-trial analysis and feedback directly into protocol development.
- Analysis of clinical outcomes of each trial will address the concerns of non-researchers, including consumers, policy makers, and news organizations.

Scenario

Chair of oncology at Gateway Medical Center, John Carter, MD, PhD, is concluding a yearlong proof-of-principle trial using OncoDrug to interfere with cell cycle progression. Clinical responses occurred, primarily in the patients whose tumor markers predicted a high susceptibility to the drug. In Dr. Carter's view, these findings form the hypothesis for a Phase III clinical trial.

Dr. Carter goes to the National Cancer Institute (NCI) Web site to access information bearing on his hypothesis and to determine whether another research team holds or is evaluating that hypothesis. He enters the criteria for his search; the resulting report draws from multiple databases. The Clinical Trials Database identifies ten past and one current clinical trial using OncoDrug to treat breast cancer, and CancerLit locates relevant published articles. The Electronic Journal of Negative Results reports on the efficacy, safety, and toxicities of past trials, including negative outcomes of OncoDrug trials. As he reads the information, Dr. Carter saves the information he will use in designing the trial. He reviews the list of people who hold the Investigational New Drug (IND) for OncoDrug and electronically signs the disclosure forms required to obtain more information, including unpublished data from the company that developed OncoDrug, PharmaCo. In addition, he notes that the Mid-Central Oncology Cooperative Group (MCOG)—to which his medical center belongs—has recently published a call for concepts consistent with his hypothesis.

Dr. Carter next uses a Web-based form to prepare a letter of intent for a multisite trial involving colleagues from three other institutions, all members of MCOG, and the URL is sent to his three research colleagues as well as MCOG staff. MCOG agrees to fund the trial and to provide him with a trial manager to help in designing the trial protocol and managing the data analysis. The three collaborators and Dr. Carter discuss their protocol plans together and with translational scientists at their individual institutions.

Once he receives the MCOG organ site subcommittee's endorsement, he accesses the authoring toolkit on the NCI Web Site and begins to design the protocol. The toolkit provides existing templates for OncoDrug trials, including eligibility criteria, inclusion/exclusion criteria, and drug schema. These templates Dr. Carter modifies as needed. Where required, he adds protocol-specific elements in his word processor. He also uses the toolkit to access an informed consent form approved for multisite trials, to identify a cooperative tissue bank for sharing with other researchers, and to request comments from basic scientists and investigators on other OncoDrug trials about his new trial.

With the input from other researchers, Dr. Carter completes any additional modifications to the protocol components and forwards it on. It is automatically routed to Melinda Jones, the trial manager assigned to him by MCOG, and to the NCI drug monitor, Dr. Paul Morris, and Sally Williams, the NCI disease coordinator.

Trial manager Jones and Dr. Morris use the toolkit to distribute portions of the protocol document to members of the review team. There is simultaneous, parallel review of different components and Dr. Carter is notified of questions from each team, making changes in a joint working document. They shepherd the protocol through all phases of the development, review, and approval process. All team members collaborate online to share questions and responses and to minimize redundant or sequential reviews. The protocol highlights all modifications and new sections for detailed intensive review, focusing the reviewers' efforts. The protocol is approved within 60 days of submission, and Dr. Carter receives NCI certification for the trial.

The design phase complete, Dr. Carter and trial manager Jones activate the trial at all four sites, including Plantation Medical Center where Elizabeth Austin, MD, is leading the trial. To identify patients eligible for the trial, Dr. Austin searches through a patient database on the Cancer Knowledge Base that contains clinical information obtained with the consent of each individual patient who has self-registered interest at Plantation Medical Center's patient work stations or from their home. Using this information, which is based on common data elements and clinical states defined by NCI consensus groups, Dr. Austin obtains the list of eligible patients in her geographic area and their primary care providers.

One of these is 55-year-old Judith Johnson. After three symptom-free years, she has just been diagnosed with a positive biopsy and with multiple nodules in both lungs and lesions in the spine and pelvis. With patient Johnson's consent, her primary care doctor, Dr. Simpson, has accessed the NCI Web site for clinicians to gather information on her prognosis and treatment options, one of which is the OncoDrug Clinical Trial, and has entered her basic clinical data into the patient database.

Dr. Austin emails Dr. Simpson to indicate that patient Johnson is eligible for the OncoDrug trial and ask him to speak with her about the trial. After he explains the benefits and risks associated with the trial, she enrolls, signs the electronic informed consent form, and authorizes the release of her patient record. Used to complete the study enrollment forms, the information also includes the organ function data and/or genetic phenotype needed to calculate the dosage of OncoDrug she will receive. Once her enrollment is confirmed, all those to be involved in the trial are notified. Judith Johnson's patient record specifies her preferences on how she wishes to receive personal information during the trial.

Clinical team members enter clinical observations and the contracted laboratory and imaging center enter results into the patient record; these are automatically populated to the clinical trial database, which is available online to password enabled individuals based on their role in the trial. The database continuously updates treatment schedules; generates reminders, alerts, and task lists for patient Johnson, Dr. Simpson, Dr. Austin, and the rest of the team; and automatically issues reimbursements.

When Judith Johnson's white blood cell count falls below expected levels to reach a grade 4 toxicity, the trial database automatically prepares an online adverse drug event (ADE) for distribution to the investigators, MCOG,

PharmaCo, and the institutional review board. Dr. Austin and Dr. Simpson review the information and decide to keep patient Johnson in the trial. PharmaCo prepares a narrative and submits the adverse event to the FDA.

On the trial database, Dr. Carter, Dr. Austin, and representatives of the NCI use key performance metrics (e.g., number of patients enrolled, number of adverse events) to evaluate the trial's progress. The institutional review board accesses real-time data for tracking and monitoring, and physicians and patients are updated via their preferred method. MCOG representatives monitor the trial by following the real-time clinical data, diminishing the need for visits to the trial sites. Since all clinical data are captured directly from the patient record, source data verification is done remotely. Monitoring mechanisms identify unusual, missing, or inconsistent data throughout the trial—and immediately notify the investigators and their trial managers.

At the conclusion of the trial, Melinda Jones validates and "locks" the database. Dr. Carter, the NCI, and PharmaCo "unblind" the study and perform data analysis. The analysis completed, the investigators prepare the clinical study report for the NCI and the FDA and publish two research articles on the trial. The three research reports are disseminated online to Judith Johnson and other patients and advocacy groups that have requested such information. Based on Dr. Carter's trial, PharmaCo presents the new indication for OncoDrug to the FDA for approval.

Trial Manager Perspective on Clinical Trials in 2004

In 2004, trial managers—the individuals who provide administrative support for the clinical trials process—will transform "data oversight" into "information insight." In cooperative groups and contract research organizations (CROs), trial managers will move beyond data and documents to create rich and usable information repositories. The *Cancer Informatics Infrastructure (CII)* will help them in their work with *Institutional Review Boards (IRBs)* to rationalize the approval process and incorporate advances in genetically customized drugs into clinical trials.

The goal is for trial managers to:

Minimize time from scientific concept to first patient accrual.

- Electronic templates will expedite protocol design and preparation, by building on existing knowledge and helping developers and reviewers focus on new questions.
- Trial managers will track multiple reviews concurrently, while ensuring that concerns are shared across review groups for collaborative resolution.
- Ancillary service providers (labs, imaging centers, etc.) will enter into standardized contracts for trials online, assured that their services will be promptly approved and reimbursed electronically.

- Web-based data entry will accelerate determination of patient eligibility while ensuring the quality of the data collected in the registration process.

Maximize patient participation in cancer clinical trials.

- Software tools—intelligent agents—will search for protocols and disseminate trial summaries, customizing information for the individual conducting the search.
- Intelligent agents will screen patients for protocols, matching patient data to protocol specifications (eligibility criteria, disease state, etc.) to identify the best possible options.
- Web-based education tools for patients will provide reliable, up-to-date information about clinical trials and support them in making decisions about cancer treatment options.

Exchange information to optimize effective studies.

- Web-based training materials will facilitate trial start-up for investigators and physicians, improve compliance with protocol requirements, and ultimately speed time to completion.
- Web-based access to data captured at the point of care will:
  - support remote monitoring of study sites
  - automate basic data analyses
  - report to stakeholders in real time when appropriate.

Facilitate translation of clinical trial results into cancer care.

- The patient-centric records used in clinical trials will:
  - capture basic treatment and outcomes data
  - populate the clinical trials database and data repository
  - be available on the Web for all authorized users.
- Patient data in the clinical trial database will provide the basis for creating new clinical guidelines.
- Automated "clinical decision trees" will collect data on individual patients and provide patient-tailored decision support.
- Web-enabled dissemination of clinical outcomes will generate hypotheses for new clinical trials.

Scenario

In his role as chair of the Mid-Central Oncology Group (MCOG), a research cooperative, Dr. Sheats ensures that the group's research is closely aligned with the priorities of the National Cancer Institute (NCI) and that affiliated investigators receive the funding and trial management services they need.

Drawing on expert advice and databases of research information, MCOG identifies projects that merit funding and research gaps that exist. Using a common development template, MCOG creates calls for concepts that are placed on the NCI Web Site. Researchers retrieve the calls and submit letters of intent online to MCOG for review. One such letter comes from Dr. Carter, who proposes a study of OncoDrug in the treatment of breast cancer. It is reviewed and funded by MCOG.

Upon the award, Dr. Sheats calls Dr. Carter to outline the clinical trail process. He reviews the services MCOG provides, describes how funding is disbursed electronically, and informs him that Melinda Jones, one of MCOG's trial managers, will be assigned to his study. When Melinda Jones receives an email from Dr. Sheats notifying her of the trial and her assignment to it, she contacts Dr. Carter online, sending the procedures for investigators conducting trials with MCOG. To assist in the authoring process she directs him to the protocol toolkit on the NCI Web site. The toolkit provides him with common protocol templates, including eligibility criteria, inclusion/exclusion criteria, drug schemas, informed consent forms, and patient accrual benchmarks.

Dr. Carter uses the toolkit to build new parts of the protocol that do not exist, such as the portion dealing with genetically linked response to OncoDrug that he is testing in this trial. The toolkit automatically highlights his changes and additions. After his initial changes are complete, he forwards the document to trial manager Jones.

Using the toolkit, trial manager Jones distributes portions of the protocol to the review team, including the Institutional Review Board (IRB), the protocol design coordinator, and the sponsor/facilitator of OncoDrug trials at NCI. Using the NCI's protocol approval tracking system (PATS), trial manager Jones is able to monitor parallel reviews of the protocol and coordinate the required changes. The online review process minimizes redundancies, as reviewers are aware of how the protocol differs from the standard templates, and can collaborate to address concerns and comments about the protocol. The highlighting of all modifications and additions allows them to focus on key issues. Within 60 days of submission, the protocol is approved by NCI and the IRB.

To activate the trial, trial manager Jones forwards the protocol online to investigators who expressed an interest in participating in the trial. Using the NCI's Web-enabled library of common data elements, she generates a data entry form, modifying and adding any necessary common data elements. An initial database structure is generated automatically as she composes the data form. Working with the biostatistician and the database manager for the OncoDrug study, she finalizes the structure of the study database, and sends a copy to Dr. Carter for his approval.

Next she activates the NCI-required fields within the study database to automatically submit data to the NCI database on a regular schedule, and finalizes the randomization plan and patient accrual schedule. To identify which service providers can best support the trial, she queries the ancillaries database for comparative information on companies that comply with NCI-supported standards for the electronic transmission of test results. After selecting a laboratory for blood work, an imaging center, and a pathology service, she emails each of them a standard ancillary-services contract for electronic signature.

Within MCOG, she notifies those responsible for quality assurance of the new trial and its participating sites. The quality assurance group analyzes the historical data for each of the facilities to verify adherence to good clinical practices and conducts brief site visits. Most subsequent quality monitoring is performed remotely, by ongoing review of the data submitted electronically from the remote sites.

To set up the training program for the trial, she consults online with MCOG's education specialist. The specialist modifies standard templates to develop Web-enabled patient education materials, as well as training sessions for investigators and research assistants. All the education materials are made available in print and online to authorized individuals.

Now ready to activate the trial, trial manager Jones forwards pertinent information to the NCI Web site, which in turn notifies participating oncology centers and oncologists of the trial's availability. Two days after the training session, an investigator enrolls the first patient using remote data entry. Trial manager Jones monitors the process, as errors in the initial data set are identified and clarification is immediately requested from the researcher entering the data. As more patients are enrolled, the trial manager continues to track the data for accuracy and completeness.

As patients are enrolled in the trial, their DNA sequences are captured and sent electronically to the packaging and supply distribution center of PharmaCo, the company that manufactures OncoDrug. Customized patient drug packages based on pharmacogenetic dosing regimens are developed and sent to the treatment site.

To ensure that the project stays on track, trial manager Jones monitors the accrual rates and compares them to the projections. For each participating investigator, she approves monthly reimbursement, based on the number of patients accrued and the quality of data collected. She also tracks ancillary charges, which are submitted and reimbursed electronically. No additional administrative paperwork is required.

Melinda Jones, MCOG's quality assurance team, and the IRB monitor the trial by searching through clinical data in real time. This "living view" of the trial results diminishes the need for visits to the trial sites. All clinical data are captured directly from the patient record and verified online. Throughout the course of the trial, monitoring mechanisms automatically alert the trial manager and the investigators to unusual, missing, or inconsistent data. To ensure that the quality of the database is maintained, she monitors database alerts and assures their prompt resolution.

Within 60 days of the last patient's enrollment, all data are submitted and the trial concluded. After cleaning and validating the data, trial manager Jones "locks" the database. Basic statistical analyses are performed automatically and forwarded to Dr. Carter. As soon as a biostatistician has performed the more complex analyses, a copy of the results goes to Dr. Carter. He reviews the results and devises additional analyses in consultation with the biostatistician. Negative results are extracted and sent to the Electronic Journal of Negative Results.

Once the results are finalized, Melinda Jones helps Dr. Carter and his co-investigators disseminate their findings. She works with Dr. Carter to finalize the trial summaries for the NCI Web site and to prepare publications. She also helps him organize and facilitate a series of online discussions, tailored specifically to investigators, oncologists, and patients and their family members. These sessions foster new investigator collaborations and generate new ideas for future trials, including recommendations expediting the use of OncoDrug in breast cancer. The sessions also improve cancer care, by making patients better informed and by developing new guidelines for treating patients.

Payer/Provider/Delivery System Perspective on Clinical Trials in 2004

In 2004 and beyond, organizations that provide prepaid healthcare services on a per member basis—HMOs, managed care organizations, insurers, HCFA, integrated delivery and financing systems—will see clear value in offering their members access to clinical trials. They will find clinical trials administratively efficient and clinically effective, and consider improved outcomes and greater control of information and decisions as protection against litigation, justification of enhanced reimbursement, and a distinct marketing advantage.

The goal is for payers to:

Provide high quality cancer treatment for their members.

- National Cancer Institute (NCI) certification of trials supported by the Cancer Information Infrastructure (CII) will ensure high quality care for trial participants.
- Members of organizations providing care on a per member per month basis will have access to clinical trials through the benefit packages provided them.
- Payers, providers, and delivery systems will have data that measure performance, support decision making, and demonstrate the value of clinical trials as a treatment option.
- Ease of access to and participation in clinical trials will promote them as a standard option for treatment of all patients.

Make a solid business case for participating in clinical trials.

- With validated quality and processes, NCI certified clinical trials will limit payers' exposure to liability for adverse events and less than optimal outcomes.
- Payers, providers, and delivery systems will use outcomes of trial-related care as a basis for supporting accreditation (e.g., National Committee on Quality Assurance).
- Providing NCI certified trials as a benefit will curtail the creation of new precedence, while allowing care options to advance.
- Documenting that the value of clinical trials accrues to payers and providers as well as patients will reinforce their viability as a treatment option.

Scenario

Founded in 1986, GoodHealth is a not-for-profit managed care organization with three million members. While increasing its membership by 10% annually, GoodHealth has kept its per-member-per-month rates in line with the national average. To enhance its reputation as a high value, customer service-oriented payer, GoodHealth—in collaboration with one of its major customers, the MidWest Employer Coalition—has extended its product line to include options with expanded clinical trial benefits for their members. In structuring these benefits, the two organizations consult with the National Cancer Institute (NCI) on issues of cost and value, under the auspices of the partnership of the American Association of Health Plans (AAHP) with NCI's parent organization, the National Institutes of Health (NIH). Benefits in place, GoodHealth is entered into the payer database for access by investigators planning trials and for patients and physicians looking to verify coverage.

Once in the database, payers access and receive a range of information on clinical trials. When trials are being launched in the geographical area GoodHealth serves, GoodHealth's medical director is sent information online for review. When he receives information about Dr. Carter's trial, the director searches the NCI cancer research database for findings from earlier OncoDrug studies. Responsible for ensuring high quality care for members and protecting GoodHealth from liability, the medical director looks to NCI certification to confer a high degree of confidence in the quality of the trial and assistance from the NCI in the event of litigation.

GoodHealth staff review cost information entered by the trial investigator during the design process estimating costs for trial-related services charged by the laboratories and diagnostic centers in NCI's ancillaries database, along with local rates for purposes of comparison. Cost data also identify the proposed level of reimbursement for participating physicians, based on number of enrollees and quality of data submitted.

Based on these data, combined with internal criteria, GoodHealth notifies Dr. Carter that they want to participate in the trial. After they negotiate and finalize a contract regarding reimbursement of patient care costs for their members enrolled in the trial, the NCI Web site on OncoDrug is updated to state that GoodHealth will be supporting the trial.

As their practice requires, GoodHealth alerts their case managers online about the OncoDrug clinical trial. After identifying the high-risk member population that might benefit from the trial, case managers notify individual members' primary care physicians and direct them to the NCI Web site for information about the OncoDrug trial, including eligibility criteria.

One such physician is Dr. Robert Simpson, who has several high-risk patients in his care, including 55-year-old Judith Johnson, who has been symptom-free since treatment for breast cancer three years earlier. Shortly after Dr. Simpson has learned about the OncoDrug trial, he sees patient Johnson in his office with a lump below her breast and back pain and orders the required diagnostic tests. After the tests, indicating the cancer has spread, patient Johnson and her husband meet with Dr. Simpson to discuss her prognosis and the courses of treatment available to her. Dr. Simpson gives them patient education information he has obtained from the NCI Web site on the OncoDrug trial and other options for them to use as they decide what treatment option to choose.

At her next visit, when Judith Johnson indicates she has decided to participate in the OncoDrug trial, Dr. Simpson performs an online eligibility check and electronically enrolls Judith in the trial. Her enrollment information is routed online to GoodHealth and to Dr. Austin, the oncologist who will be treating patient Johnson during the trial.

From this point on, all the clinical information related to patient Johnson's treatment is entered directly into her Web-based patient record and the trial database. That record electronically authorizes all services called for by the protocol, including those provided by GoodHealth and those by ancillary facilities contracted for the trial. The entry of the clinical data from required services automatically triggers payment, speeding reimbursement and lessening administrative paperwork for GoodHealth, its providers, and members. Dr. Simpson is freed of the need to write out paper referrals and authorizations for patient Johnson, who is assured that all services she receives under the protocol are covered by GoodHealth.

Once the trial is complete and data have been analyzed, while preserving the confidentiality of patient data, the results are shared with its participants at GoodHealth, including primary care physicians like Dr. Simpson and patients like Judith Johnson. They receive information on the trial's findings, prepared for them as physicians or patients, and GoodHealth incorporates the information into their disease management program for cancer. In addition, GoodHealth receives trial data to use in documenting their performance as a managed care organization in treating cancer, as required by Health Employer Data and Information Set (HEDIS) and the Foundation for Accountability (FACCT).

To document patient satisfaction and outcomes, GoodHealth surveys Judith Johnson and other members involved in the trial using several instruments, including the standard report known as Short Form-36 (SF-36). GoodHealth shares the feedback they receive with NCI, for use in improving NCI-sponsored investigator training and educational programs. GoodHealth also sends reports on trial findings and patient satisfaction to large employer groups, like the MidWest Employer Coalition, interested in clinical trial options for their members as a component of quality care.

Acknowledgments. Throughout its deliberations, the Long Range Planning Committee drew upon expertise within the National Cancer Institute, including many NCI staffers in its meetings. In addition, the LRPC also consulted with experts from academia and the private sector. A small "tiger team," including Marion Ball, Michael Becich, Christopher Chute, Judith Douglas, Michael Glodé, Curtis Langlotz, and William Scherlis, assisted in developing the final report. The tiger team was briefed by representatives from Oracle and worked with a team from First Consulting Group led by C. David Hardison during phase 2 activities.

National Cancer Institute Long Range Planning Committee (LRPC) Members*. Marion J. Ball, First Consulting Group and Johns Hopkins University; Michael J. Becich, University of Pittsburgh School of Medicine; Douglas W. Blayney, Pomona Valley Hospital Medical Center; David N. Campbell; Christopher G. Chute, Mayo Foundation; Morris F. Collen, Kaiser Permanente; Don E. Detmer, University of Virginia; Alan Dowling, Ernst & Young; John P. Fanning, Department of Health and Human Services; L. Michael Glodé, University of Colorado Health Sciences Center; David Harrington, Dana-Farber Cancer Institute; Robert A. Hiatt, National Cancer Institute; Curtis P. Langlotz, University of Pennsylvania and EDICT Systems; Nancy M. Lorenzi, University of Cincinnati Medical Center; William L. Scherlis, Carnegie Mellon University; Eleanor McFadden, Frontier Science and Technology Research Association; Mitchell Morris, MD Anderson Cancer Center; Joyce Niland, City of Hope National Medical Center and Beckman Research Institute; Jane Reese-Coulbourne, National Cancer Institute; Howard R. Soule, CaPCURE; Juilian Smith, National Cancer Institute; Robert E. Wittes, National Cancer Institute; Jay M. Tenenbaum, Veo Systems; Yelena Yesha, University of Maryland Baltimore County.

*Affiliations are those held by members during the committee's deliberations.

3
Clinical Trials in Practice

L. MICHAEL GLODÉ

For the past three decades, individuals and organizations that conduct clinical trials have struggled to increase patient enrollment. As the number of patients required for the average clinical trial has increased, recruitment has become the primary obstacle to fast, efficient trial completion, consuming close to 30% of clinical development time. To expedite trials, we must identify the factors that complicate patient recruitment and implement solutions like improved trial design and e-enabled enrollment. In this chapter, we explore our progress to date, summarizing research on clinical trial participation and describing current efforts to solve the recruitment problem.

The Challenge

Various studies have identified barriers to and success factors for increased trial participation. For example, Albrecht et al. examined videotapes of physician–patient interactions and discovered that oral communication of the elements in a consent form, whether legalistic or more socially oriented, improved trial participation rates (Albrecht, 1999). Ellis (1999) evaluated Australian oncologists and reported that "...barriers to participation in current breast cancer trials were lack of resources (44%) or issues related to specific trials (...e.g. relevance of the research questions or choice of standard therapies)."

A study of Eastern Cooperative Oncology Group (ECOG) physicians and members of the National Medical Association (NMA) uncovered other barriers and potential solutions. A significant percentage—69% of NMA members and 43% of ECOG physicians—reported a lack of information about specific clinical trials, and 47% of NMA physicians and 4% of ECOG physicians cited the scarcity of minority investigators. As solutions, both groups suggested improving communication (73%) and providing patients with culturally relevant educational materials (40%). Other potential solutions met with different responses from the two groups. A greater number of ECOG physicians endorsed the addition of more minority outreach staff (22% versus 6% of NMA physicians), and far more NMA members suggested increasing the involvement of referring physicians (44% versus 4% of ECOG physicians) (McCaskill-Stevens, 1999).

Finally, a Scandanavian survey by Hjorth collected physicians' opinions on crucial factors for patient participation. According to the study, the physicians "considered the scientific purpose of a trial to be the most important factor for patient accrual, followed by the simplicity of study protocol, the rightness of ethical aspects, the quality of communication with the study organization, and the degree of participation in investigator meetings" (Hjorth, 1996).

To fully evaluate these and other variables associated with clinical trials accrual, Dr. Alan Lichter initiated a series of studies by the American Society of Clinical Oncology (ASCO) (Emanuel et al., 1999). Survey questionnaires were mailed to 8,093 practicing oncologists, and replies were received from 3,550 (43.9%). Eighty percent of oncologists had participated in clinical trials within the previous three years. They reported that 29.5% of their patients were eligible for a trial, 22.6% had been approached, and 14.3% were actually enrolled. The key factors that prevented higher enrollment included:

- Restrictive eligibility criteria
- Lack of protected time
- Pressure to generate revenue
- Excessive paperwork
- Lack of availability of research nurses and data managers.

When asked what factors would help enroll patients, respondents provided the data in Table 3.1.

In a companion study of industry trends, 116 companies reported 267 compounds in 647 clinical trials. Thirty-two (28%) of the companies

Table 3.1. Factors identified as helpful to enroll patients

Reduced paperwork for enrolling	86.9%
Reduced paperwork for reporting	85.4%
Assured reimbursement of clinical costs	83.1%
More data management help	80.7%
New drugs at low cost	79.7%
Increase in enrollment reimbursement	77.5%
Internet list of protocols	61.3%
Coordination of cooperative groups	60.5%
National enrollment center	46.7%

Source: Adapted with permission from Schnipper, L. 1999. Presidential Symposium: Report of the Clinical Trials Subcommittee. (ASCO Virtual Meeting, p.13. *http://www.conference-cast.-com/asco/default_vm99.htm*)

provided responses to questionnaires and reported that oncology trials ranked as the fourth largest category of their research, comprising 9% of ongoing trials. (Other areas were cardiovascular, 25%; central nervous system [CNS], 17%; and respiratory, 14%.) These studies accounted for 13,321 patients, which, when combined with the known 20,000 patients in government trials and 7,000 patients in other types of trials, matches the overall estimate that less than 3% of oncology patients participate in clinical trials (Schnipper, 1999).

Studies of clinical trial sites found that conducting a 20-patient trial of moderate intensity requires almost two full time equivalent persons (FTEs). This translates to over 200 staff hours per patient, with academic and freestanding centers reporting the highest time requirements, at 389 to 455 hours per patient, and group practices reporting the lowest, at 136 to 141 hours per patient (Schnipper, 1999). Data management and nursing occupied the bulk of this time.

When deciding whether to participate in a clinical trial, sites reported that their ability to bring therapy to patients and the importance of the research question were the most important contributing factors, as shown in Figure 3.1.

The survey also enumerated the activities required to conduct a clinical research trial. These are:

- Pre-Institutional Review Board (IRB) submission
- Study initiation

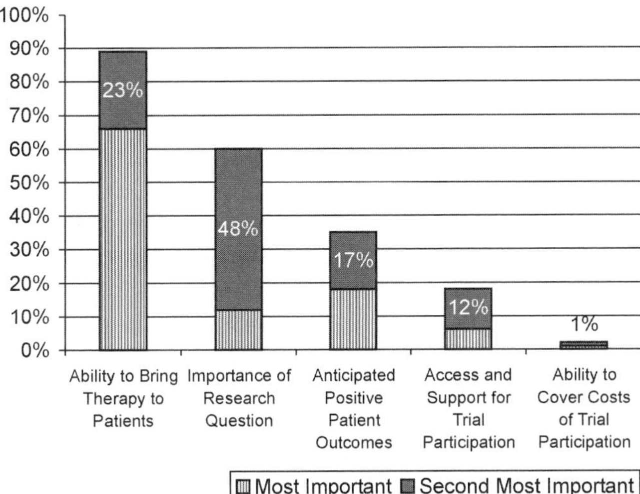

Figure 3.1. Sites' most important factors in reaching a decision about clinical trial participation. (Adapted with permission from Schnipper, L. 1999. Presidential Symposium: Report of the Clinical Trials Subcommittee. ASCO Virtual Meeting. http://www.conference-cast.com/asco/default_vm99.htm)

- Recruitment
- Randomization
- Supply management/dispensing
- Office visit—study drug
- Office visit—follow-up
- Adverse events (severe, moderate)
- Data management and analysis
- Audits and monitoring visits
- Communications with sponsor
- Post-study followup
- Post-study investigator meetings (Schnipper, 1999).

Solving the Recruitment Problem

Taken together, these studies highlight the need to improve patient accrual for trials. In the ASCO study, the patient recruitment and consent process was nearly as time-consuming and costly as office visits and data management/analysis. Numerous investigators have suggested solutions, and reports are available for public scrutiny.

Technology-related solutions may meet some of the challenges outlined in the preceding studies. Substituting an efficient electronic system can reduce paperwork for enrolling and reporting patients, the top two items on the ASCO survey list shown in Table 3.1. Other items on the list—more data management help, Internet listing of protocols, coordination of cooperative groups, and a national enrollment center—present direct challenges to the technical community and the National Cancer Institute (NCI) Informatics Infrastructure.

To address the remaining challenges, including reduced paperwork for enrolling and reporting patients, the NCI Cancer Informatics Infrastructure effort has concluded that universal medical language standards will effect the greatest contribution from public and private sectors. All involved parties, whether they are pharmaceutical companies, cooperative groups, or NCI-sponsored studies, should use common patient registration and reporting forms.

Various groups maintain efforts to help researchers conduct clinical trials with the aid of technology. The following are some examples.

The NCI CancerTrials Web Site

The NCI CancerTrials Web site (http://cancertrials.nci.nih.gov; see Figure 3.2), which participates in the larger government effort known as ClinicalTrials.gov, has already addressed the Internet list of protocols. Intense use of similar Internet addresses compromises both of these sites. The University of Virginia uses "cancertrials.com" for its melanoma clinical

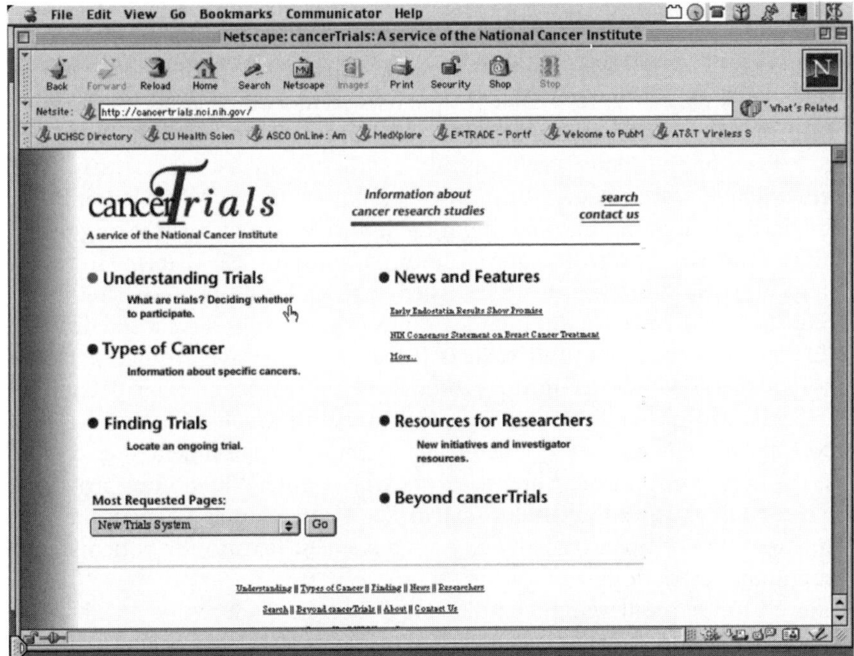

FIGURE 3.2. http://cancertrials.nci.nih.gov

patient recruitment site (http://www.cancertrials.com/), and "clinicaltrials.org" (http://www.clinicaltrials.org) is an M.D. Anderson Web site that educates patients and physicians about cancer research at that institution. While Pharmaceutical Research Plus, Inc., a for-profit company with an incomplete resource library, uses "clinicaltrials.com," Clinicaltrials.gov (http://clinicaltrials.gov), the subject of Alexa McCray's contribution to this volume, contains in-depth information for cancer patients interested in all types of clinical trials.

The NCI staff designed the CancerTrials Web site to provide professionals and patients with information about ongoing trials. Its sections contain information on understanding trials, news listings on specific types of cancer (mostly from NCI resources), and the Physician Data Query (PDQ) search system, organized into a filtered system much like PubMed. Professionals or patients can enter filters for type of study (e.g., Phase I, II, III, adjuvant), location in the country by state, and approach (e.g., angiogenesis, vaccine, chemotherapy), and then submit for a complete listing of trials meeting the criteria. For the more sophisticated user, the CancerTrials Web site offers more than the other major government Web site, ClinicalTrials.gov. The latter system currently lists 1,960 open cancer trials, but users may find it more difficult to search by trial type because the filtering system covers broader applications, like searching for antibiotic trials in otitis media.

CenterWatch

On the commercial side, the most comprehensive response to the clinical trials challenge is CenterWatch (http://www.centerwatch.com). A Boston-based publishing and information services company founded in 1994, this site focuses on the clinical trials industry, with an emphasis on industry. The CenterWatch search system bears some similarity to the NCI CancerTrials system, but it suffers somewhat from the industry system for tracking trials.

For example, "prostate cancer" returns a list of 136 trials. However, many of these are the same trial listed with different protocol numbers, because they are open in different locations (e.g., 26 sites have a zoledronate infusion protocol open, and each is listed as a separate protocol). Using another method—searching for protocols open, for example, in Kentucky for breast cancer—only one listing appears, even though ClinicalTrials.gov and CancerTrials.gov list 18 open trials. Although government sites do not list the industry-sponsored breast cancer trial, CenterWatch does provide a link to NCI trials via the patient screen. The CenterWatch gateway can also generate a list of open trials by city, a convenient feature for patients with geographic restrictions.

Several other emerging commercial Web sites address clinical trials infrastructure and recruitment issues, and CenterWatch maintains a symbiotic relationship with one. Among the largest of the "dot.com" health companies, WebMD (http://webmd.com/) uses the CenterWatch site as a gateway to cancer clinical trials. Like CenterWatch it reprocesses the trials using a separate gateway that ensures both WebMD and CenterWatch "branding" of the information generated.

Lifemetrix.com

Lutz and Henkind reviewed several other websites dealing with clinical trials infrastructure and recruitment (Lutz & Henkind, 2000). Noting that the paper-choked system demands a new patient recruiting environment, they listed a number of Internet sites, as reviewed in Table 3.2.

Table 3.2. Commerical Internet sites offering clinical trials search capabilities

Internet Site	Content
www.oncology.com	Searches use same database as Center Watch, licenced by Acuarian
www.ecancertrials.com	Uses four step search process
www.canceredication.com	Searches use the NCI Cancer Trials database plus cooperative groups
www.cancerfacts.com	Searches use same database as Center Watch
www.oncolink.com	Searches use the NCI CancerTrials database plus cooperative groups and University of Pennsylvania protocols
www.cancersource.com	Search strategy is "under construction"
www.cancerpage.com	Connects to TrialMatch™, a service of LifeMatrix.com (see text)

Among these sites, the most innovative for average patient use is probably the TrialMatch™ system developed by Lifemetrix.com, a business-to-business disease management company specializing in oncology, asthma, congestive heart failure, HIV/AIDS, high-risk pregnancy, and diabetes. To help manage such patients, Lifemetrix developed TrialMatch, which adds granularity to trial searches. For example, if a prostate cancer patient has a rising prostate-specific anitgen level, screens direct him to answer questions like whether he has tried antiandrogens or has had chemotherapy.

This capability allows patients to fill out their own eligibility page. A submission form offers guidance from an RN and a pledge to try to return inquiries within 24 hours. TrialMatch asks patients if they wish to be contacted, assures confidentiality, and passes authorized email addresses to a CRO or pharmaceutical company if a patient is eligible. TrialMatch is willing to list new pharmaceutical protocols for a fee and has a special interest in oncology. They will also list IRB-approved protocols from individual investigators, using eligibility criteria to match the protocol to the question area for patient response.

Managed Health Organizations

Large managed healthcare organizations conduct other patient recruitment efforts. One prominent oncology example is U.S. Oncology, covered elsewhere in this book. A second example is Health Benchmarks, Inc. (HBI), an organization that reports detailed access to over 5 million members of contracted provider groups in California and the northeastern United States (http://www.healthbenchmarks.com/clinical.asp). HBI offers a general form for patients interested in a particular disease category and a separate questionnaire for prospective investigators to fill out. Then they match the care providers, pharmaceutical (or other) trial initiators, and appropriate patients to the clinical trials.

The American Society of Clinical Oncology

The largest professional society of oncologists in the world, ASCO has entered the field of cancer informatics with its own Web site, ASCO OnLine (http://www.asco.org). When the society first considered launching a Web site in 1995, there were few oncology-oriented Internet resources. Notable among them, however, were the NCI Web site that offered the physician's data query materials (now CancerTrials) and Oncolink, the University of Pennsylvania site that was the forerunner of many organizational, commercial, and cancer center sources of Internet information. Developing a human infrastructure to create an electronic outlet for ASCO was a novel and somewhat threatening undertaking. Concerns raised in initial discussions included the relationships (if any) between the society's print publication and the electronic medium, its potential to affect revenues at the annual meeting by competing for pharmaceutical advertising, and methods of controlling content generation and postings.

With board approval, physician volunteers and interested members of the ASCO staff formed an ad hoc committee to develop the Web site. None of them had experience with either the technical issues or the hierarchical approaches necessary to build and maintain an electronic "mirror" of ASCO's daily operation. Following a request for proposal, they chose a vendor with technical expertise in Web site creation and selected an open architecture that used the World Wide Web over a members-only software system similar to America Online. After three months of extensive programming, ASCO OnLine was officially launched on January 1, 1997.

ASCO OnLine, pictured in Figure 3.3, has grown dramatically in both content and use. Peak utilization months are May (reflecting the interest in the annual meeting) and November (reflecting abstract submission, the fall meeting, and registration for the annual meeting). In these months, about 6,000 users per day visit the site, and there are now more than 27,000 files and directories. In January 2000, ASCO redesigned the Web site to ease navigation. Figure 3.3 displays a pivotal part of this redesign, with dropdown screens allowing immediate access to features like oncologist locators and search tools for disease-specific information.

ASCO OnLine offers the results of clinical trials in the form of abstracts presented at its annual meeting. Many of these presentations are available

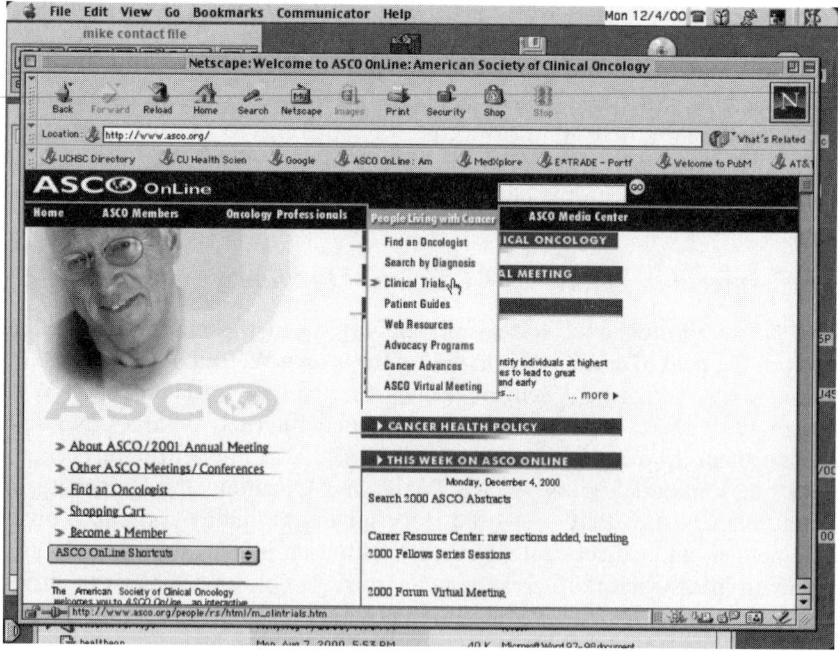

Figure 3.3. ASCO Online. (Reprinted with permission from ASCO.org)

on the Web site as slide or audio presentations. As with many other Web sites, one section provides patients with general information on clinical trials and links to many of the resources cited above, particularly the NCI CancerTrials Web site. Ongoing efforts will determine whether methods like those used for PubMed's "related articles" could be used to direct users to related protocols when they are viewing an abstract.

The American Cancer Society

The American Cancer Society (http://www.cancer.org/) has continually redesigned its Web site to meet the needs of cancer patients. The society has subscribed to the Cancer Profiler™, a software module that allows a patient to create a personalized, confidential account; enter his or her diagnosis and status (e.g., stage, previous treatment) and compare relevant treatment options and outcomes based on published clinical research. The results can be read on screen or printed for discussion with family or care providers.

Nexcura, the company that operates the http://www.cancerfacts.com Web site, supplies the software that makes this possible. A start-up company listed in the Arch Venture Partners portfolio, Nexcura lists a medical advisory board and a separate medical board of well-known leaders in the cancer field, both academic and private practice. The Nexcura software leads patients through a general and disease-specific questionnaire, including Java script to help with conflicting information. It reviews the patient's entries in a format like the one below, returned for a hypothetical patient with bladder cancer.

- You are in good health.
- You do not have severe bladder symptoms.
- Your kidneys are functioning well.
- You are not having severe bone pain.
- You have not answered the question about spread of the cancer. If you have this information, please return to the previous page and answer this question.
- You had your bladder removed to treat your most recent bladder cancer occurrence.

The Nexcura software then compares the patient's information to a database of clinical research and returns a list of relevant treatment options, along with possible side effects, and outcomes. Clicking on the treatment name provides a description of the treatment, along with questions to ask the physician. For each of the two treatment options, radiation therapy and chemotherapy relevant for our hypothetical patient, the site lists possible side effects as shown in Figure 3.4.

The American Cancer Society Web site offers a wealth of other information, including general information on clinical trials, links to the

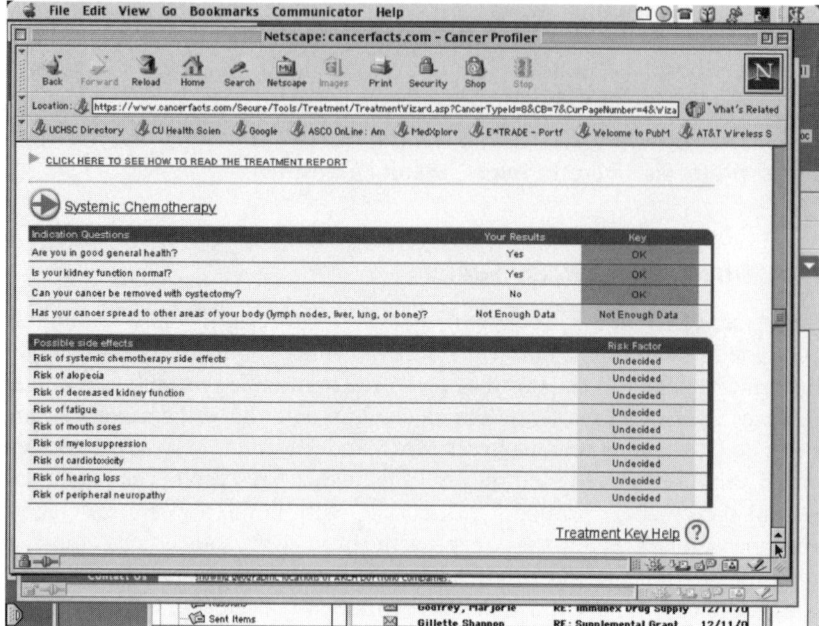

FIGURE 3.4. Treatment options. (Reprinted with permission from cancerfacts.com)

NCI ClinicalTrials Web site, and questions about trials for patients to ask their care providers.

Each of the preceding approaches has its strengths and weaknesses. For example, the NCI has a clear role and expertise in clinical trials execution, but it must rely on physician volunteers to conduct extramural recruitment. For-profit Internet entities like WebMD and the commercial Web site Medscape (http://www.medscape.com), which links to the NCI site and offers educational materials, have no expertise in clinical trials management but may attract the largest number of patients through heavy advertising and promotion. HBI must rely on pharmaceutical or other initiatives to develop the ideas and agents for clinical trials, but through contractual agreements, it can analyze the costs of such trials. Merging these diverse strengths and interests into an effective Cancer Informatics Infrastructure remains a challenge.

Looking Ahead

As discussed elsewhere in this volume, none of these initiatives achieves the paradigm of an ideal, comprehensive cancer informatics system:

initiation → approval → recruitment → reimbursement → reporting

The best examples of this paradigm are systems like iKnowmed (http://www.iknowmed.com/), discussed in another chapter, and competitors like IMPAC (http://www.impac.com/), which initially focused on radiation oncology management software. These companies have begun to accrue outcomes data that is stripped of individual identifiers but can approach the questions of specific treatment outcomes, including those for patients treated in specific trials.

The large databases of IMPAC and Lifemetrix provide insight into the future of protocol development. Fusing clinical research with commercial business-to-business outcomes and disease management software may enable an interface ideal for improving clinical trials participation. As reimbursement parties use such software to help decide which treatments to support, the evolution toward a common data dictionary like the one proposed in this book will ease comparison of protocol and non-protocol patients. Naturally, flowing from these efforts will be the desire to compare many different forms of treatment, a form of ad hoc clinical trial that needs only prospective planning to represent true Phase III protocol design and execution.

References

Albrecht TL, Blanchard C, Ruckdeschal JC, Coovert M, Strongbow R. 1999. Strategic Physician Communication and Oncology Clinical Trials. J Clin Oncol 17(10):3324–32.

Ellis PM, Butow PN, Simes RJ, TaHersall MH, Dunn SM. 1999. Barriers to Participation in Randomized Clinical Trials for Early Breast Cancer Among Australian Cancer Specialists. Aust N Z J Surg 69(7):486–91.

Emanuel E. 1999. Presidential Symposium: Report of the Clinical Trials Subcommittee. ASCO Virtual Meeting. http://www.conference-cast.com/asco/default_vm99.htm.

Hjorth M, Holmberg E, Rodjer S, Taube A, Westin J. 1996. Physicians' Attitudes Toward Clinical Trials and Their Relationship to Patient Accrual in a Nordic Multicenter Study on Melanoma. Control Clin Trials 17(5):372–86.

Lutz S, Henkind SJ. 2000. Recruiting for Clinical Trials on the Web. Healthplan 2000 41(5):36–43.

McCaskill-Stevens W, Pinto H, Marcus AC, Comis R, Morgan R, Plomer K, Schoentgen S. 1999. Recruiting Minority Cancer Patients into Cancer Clinical Trials: A Pilot Project Involving the Eastern Cooperative Oncology Group and the National Medical Association. J Clin Oncol 17(3):1029–39.

Schnipper L. 1999. Presidential Symposium: Report of the Clinical Trials Subcommittee. ASCO Virtual Meeting. http://www.conference-cast.com/asco/default_vm99.htm.

Section 2
The Infrastructure

William L. Scherlis
Section Editor

Introduction
Developing and Improving the Informatics Infrastructure to Support Clinical Research

William L. Scherlis

In this section we address some of the challenges of creating technological infrastructure to support clinical cancer research. The conduct of clinical trials is a highly complex and distributed enterprise. Any such infrastructure must support rapid ongoing evolution in the clinical practices and trial processes it supports and in its many technological elements. These range from the underlying communications and information technologies to the processes, protocols, and standards adopted to support clinical trials. The infrastructure must support a broad community of users, including individuals and institutions, with diverse and often conflicting interests. The infrastructure must also operate within a complex and evolving legal, regulatory, and procedural framework.

The benefits and challenges of developing computer-based patient records (CPR) systems are well-documented, as are the broader socioeconomic benefits of the developing Internet-based information infrastructure. Our focus is on the considerations that must be addressed to integrate these two huge enterprises in the service of cancer clinical trials—to create, in other words, a Cancer Informatics Infrastructure (CII).

Just as carefully designed common protocols are essential to the function of the Internet, so are common information elements crucial to an informatics substrate for clinical trials. Indeed, common protocol and information elements are what allowed, more than two decades ago, the inter-networking of diverse separate networks to create today's Internet. Common information elements include such items as nomenclature, scales, data elements, and protocol process descriptions. (These are addressed later in the book.) Common data elements evolve as understanding evolves, and it is desirable to uncouple this evolution of content from the evolution of the representational and process-support schemes underlying the content. Simply put, the decision to adopt, for example, XML-based information interchange is separate from the design of particular categories of common data elements. Decisions of representation and process support are engineering decisions, based partly on the technical merit of candidate technologies and partly on consistency with engineering choices made in the broader IT community. This latter "bandwagon" criterion addresses hard-to-quantify issues such as engineering risk, overall design flexibility, potential for interoperation, and architectural robustness. This criterion also includes issues related to standards adoption and market tipping (Shapiro & Varian, 1998).

Underlying the mechanisms for representation and process support is a base of core technologies that provide capabilities such as information management, metadata management, transaction support, security and authentication, and data communications. It is tempting to assert that in applying these underlying technologies to a Cancer Informatics Infrastructure, choices can be made simply by following the marketplace. This would mean, roughly, that the trials community adopts a baseline selection of infrastructural choices, such as Web-based information sharing, XML-based data representations, Internet-based data communication, relational database engines, and Web-based security and authentication. This scenario has the benefit that the community becomes able, almost by default, to "ride" the technology growth curves, including, for example, Moore's law for computer processing power and the growing set of consensus standards for XML representations of elements for electronic commerce transactions. The choice also appears expedient because it limits the extent of education required about the engineering and implementation details of these underlying technologies, because so many are offered as turnkey solutions.

The chapters in this section highlight the dangers of blindly following this baseline approach. Although there is nothing wrong with the any of the individual choices noted above, potential dangers lurk in their combination and in their mode of deployment. In this regard, careful attention must be given to the specific requirements of cancer clinical trials, ranging from aggregation over computer-based patient records, selection of common clinical data elements, and end-to-end security management for the large number of participants representing the diverse interests who merit access to various portions of the shared data. The integration challenge is how to address these diverse trial-specific needs while ensuring that the overall capability can evolve rapidly, both as the underlying infrastructure grows and as the tools, data elements, and processes for managing trials all improve.

The Internet underlies nearly all proposed solutions. In developing and improving an informatics infrastructure to support cancer trials, the Internet is worthy of study for two reasons. First, it is a critical and, arguably, unavoidable infrastructural element for any large-scale informatics enterprise. Second, the Internet can itself be taken as a successful and instructive example of a rapidly evolving suite of inter-related standards. It is a socio-technical system that has successfully withstood three decades of use and nine orders of magnitude in growth. It is also community-based in the sense that it is fundamentally not under the control of any single organization. In other words, the processes by which the Internet evolves are significant not only because of their impact on trials infrastructure, but also because they are instructive in how evolution can be managed for the trials infrastructure itself, which resides above the base set of Internet services.

Through what mechanism can a decision be made to accept the Internet as the critical infrastructure for cancer trials? A study of the processes and practices of Internet growth and evolution indicates that risks are carefully managed through a variety of mechanisms, despite the large number and high interdependency of standards.

There is rapid evolution of our understanding of cancer diagnosis and treatment and of best practices for the conduct of trials. This evolution will necessarily be more rapid than that of the architecture for trials support, with its huge number and diversity of stakeholders. The evolution of the Internet (and the principles of operation of organizations such as the Internet Engineering Task Force) offers lessons in how these processes can be managed in the cancer trials community.

Chapter 4, by Jay M. Tenenbaum, juxtaposes the design of the infrastructure for cancer trials with that for distributed e-business enterprises. Both deal with highly structured shared documents, online services of various kinds, location directories and registries, process and protocol support, and other distributed activities. The role of XML is highlighted, focusing on how a simple structural representation can provide a basis for codifying a diverse array of representational standards.

Chapter 5, by Clifford Neuman, focuses on issues of security and privacy. The diversity of stakeholders and their requirements for access to trials data creates a complex set of requirements for protection of information. The complexity is magnified by the changing legislative and regulatory environment, as well as by the diversity of policies among sets of trials. For particular elements of shared microdata, there are issues of confidentiality, integrity, and conformance with change protocols. Access by individuals and organizations to the trial data must be authenticated, and there must be non-repudiation for transactions on the data. How can developers of institutional segments of the overall Cancer Informatics Infrastructure make good technology choices without threatening the security and privacy attributes of an entire trials database? Neuman examines technologies such as firewalls, secure socket layer, the security system, digital signatures, authentication, and audit.

Chapter 6, by Ron Larsen and Jean Scholtz, moves beyond the conduct of trials into the scientific dissemination process that follows. Effective dissemination of information is essential for all stakeholders in the process of cancer clinical trials. The National Library of Medicine made pioneering steps in providing effective online access to medical information, effectively creating a highly efficient digital library for the entire healthcare community. Larsen and Scholtz consider what are next steps for digital libraries and organizational information sharing systems. They identify particular design attributes and consider various architectural approaches.

References

Shapiro C, Varian HR. 1998. Information Rules: A Strategic Guide to the Network Economy. Boston: Harvard Business School Press.

4
Cancer Informatics: Lessons from the World of e-Business

Jay M. Tenenbaum

American medical technology may be the envy of the world, but the US health care industry is downright backward with it comes to running its own business.

While banks, airlines and other service businesses long ago embraced automation to perform routine tasks, technology has been slow to take hold in health care. The US medical system of mostly independent doctors is highly fragmented. Administrative and clinical procedures are rarely standardized. And insurers' different rules for everything from drug coverage to claims forms have created barriers to the kind of connectivity that would bring health care into the digital age....

But thanks to the Internet, ...technology is slowly starting to simplify the business of health.

(Source: Rundle RL. 2000. The Wall Street Journal.)

Like the rest of health care, cancer research is a highly fragmented enterprise with complex paper-based processes that are inefficient, error prone, and often redundant. Few standards exist for these processes or the data they generate. These shortcomings have a negative impact on the cost, timeframe, and quality of clinical trials. They also impede collaborative research and slow the dissemination of research results into clinical practice.

Fortunately, Internet-based integration frameworks have helped solve similar problems in the business world, and there is good reason to believe that they will be equally effective in the healthcare domain. Our optimism stems from the belief that the same integration challenges arise in both domains, namely:

- Sharing data and information among heterogeneous systems that were never designed to interoperate
- Automating and integrating ad hoc paper-based processes within and across organizations.

This chapter explores the parallels between cancer informatics and e-commerce and concludes that there is indeed a substantial opportunity to leverage both expertise and technology from the business world. We first discuss the major integration challenges encountered in e-business and how they are being addressed through e-marketplaces and business networks. We then outline the design for a Cancer Informatics Infrastructure (CII) based on these models and discuss the necessary incremental developments. We conclude by speculating about the implications of e-business integration for cancer informatics and healthcare networks in the future.

The Business-to-Business (B2B) Integration Problem

The fundamental challenge of ecommerce is enabling companies to do business across a network despite differences in their business processes and computer systems. Traditionally, these problems were overcome through custom point-to-point integration or Electronic Data Interchange (EDI) networks. Both approaches are expensive and time consuming to implement, and therefore make economic sense only when companies do a lot of business together. The Internet, by contrast, promises an open marketplace where companies can do business spontaneously with anyone, anywhere, anytime. Fulfilling this promise requires a radically new integration solution, equally applicable to cancer informatics.

How can business systems from multiple vendors be connected if they were never designed to interact? In the absence of universal standards, integration must proceed incrementally. Internet marketplaces first standardize the processes and data formats within a particular business sector, such as automobiles or chemicals. Companies in that sector can connect once and immediately do business with anyone there. Next, industry exchanges and regional hubs integrate these specialized marketplaces, to enable cross-market trades. Since 1999, about 1,000 net markets and 75 industry and regional exchanges emerged, transforming the Internet into a global marketplace.

An Example

The personal computer (PC) industry illustrates this solution. As shown in Figure 4.1, the industry first relied on custom integration and EDI solutions to create two-tier distribution chains to connect manufacturers, distributors, and resellers. Companies such as Compaq and Ingram, which do hundreds of millions of dollars of business together each year, could easily justify the expense.

However, as suggested in Figure 4.2, such point-to-point integration solutions cannot scale. Overall, the PC industry includes 5,000 to 10,000 manufacturers and as many as 100,000 resellers. Even a huge distributor like Ingram, with 50% of the market share, can integrate directly with only a small fraction of its trading partners, limiting its ability to forecast demand and track inventory as it moves through the channel. This lack of channel visibility makes it difficult for traditional manufacturers like Compaq to compete with direct sellers like Dell and Gateway, that bypass distributors and build to order.

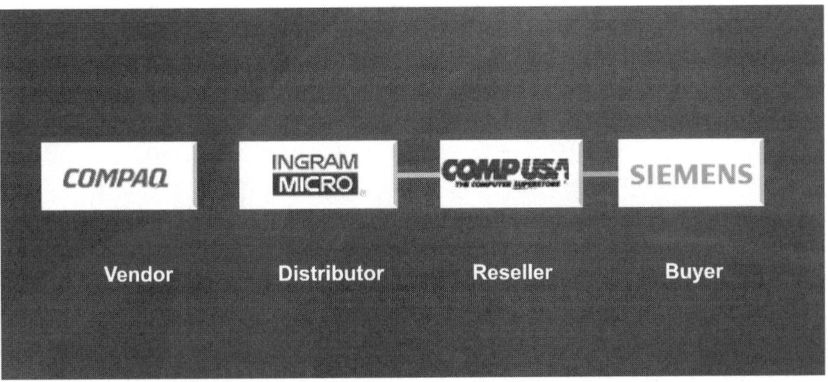

FIGURE 4.1. Basic two-tier distribution channel.

The solution, shown in Figure 4.3, replaces rigid supply chains with open "business webs." Companies share information with trading partners by displaying it on their Web sites, from product data and price lists to production and shipping schedules. Formatting the information using XML tags enables it to be understood by computers as well as viewed manually using a browser. The resulting visibility makes supply chain problems easy to solve. For example, Compaq could avoid over- and under-stocking by periodically polling each distributor and reseller to obtain current inventory levels.

The information posted by IT supply chain participants is enabling e-markets to offer valuable new services, ranging from intelligently matching buyers and sellers to optimizing inventory and production across an entire industry. There is indeed a direct analogy between how the advent of

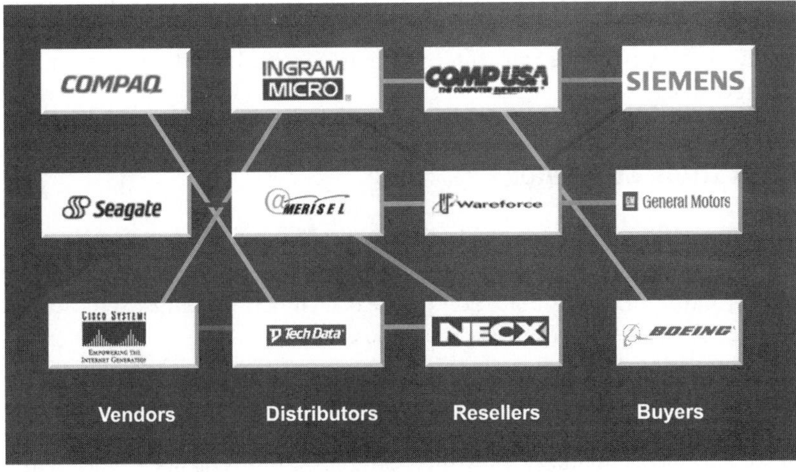

FIGURE 4.2. Industry-wide supply chain.

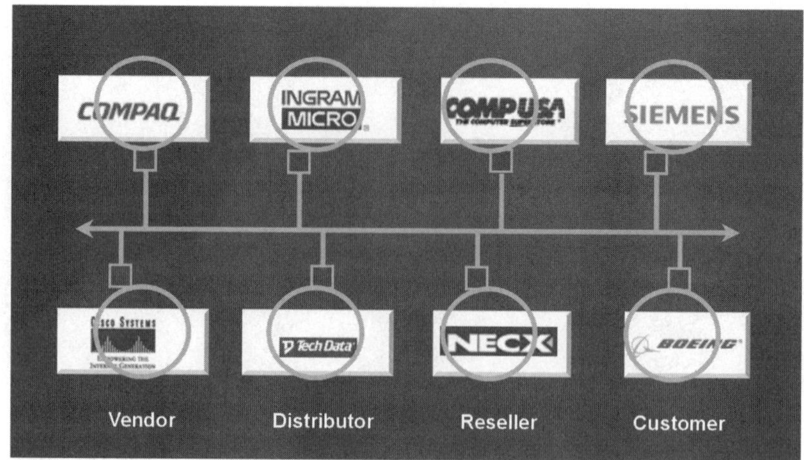

FIGURE 4.3. Industry-wide business web.

relational databases in the 1980s enabled Enterprise Resource Planning (ERP) applications and how business webs are now enabling this new class of Inter-Enterprise Resource Planning (I-ERP) applications: Whereas relational databases rationalized the data across an enterprise, the web rationalizes data across an industry.

Like opportunities abound in any industry with a fragmented value chain, including health care, and they even extend beyond industry boundaries. For example, a car company in the auto industry exchange should be able to purchase components from an electronics industry exchange, as well as obtain financing from a financial exchange.

The author's company, Commerce One, has integrated nearly 150 such e-marketplaces into a global trading web representing over 2 trillion dollars of aggregated spending. We believe that, within a few years, integration frameworks will make all Internet markets and trading communities interoperable.

Integration Technology

The principal job of an integration framework is enabling companies to do business with each other, regardless of their internal e-commerce systems, data formats, and communication protocols. Integration must thus occur at the level of business processes rather than systems.

Although there is still no universal architecture for e-business process integration, most of today's leading commercial solutions trace their roots to eCo System, a framework proposed in 1995 by the CommerceNet consortium (Tenenbaum, Chowdhry, Hughes, 1997; Glushko, Tenenbaum, Meltzer, 1999). Although Ariba, Web Methods, and other leading vendors are moving toward similar architecture and data models, Commerce One's implementation remains most faithful to the original eCo vision.

Services

To rise above system implementation details, the eCo framework introduced the abstraction of companies interacting with their trading partners through Web-based services. In distributed computing frameworks, services have long been used to provide simple ways of accessing a company's core processes—for example, to search a manufacturing company's catalog, track an order, request a rate quote, or schedule a pickup from a transportation company. However, such services were traditionally accessed through application programming interfaces (APIs). APIs tend to be complex and proprietary, because they're designed to integrate idiosyncratic computer systems rather than generic business processes, making systems integration costly and time-consuming.

Documents

A breakthrough occurred in 1997 with the realization that a better way to integrate business services was not through APIs but by exchanging business documents: purchase orders, invoices, shipping schedules, and the like. Documents are an ideal interface to business services for several reasons. First, that is how businesses communicate today, routinely exchanging documents via mail, email, the Web, EDI, and fax. Second, documents, unlike APIs, are easy for people to understand. Third, documents contain information in a declarative form that is also easy for machines to process. Documents thus provide an intuitive way of integrating people and services over a network.

When a document is sent to a service, a parser extracts information and applies business rules, triggering one or more of the following actions:

- The document is processed manually using an email client or Web browser
- Information from the document is passed through a traditional API to a local business application (e.g., an order entry system)
- The document, or one derived from it, is routed over the Internet to another service.

Rules can also trigger scripts that choreograph these basic actions into complete business processes. When a purchase order arrives at a distributor's ordering service, for example, the customer's name and address go to an internal account database for verification or updating, and information about part numbers and quantities is copied to a request for quotation form and sent to suppliers. If suppliers have an adequate quantity in stock at the right price, the vendor accepts and forwards it to an order entry system.

Otherwise, the purchase order is routed to a customer service representative for manual processing.

Registries

Registries are Web sites, public or private, where companies tell potential trading partners how to do business with them. On the registry, a company can publish its online services and state which documents to use when interacting with those services and in what order. For example, company X might register a sales service that accepts purchase orders conforming to X.12 850, UN-EDIFACT, or OBI specifications and then returns the corresponding purchase acknowledgment forms.

Public registries facilitate spontaneous commerce between trading partners without custom integration or prior agreement on industry-wide standards. Companies consult the registry to learn how to communicate with a particular trading partner, or search it to find trading partners who can accept their documents. Registries also accelerate the trend from legislated to market-driven standards. While companies will naturally gravitate toward popular document standards that bring them the most business, aggressive companies may opt to differentiate themselves by also accepting other formats, thus making it easier to do business with them.

In the absence of industry-wide standards for service registries, Commerce One recently joined with other leading vendors, including Ariba, IBM, and Microsoft to develop Universal Definition, Discovery, and Integration. Known as UDDI and detailed on the Web site (http://www.uddi.org), this common registry/directory service allows users to search for companies by name or service type—the traditional white and yellow pages—as well as offering "green pages" explaining how to interface to services through documents or traditional APIs.

Discussion

An integration framework based on services, documents, and registries has fundamental advantages over traditional solutions. These advantages include the following.

- **Loose coupling.** Integrating business services through the exchange of documents is fundamentally simpler than coupling them through APIs. Companies need only agree on the information a document contains, which for commercial documents is already highly standardized, not on how that information is processed. Each company can exploit the information in accordance with its own business rules and processes.
- **Incremental automation.** All organizations can participate. Those still employing manual, paper-based processes can begin by converting paper documents to Web-based forms. Upgrading to electronic documents provides immediate productivity gains by reducing delays and errors associated with moving paper. It also lays the groundwork for subsequent

automation, since business rules can be applied to generate routine responses or route documents to other services. Services can be automated independently, one task at a time, and users need never know whether a service they request is delivered manually or automatically.

- **Ease of programming.** Rule-based programming and scripting are programming styles most people find highly intuitive. Anyone who can format a PowerPoint slide master or an Excel spreadsheet should be capable of automating routine tasks and processes, particularly when given generic templates to customize.
- **Elimination of organizational boundaries.** The transaction costs of accessing a networked service are essentially the same whether that service is provided within a company or outsourced over the Internet. As Nobelist Ronald H. Coase observed, such a situation will drive companies to focus on core competencies where they are truly competitive, offering those services to the marketplace and outsourcing all others (Coase, 1988).
- **Plug and play commerce.** The eCo framework encourages businesses to build on each other's services, using them as components to create virtual companies, markets, and trading communities. The ability to rapidly design and implement innovative services that others can build on is sparking an explosion of entrepreneurial services in the B2B sector, one that is rivaling the growth of the Web itself.

We find these advantages compelling for e-business, and we believe the eCo framework can offer similar benefits to the cancer informatics community.

*The Role of eXtensible Markup Language (XML)**

The above discussion glosses over a crucial question: in the absence of universally adopted standards, how can corporate computer systems make sense of one another's documents? The answer begins with extensible Markup Language (XML), a simplified meta-language derived from SGML. Rapidly emerging as the standard for self-describing data exchange in Internet applications, XML provides "tags" that allow computers to understand the meaning of data (i.e., whether a number represents a price, a date, or a quantity). This significantly increases the functionality of Web commerce applications because they can do much more than simply display the data. For example, items in an XML-encoded catalog can be sorted by price, availability, or size.

The real power of XML, however, lies in its extensibility and ubiquity. Anyone can invent new tags for subject areas, define them in Document Type Definitions (DTDs), and post the DTDs on the Web or in a registry.

---

*Source: Adapted from Glusko, RJ, Meltzer B. Eco system: An XML Framework for Agent-Based E-Commerce. Communication of the ACM 42:3 (March 1999): 106–114.

```
<Catalog>
    <Computer Type="laptop">
        <Manufacturer>IBM</Manufacturer>
        <ProductLine>Thinkpad</ProductLine>
        <Model>560X</Model>
        <Specifications>
        <Speed>233 Mhz</Speed>
        <Memory>32 MB Memory</Memory>
        <Disk>4 MB Disk</Disk>
        <Weight>4.1 pounds</Weight>
        <Price Currency="US">$3,200</Price>
        </Specifications>
    </Computer>
</Catalog>
```

FIGURE **4.4.** Laptop description in XML.

As a result, everyone can validate and interpret documents conforming to published DTDs or create new document types.

Figure 4.4 shows a simplified example of an XML-encoded catalog entry for a laptop computer. The example begs two important questions: where do the tags come from, and what happens when two companies want to do business but use different tags? XML is only part of the story. A complete business integration solution also requires:

- Standardized tags or metadata for particular commerce communities
- A means for mapping between different metadata descriptions
- A server for processing XML documents and invoking appropriate applications and services.

The XML Common Business Library (xCBL)

If every business invented its own XML definitions, the Web would be scarcely more usable as a platform for agents and other automated processes than it is today. Recognizing this, many companies are collaborating on initiatives that focus on XML standards for particular industries or business processes, as shown in Table 4.1.

These independent initiatives do little to facilitate interactions across industry and functional boundaries. What purchase form should a company like Office Depot, a member of the Open Buying on the Internet (OBI) consortium, use to order computers from Compaq, a participant in RosettaNet? A company participating in only a few trading communities may opt to support several document standards, but companies like Office Depot and Compaq that do business in many marketplaces require a solution that can scale.

Scalable solutions require a library of document components and templates common to many business domains. Each trading community

TABLE 4.1. Domain-specific commerce languages

The power of XML to enable interoperability and simplify the sharing and reuse of information between business domains has encouraged many companies to work together to develop XML-based specifications for the information they most often need to exchange. Some examples:

- **Open Trading Protocol (OTP)**, a consortium of banking, paymenlt and technology companies, is specifying the information requirements for payment, receipts, delivery, and customer support (http://www.otp.org). OTP's goal is to enable the efficient exchange of information when the merchant, the payment handler, the deliverer of goods or services, and the provider of customer support are different entities.
- **XML/EDI**, a group jointly chartered by CommerceNet, ANSI X12, and the Graphics Communication Association, that is defining how traditional X12 EDI business data elements should be represented using XML (http://www.xmledi.com).
- **RosettaNet**, an Information Technology industry initiative designed to facilitate the exchange of product catalogs and transactions between manufacturers, distributors, and resellers of personal computers (http://www.rosettanet.org).
- **Open Buying on the Internet (OBI)**, an initiative started by American Express and major vendot and buying organizations (e.g., Office Depot, Ford) to automate corporate procurement (http://www.openbuy.org).
- **Information and Content Exchange (ICE)**, an initiative organized by Vignettte, News Corp, CNET, and many other "content companies" to enable the efficient creation and management of online networked relationships such as syndicated publishing networks, Web superstores, and online reseller channels (http://www.w3.org/TR/1998/NOTE-ice-19981026).
- **Open Financial Exchange (OFX)**, originally proposed by CheckFree, Intuit, and Microsoft for the electronic exchange of financial data among consumers, small businesses, and financial institutitons to support banking, bill payment, investment, and financial planning activities (http://www.ofx.net).

(*Source:* Glusko, Tenenbaum, Meltzer © 1999 ACM Inc. Reprinted with permission)

maps its documents to these elements, a one-time process that takes days to accomplish. After this is done, members of that community can do business with every other community that has completed the same mapping process. Imagine thousands of OBI merchants doing business with thousands of RosettaNet suppliers, creating millions of new trading opportunities. This was our inspiration for developing the XML Common Business Library (xCBL), shown in Figure 4.5, which contains information models for generic business concepts, including:

- Business description primitives like companies, services, and products
- Business forms like catalogs, purchase orders, and invoices
- Standard measurements, date and time, location, and classification codes.

The information is represented as an extensible, public set of XML building blocks that companies can customize and assemble to develop XML applications.

Seeded with industry-standard messaging conventions, the xCBL includes ISO codes for countries, currencies, time, etc., as well as elements from EDI and XML standards initiatives (such as ebXML, OBI, RosettaNet).

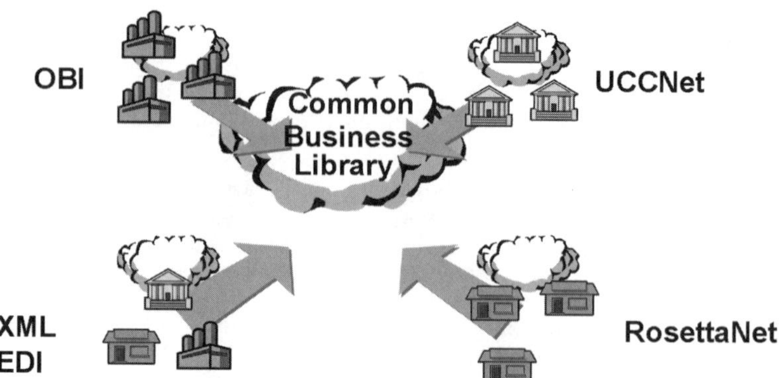

FIGURE 4.5. XML Common Business Library (xCBL).

Document components are mapped to each other using dictionaries of generic business terms and data elements.

While originally intended for mapping XML dialects, xCBL document elements have an equally important role in developing new XML document models. Reuse of semantic components reduces time to market, increasing the likelihood of the new model becoming a de facto standard; in addition, reuse ensures interoperability with all models built from or mapped into those components.

The eCo architecture is based on the premise that there will be many standards, not one single standard, for e-commerce. Accordingly, xCBL is not a standard per se, but rather a collection of business elements common to all EDI and Internet commerce protocols. Its reusable components speed the implementation of standards and facilitate interoperation by providing a common semantic framework. This approach is fundamentally different from the usual one taken by standards organizations and software vendors. It occupies an "openness high ground" that embraces all the competing standards developed to take advantage of XML.

The XML Commerce Connector

The core of the integration framework is the XML Commerce Connector (XCC) as portrayed in Figure 4.6. This software authenticates and parses incoming documents and validates that they conform to their published DTDs. It then routes them in accordance with business rules to relevant business services, for example, routing a request for product data to a catalog server or forwarding a purchase order to a supplier's ERP system. The XCC server also handles translation tasks, mapping the information from a company's XML documents onto document formats trading partners use and into data formats its legacy systems require.

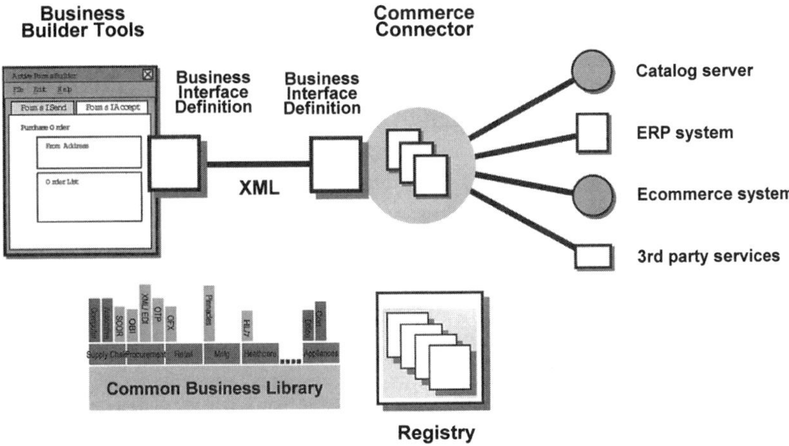

FIGURE 4.6. XML commerce connector.

Plug and Play Commerce

As shown in Figure 4.7, XCC document routers are the glue that binds a set of internal and external business services to create a virtual enterprise or trading community. XCC routers can:

- Link companies with their customers and suppliers to create a virtual company
- Link a distributor with its customers and suppliers to create an online trading community

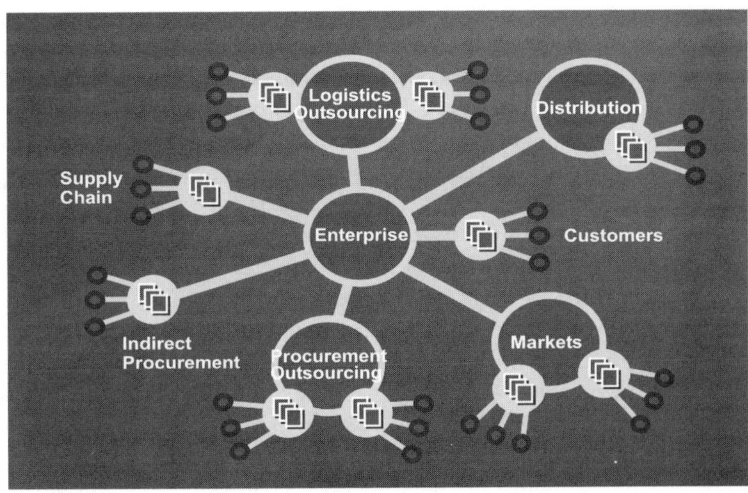

FIGURE 4.7. Plug-and-play commerce.

- Create Internet markets and exchanges
- Integrate third-party services into outsourced solutions.

The resulting business entities, created through the exchange of XML documents, are themselves building blocks that be further combined. Reroute a few XML documents and instantly plug the virtual company in Figure 4.7 into the online distribution channel or marketplace, or outsource its procurement and logistics functions. XCCs make it possible to build virtual companies from component services, much as a child might assemble structures using Tinker Toys.

Content Aggregation

We have thus far focused on the document-based integration of business processes and transactions. A complementary set of issues concerns the integration of product data and catalogs. Because competing suppliers describe identical or comparable products in unique ways, buyers find it difficult to aggregate catalogs and search for products across multiple vendors. Since there are many more suppliers and products than transaction documents, catalog aggregation has proved to be the major bottleneck in creating online trading communities.

The e-commerce industry has responded by establishing content factories. The factories acquire raw supplier content in diverse forms ranging from paper catalogs to Excel spreadsheets to proprietary databases. They then create a database containing normalized product descriptions, classified according to a standardized taxonomy such as the United Nations Standard Product and Classification Code (UNSPSC). The process is labor intensive and error prone and therefore not scaleable. Moreover, many vendors object to having their content aggregated because it limits their ability to differentiate themselves from competitors.

Within Commerce One's integration framework, a virtual catalog service named iMerge allows buyers and sellers to manage their own content as they see fit. It achieves interoperability by defining a common product taxonomy and content schemas. Companies map their proprietary data to the common format in a one-time effort, as they would map proprietary transaction documents to xCBL schema. The virtual catalog forwards product queries to appropriate vendors in their preferred format, maps responses back into the standard format, integrates them, and presents them to the user.

Figure 4.8 portrays a hypothetical iMerge catalog network for the PC supply chain discussed earlier in this chapter. Any company can publish its catalogs and product datasheets on the network by mapping them to the common industry format. Other companies can subscribe to this data to create their own virtual catalogs. Because most product data originates with manufacturers, the publishing process begins with them. To create their own catalogs, distributors subscribe to a manufacturer's content and add value by embellishing the description or combining it with data from other

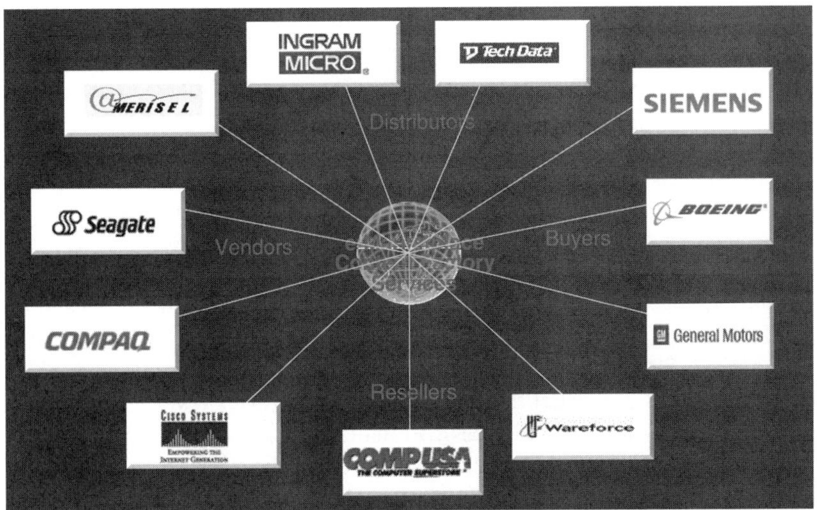

FIGURE 4.8. Content services (iMerge).

manufacturers to describe a system (e.g., a Compaq PC bundled with an HP printer). Similarly, resellers build their catalogs by subscribing and adding value to distributor catalogs. Outside the PC industry, buyers like GM, Boeing, and Siemens build their own corporate virtual catalogs by subscribing to selected reseller catalogs or the entire network.

Business Integration Frameworks

A complete integration framework encompasses both transactions and data, each of which involves mapping documents to a common schema. Mapping catalog pages to transaction documents completes the picture.

A typical procurement process might begin by searching a distributed catalog. The resulting product description can then be inserted onto a purchase requisition and routed through an internal approval process. Upon approval, the product information might be mapped into a preferred supplier's nomenclature and copied onto a purchase order, which then goes to the supplier. These simple operations—document mapping, copying, and routing—are the essence of the business integration framework.

Using the preceding framework, Commerce One is building a global Web of interoperable e-markets, industry exchanges, and commerce networks. As of this writing, nearly 100 entities have been integrated, creating the world's largest online trading community. It includes thousands of buyers and suppliers, with a potential aggregate annual expenditure in excess of 2 trillion dollars. To convey a sense for the openness and scalability of document-based integration, we shall briefly trace the evolution of this global trading community.

The Global Trading Web (GTW) began in March 1999 with a single node, a marketplace known as MarketSite.net connecting a few dozen U.S. buyers and sellers of general-purpose business products and services. Buyers and suppliers could integrate once using XML documents and do business with every other participant, as could providers of value-added business services such as FedEx or Citigroup. Most importantly, other XML-based marketplaces could connect to MarketSite.net, enabling their buyers to trade with any MarketSite.net supplier, and vice versa.

By June of 1999, the GTW had expanded to three nodes with the addition of regional MarketSites, operated by NTT in Japan and British Telecom in the UK. This union created the first truly global Internet trading community. While buyers and suppliers could now exchange XML documents across markets, such transactions grew slowly because there were not yet value-added services to facilitate international trade.

The next year brought further expansion and development. In the fall of 1999, the first vertical industry marketplaces joined the network, most notably General Motors' Trade Exchange for the automotive industry. Each of these exchanges brought thousands of new companies into the GTW, expanding the community an industry at a time. During 2000, the GTW continued to grow rapidly, as over two dozen regional exchanges and 75 large and small vertical exchanges joined the network. At the start of 2001, the pace of integration was continuing unabated, posing significant scaling challenges.

In the coming year, the GTW is expected to add hundreds, perhaps thousands, of new marketplaces. Many of these will be private exchanges, created by companies to tightly integrate their supply and distribution chains. Companies will rapidly assemble these virtual trading communities from the thousands of published GTW services, using plug and play commerce tools. Thousands of other companies will join the GTW through gateways to established electronic trading networks, such as EDI Value Added Networks (VANs).

To avoid communication bottlenecks, the architecture of the GTW will evolve into a hierarchical peer-to-peer network. Corporate private exchanges like Firestone will connect to an appropriate vertical marketplace like Tires, which in turn will connect to a relevant industry (auto) or regional hub (Indonesia). The majority of transactions at any level will take place directly between peers through email or the Web. Documents will pass through marketplaces and exchanges only when they add value—providing a matchmaking service, for example, or routing the document to another trading community.

The GTW's expansion places a premium on services that help trading partners in different marketplaces find and trust each other. Basic matchmaking services, such as catalogs and auctions, are already being linked across markets into GTW-wide services. They are also being augmented with additional value-added services to create complete sourcing solutions. By the end of 2000, for example, a GTW-wide catalog service will allow buyers to locate the nearest supplier of an urgently needed product anywhere in the world and obtain information about its price, availability, and delivery. Alternatively, buyers can run multi-marketplace reverse auctions and rely on a suite of services to complete trades safely, including supplier qualification, escrow, insurance, logistics, credit, and currency hedging.

The GTW's evolution from a single centralized marketplace to thousands of peer-to-peer trading communities underscores the scalability of a business integration framework based on XML documents and services. The versatility of the approach is borne out in the ability to create global catalog and auction services, and to integrate them with value-added services like escrow and logistics to create end-end trading solutions. Moreover, as we are about to see, the framework is applicable to virtually any domain and business process.

Lessons for Cancer Informatics

We believe that the B2B integration framework discussed here can be readily adapted for use in cancer informatics. The framework is based on generic architectural elements that are domain- and process-independent: services, XML documents, and common data models. Software that routes documents through services operates the same, whether sending a purchase order to an order entry service or a lab result to a patient data service.

Adapting the integration framework involves three efforts:

- Defining the appropriate services and documents
- Creating the requisite infrastructure for interoperation, namely registries for defining and locating services and common data models for mapping documents and data
- Defining processes in terms of the decision rules that govern the flow of documents through services.

Core Services

The first step is encouraging everyone in the cancer research community, from university laboratories to government regulators, to develop Web-based services that allow access to their information and processes. The most basic services fall into three broad categories: documentation, information, and shared services.

• **Documentation services.** These automate the creation, submission, routing, and processing of the many forms and documents involved in a clinical trial, including appointment schedules, patient data records, protocol specifications, and FDA filings. Such services reduce the time, cost, and error associated with today's manual paper-based processes.

• **Information services.** These support the storage, analysis, retrieval, and sharing of the diverse data sets used in clinical trials. Providing Web access to patient data, for example, will reduce redundant tests and facilitate second opinions, thus encouraging patient participation in trials. Aggregating patient data from multiple trials can improve the accuracy of statistical data analysis and pattern discovery.

• **Shared services.** These represent core competencies for clinical trials, such as protocol design, patient recruitment, statistical analysis, compliance monitoring, and securing FDA approvals. Organizations that excel at one or more of these functions can offer their services to others over the Internet. In turn, they are able to outsource functions that others can perform better or cheaper. Outsourcing improves the cost effectiveness of all clinical trials by promoting centers of excellence and economies of scale. It also encourages greater cooperation among trials and between centers.

Value-Added Services

Core services provide the foundation on which other services can build and add value. The possibilities for value-added services are limited only by the imagination of cancer researchers and healthcare informatics entrepreneurs. Three examples of services that fulfill clear market needs and are likely to emerge in the near term follow:

- **Efficient marketplaces for clinical trials and related services.** Examples include markets that match patients with trials and markets that help principal investigators locate contract research organizations.
- **iKnowMed.** This service manages complex protocols by tracking a patient's progress through a trial, ensuring at each step that the patient has completed all prerequisite tests, procedures, and approvals (see www.iknowmed.com).
- **Active Health.** By applying standard-of-care rules, this service offers "second opinions" on the appropriateness of a test or treatment.

Startups like iKnowMed and Active Health are already developing the services that bear their names. The question is whether such services will be deployed as standalone applications or interoperable Internet services that others can easily integrate and expand. A clinical trials marketplace, for instance, might well use a service like Active Health to check the appropriateness of its patient assignments. Only if services can interoperate will health care experience the same intensity of entrepreneurial activity that evolved in the B2B sector.

Infrastructure

Making CII services interoperable requires an investment to create the requisite infrastructure. Fortunately, the incremental investment is modest, because the CII can directly leverage existing elements of infrastructure and technology from the B2B and healthcare worlds. These elements include:

- **XML documents.** Standard documents for patient registration, patient data records, insurance reimbursement, and myriad other forms involved in the day-to-day conduct of trials. The documents can build on HL7 and other XML healthcare initiatives.
- **Registry service.** An online directory where providers can publish the availability of services and users can locate services they need.
- **Schema library.** A library of reusable data elements and document templates, analogous to xCBL, for creating and mapping documents. The medical research community has led efforts to standardize terms and taxonomies, ranging from the National Library of Medicine's MeSH taxonomy of medical terms to the NCI's Common Data Elements. Seeded with these assets, the library will quickly become operational.
- **Virtual database service.** A service that can aggregate and search data from the multiple heterogeneous databases maintained by organizations participating in a clinical trial or research program. Such a service can be implemented quickly using the same technology that iMerge employs to search multiple vendor-managed catalogs. Each organization controls its own data but provides selective access through a distributed query service.
- **Connectors.** Middleware that connects XML document routers to legacy healthcare applications.

Investing in a network of shared services and infrastructure has transformed the B2B world in profound and unpredictable ways. In coming decades, it will have a similar impact on the cancer trials community.

Conclusion

The Internet is transforming the business world through Web-based services that enable companies to integrate their business processes and systems. Companies access each other's services using self-defining XML business documents that both people and computers can understand. Service registries tell potential trading partners what business services a company offers and what documents to use when invoking those services. The Common Business Library (CBL), a repository of data elements common to many business domains, speeds the implementation of XML standards and facilitates their interoperation by providing a common semantic framework.

Integrating businesses through services and documents overcomes two longstanding barriers to electronic commerce. It facilitates spontaneous commerce between trading partners without custom integration or prior agreement on industry-wide standards, and it encourages an incremental path to business automation in which browser-based tasks are gradually transferred to computer agents. These advances eliminate much of the time, cost, and risk of traditional systems integration and EDI, replacing them with a simple, affordable, and open solution. They nourish entrepreneurial activity by encouraging companies to build on each other's services and to create innovative new services and structures.

In this chapter, we posit that this loosely coupled, incremental approach to B2B integration is also the right way to build the Cancer Informatics Infrastructure (CII). Starting with a single trial, the approach can effect immediate benefits by improving the speed and accuracy of paper-based processes like scheduling appointments, verifying insurance eligibility, obtaining patient records, filing reports, and billing. As additional trials join the network, they can begin sharing and building on each other's services. Markets will emerge to match service users and providers, accelerating outsourcing and attracting new value-added services from the commercial sector. The resulting efficiencies and economies of scale will advance productivity and innovation in unforeseeable ways, ultimately transforming the very nature of clinical trials.

Looking Ahead

How, exactly, might the CII transform clinical trials? We offer this vision not as a prediction, but as a goal to guide future work. We picture today's isolated stovepipe trials replaced with a community-wide network of shared services encompassing all experiments, institutions, and cancers. Eliminating boundaries will foster innovative services—and more importantly, encourage a new way of thinking about trials that benefits the key stakeholders.

- **Patients.** By comparing their profiles—current clinical state, personal and medical data, previous treatments, etc.—with those of responders and non-responders, patients can be assigned to the trials most likely to benefit them. Based on what was learned during the trial, those who fail to respond can be rationally reassigned to another trial.
- **Researchers.** Access to a vastly larger and richer pool of data about patients, diseases, and treatment outcomes, as well as sophisticated statistical analysis services, will greatly improve research. For example, Bayesian decision services will provide earlier indications of a treatment's efficacy (Economist, 2000). Moreover, by sharing data, the research community can make more effective use of a limited pool of patients. Patients desiring a specific experimental treatment might, for instance, be spared the anxiety of being assigned to a control group if the trial they enter is able to identify suitably matched controls from other trials.
- **Principal investigators.** By reusing proven forms, protocols, procedures, analysis tools, and services from previous trials, investigators will be able to quickly design new trials. Once approved, a trial will benefit from the use of e-markets to quickly recruit centers, doctors, and patients.

Because the Internet knows no boundaries, clinical trials networks will soon link with networks from related communities like biotechnology and health care, creating one vast universe of services. Bioinformatics companies, for example, will offer sophisticated pattern discovery services that use gene and protein arrays to find sensitive new markers for detecting disease onset, monitoring progression, and assessing treatment effectiveness. Pharmaceutical companies will use the same data to identify and prioritize promising drug leads, leading to a dramatic increase in the success rate of trials. Healthcare providers will find it easier to participate in clinical trials and locate appropriate trials for their patients.

The Internet will not cure cancer, but it will help improve and accelerate the research leading to breakthrough treatments. In the meantime, its crucial role in integrating clinical trials into mainstream medicine will revolutionize health care.

References

Coase RH. 1988. The Nature of the Firm. In The Firm, The Market, and the Law. Chicago: University of Chicago Press, 33–55.

The Economist. 2000. In Praise of Bayes, September 30.

Glushko RJ, Tenenbaum JM, Meltzer B. 1999. An XML Framework for Agent-Based E-commerce. Communications of the ACM 42(3).

Rundle RL. 2000. E-Business: High-Tech Bypass for a Clogged Health-Care System. In The Wall Street Journal, October 23, p. B1.

Tenenbaum JM, Chowdhry TS, Hughes K. 1997. Eco System: An Internet Commerce Architecture. IEEE Computer 30(5):48–55.

5
Security and Privacy

Clifford Neuman

In an ideal environment, physicians and others involved in cancer research and patient care would have easy access to needed information. Common sense, the Health Information Portability and Accountability Act (HIPAA), and related regulations demand that we defend such information from inappropriate modification and retrieval, thus protecting patient safety, the integrity of study results, and the privacy of patient health records. The challenge is deciding which information to protect, what kinds of protection to establish for each type of information, and who should have access to or permission to modify the data. Only when we establish such policies can we apply technical measures to provide appropriate safeguards.

In this chapter, we examine the sources of information and the ultimate use of that information. We discuss issues to consider when setting policies for system access, explore the kinds of policies that might apply, and consider some security technologies—existing or in development—needed to implement and enforce such policies. We end with a discussion of management issues that will arise when we deploy these technologies in the context of medical informatics.

Managed Information

The goal of a medical informatics system is to help researchers and practitioners access medical information. Because of the kinds of data managed in such systems and the different players who need access to the information, defining access policies is difficult. Here, we describe what kinds of information each player requires and the challenges they may face.

Researchers need to identify trends and extract summary information regarding family and patient histories, diagnoses, treatments, and results of treatments across large populations and over extended periods. They may need to correlate these results with patient characteristics and track individual results and treatment scenarios over time.

Most researchers will not need to access identifying information about patients, except to correlate the data mentioned above. Though they might not need identifying information, they may be able to infer it from other data in a record. The level of detail at which summary and statistical information should be available may vary, depending on the researcher and any relationship with a particular study. Thus, the need to offer as much information as possible to researchers other than those who collected the data conflicts with the need to protect the privacy of patients and study participants.

Practitioners require access to detailed histories of their own patients, as well as family histories. They usually need only high-level processed data from studies, usually in the form of published results. Practitioners participating in studies will generate data (e.g., symptoms, results) that the researchers will use, but the practitioners might not know which patients received experimental treatments and which were in a control group.

Practitioners also need to access information about drugs and other treatments, known side effects, and interactions. They may be able to derive information about new or previously unknown side effects from information other practitioners have entered, but the derived information might not be immediately available. In fact, given the high stakes of drug trial results and of discovering complications from previously approved drugs, the availability of such information may need to be limited until conclusive findings are published.

Public health officials need to access statistical data about diseases so they can spot trends and identify environmental factors that may need attention. Given the potential impact of such data and the financial stakes of those involved, the integrity and permanence of the data is crucial. Some parties may stand to gain from modifying or destroying such data.

Drug manufacturers require access to data from studies, but data integrity must be protected. Some may have incentives for changing the data to make trial results seem more positive.

In general healthcare systems, insurers need information about procedures performed to make payments. Patient privacy is crucial so that insurers cannot profile patients by family history or genetic factors and discriminate against higher risk individuals.

Patients should, in general, have access to their own medical records, but certain information might not be available to them, especially during blind trials. Patients should have the authority to control access to the detailed information in their files, identifying organizations, individuals, or classes of individuals who should have access. In some circumstances, laws may override the patient's choice and allow certain individuals to access the record, and records must be accessible when the patient is incapacitated. Ideally, policies should specify guidelines for such access in advance. When organizations make exceptions to access policies, they must appropriately document them for audit.

HIPAA and Appropriate Access Policies

The HIPAA legislation, discussed by Braithwaite in Chapter 15, and subsequent regulations implementing the act impose requirements on the security of medical information. These regulations dictate policies that the systems covered in this book must enforce, and security systems should allow the policies dictated by HIPAA to override any discretionary policies applied to such data.

As a cancer information system evolves, policies for data access must be specified with enough detail to identify not only records for individual patients, but also subsets of information within each record. In existing systems, data segregation usually enforces these policies—i.e., certain data exist on separate systems, and external queries require manual intervention to generate summary data that excludes unauthorized information. Medical informatics systems must eliminate the manual step, so the policies restricting access to particular fields must be suitable for automation.

The characteristics of the requesters will shape the policies pertaining to medical data access. The system must reliably identify the data requester to ascertain permissions granted, generate an audit trail, and permit identification of system abuses, especially where access was granted on an exception basis. Policies depend not only on the requester's identity, but also on his or her affiliations and role certifications (e.g., physician, administrator, researcher, principal investigator). Policies may also depend on specific permissions that the subject of the data had granted. These rights may be granted to the primary care physician and delegated to specialists, laboratories, or other staff requiring access to the data.

For example, a typical policy might give the patient access to all records regarding treatment, except certain information legally or contractually excepted from disclosure (e.g., whether a patient in a trial is receiving treatment or is in a control group). The patient may delegate authority to access the records to the primary care physician, who must present physician credentials plus the patient's delegated authority to access the records. The physician might further delegate specific parts of the record to specialists, who also need to present their specialist credentials and the delegated authorizations to access the records. Emergency room personnel might have special credentials that allow them to override access controls and read most patient records. However, such credentials would embed special instructions to notify the patient of overrides, providing a strong disincentive against misuse of that authority.

The system might also help generate summary data with patient identifying information removed. Such data might have different constraints associated with it than the specific patient data does. Including patient data in these summaries might depend on policies associated with the data, but certain legal reporting requirements might override the patient's ability to avoid some kinds of reporting.

Security Technologies

The capabilities of a cancer informatics system will evolve over time. The security services deployed to protect the system will evolve with it, as the kinds of required access demand policies that use security infrastructure services. Initial deployments of such a system might use segregation to protect the integrity and privacy of data. There might be relatively few classes of data: that which is public and requires primarily integrity protection, and that which is private, retained solely on internal systems, and not published for the broader community.

This first-phase system will likely depend on Secure Socket Layer (SSL) encryption and widely deployed technologies like firewalls to protect data privacy, and on digital signatures to protect the integrity of published data. Users of such a system will fall into several classes: those who have access to most of the data, those with access only to data pertaining to a smaller set of subjects (e.g., their own patients), or those with access only to published results.

Only when we deploy later stage systems will we see policies supporting delegation of authority and automatic exception processing. The later phases of the system will likely depend on newer security technologies that require tighter integration with applications and the system. Authentication technologies, digital signatures, and audit services are more important in this phase as more users gain access to data based on more detailed policies.

Here, we describe some security technologies that are important in both the early and later phases of a cancer informatics system.

Firewalls

Private data reside on computer systems connected to networks. Certain vulnerabilities within the systems might allow intruders to breach security and discover private data, bypassing the specialized interfaces that prevent unauthorized access. Many systems on which data are processed may provide relatively open access to a pre-screened set of researchers, but security measures must keep outsiders from gaining the same access.

A firewall is like a security guard posted at the door of a facility to keep outsiders from walking in. Within a computer network, a firewall is a special computer placed between the Internet and a private network to which sensitive computers are connected and may be accessed. It serves as a filter, allowing only messages that conform to policy to pass from outside to inside and vice versa. Users sending data across the firewall might have to prove their identity before establishing a connection (Cheswick & Bellovin, 1994).

Compared to other security techniques, a firewall is easy to deploy, but it provides limited protection. Because it is not integrated with internal applications, the access policies a firewall can enforce have relatively coarse granularity. A firewall can allow access or deny it, but it often cannot limit the access to certain data. Another limitation is that many administrators incorrectly assume that firewalls eliminate the need for other security measures. If an attacker manages to access a system on the inside—either because of the openings left in the firewall or through an alternate communication channel—that individual has full access to other systems on the internal network.

Secure Socket Layer

A Web page often provides controlled access for outside users, who log in and access specifically designated information (e.g., information about specific patients, or for patients, information about themselves). Usually, users can access very limited information available through such an interface. Secure access to information provided through a Web interface depends upon:

- Identifying a user
- Determining which records should be accessible
- Returning the data or accepting updates through a secure channel protected from eavesdropping and modification by other users.

The Secure Socket Layer (SSL) protocol, supported today by almost all Web browsers, is an easily deployed way to ensure these protections. This protocol typically allows users to know they are communicating with the Web server, and it protects the integrity and confidentiality of the communications channel. Servers can maintain lists of accounts, send passwords across the protected connection, and compare passwords with the ones stored in the account record. Once users establish a protected connection, they may send data in both directions. The receiving party knows that the data was not modified or disclosed to others as it traversed the Internet (Dierks & Allen, 1999).

The limitation of an SSL is that it usually depends on local means within each application (e.g., a locally maintained password file) to identify the user. Although an SSL can protect communication with a server, the server still must manage and enforce the security policies that apply to application data access.

IPSec and Virtual Private Network

The Internet Protocol Security (IPSec) system helps protect the integrity and confidentiality of network messages at a lower layer in the protocol stack than does SSL (Kent & Atkinson, 1998). This means that a system supporting IPSec can protect file transfers, other services, and the Web without having to modify individual applications. A per-host policy file can specify policies regarding the level of protection each service needs. Like SSL, IPSec usually does not identify the user of a service, only the host from which a message originates (or in some cases, only the network from which it originates). It facilitates the integrity and confidentiality of the channel used for communication.

IPSec can be used in several ways. On end systems (the client and the server systems), it identifies the end hosts and protects communication between those two hosts. However, IPSec deployment between end hosts requires support for the operating systems running on each host, support that is not universally available. More commonly, IPSec is used to implement a Virtual Private Network. In this mode, the IPSec protocol runs between firewalls or between a user's laptop and a firewall. The integrity and confidentiality of communications is protected when transiting the network outside the Virtual Private Network, but the communication is decrypted and placed on the network inside the firewall for communication with internal systems.

Regardless of the mode of IPSec deployment, the application must still authenticate the user if his or her identity is needed for access control decisions.

Digital Signatures and Certification Authorities

Digital signatures generated by a mathematical algorithm can help protect the integrity of submitted and published data. The first step in most digital signature algorithms is to compute a checksum (or "message digest") of the data and scramble it using a special "private" encryption key. The verifier of the signature unscrambles the value using a publicly known encryption key and compares it with a new checksum calculated over the data received. If data change after a digital signature is applied, the checksum does not match, and the verifier knows that the message is not authentic (Diffie & Hellman, 1976).

To validate a digital signature, the verifier must know the public key of the person who signed the message. This key may be distributed in advance, but the most common way to obtain it is to read it from a certificate, which the verifier retrieves from a directory server (CCITT, 1998; Wahl et al., 1997) or receives as an attachment to the signed document. A certificate, signed by a special entity called a certification authority (CA), is a document that certifies the association of a public key with a named individual. The verifier still must know the public key of the certification authority in advance (perhaps learning it from other certificates), but knowing this single key allows the verifier to learn the public key of other individuals for whom the CA has issued certificates.

Digital signatures serve two purposes in a medical informatics system. First, they help determine when someone has modified a document. This is important in clinical studies, where reports generated by physicians must not be modified by other "interested parties." Digital signatures also provide a limited form of "non-repudiation"; if verified, the message definitely came from someone with the private key used to generate the signature. Because this key is known only to the party whose signature it generates, the signature is proof of the individual's concurrence, assuming that the private key was not lost or stolen.

The principal difficulty with digital signatures is management. Users who must validate the integrity of signed documents must receive the public keys of the CAs needed to verify certificates. Which CAs should be trusted to certify keys is a matter of policy, and those CAs must issue certificates to signers according to another specified policy.

Authentication Technologies

Many data access policies depend on knowing the identity of the user. An application or server may determine identities locally or request a user name and password, but this requires managing an authentication (password) database on each server. Authentication services verify identity on a systemwide basis. Examples of authentication services include the Kerberos (Neuman & Ts'o, 1994) system developed at MIT, which is now distributed with Microsoft's Windows 2000 as the principal method for network authentication.

In the Kerberos system, users register with a central server for their site and log in to the network at the beginning of a session. During this phase, users retrieve credentials from the Kerberos authentication server and use them later to prove their identity to other network services when retrieving information. The authentication protocol uses encryption key, much as digital signatures prove that someone with knowledge of a private encryption key has generated a message.

As with digital signatures, management is the major difficulty for network authentication technologies. Although more easily and securely managed than password distribution to all servers, a central authority must still register users and manage password changes when they are forgotten or stolen. Both the Kerberos system for network authentication and digital signatures allow this management function to be distributed across multiple organizations, but policies must regulate the kinds of access across organizational boundaries.

Audit Functions

Because of the high stakes of medical information systems, maintaining an audit trail is critical. As a deterrent against privacy invasions, the system must be able to trace the origin of changes to records and log the origin of queries to private data. The system should also log any emergency access and immediately bring it to the attention of administrators so they can detect potential patterns of abuse. To detect attacks, intrusion detection systems (Proctor, 2000) should be integrated with the audit functions. Intrusion detection systems available today are somewhat primitive, primarily detecting known attacks on networks or systems. In time, these systems will accept data from application-based audit functions, and they will highlight patterns of access that violate high-level access policies.

Denial of Service

Because their stakes are so high, medical informatics systems must continue to operate even when concerted attacks are trying to disable them. Such denial of service attacks are difficult to prevent. It will likely take several years to develop real defenses to them (if such defenses are even possible), but redundancy can help to mitigate their effects. Critical databases should exist in multiple places so their data are still available if parts of the network are shut down. Another possibility is designing systems that queue updates rather than lose them if the system accepting updates is not reachable or does not confirm receipt. Above all, these systems must not have a single point of failure—i.e., they should not have a single component like an authentication server that leaves the system unusable if the component is not available.

Policy Management

The security services we describe in this chapter implement security policies. In today's systems, these policies tend to be "coarse grained"; for example, firewalls may pass connections from the outside network only to certain systems and ports on the internal network. As we move forward, systems will begin to implement "finer grained" policies based on the identities of users and their roles and group affiliations. The systems will grant access to individual application level objects and records within those objects.

These policies will work only if the applications managing the data explicitly understand them. Current work in the computer security research community focuses on languages to represent such policies and on procedural interfaces to enforce them. Research in this area includes the Generic Authorization and Access Control Application Programming Interface (GAA-API) (Ryutov & Neuman, 2000) and Keynote system (Blaze et al., 1999). The results of these efforts might help integrate policy management mechanisms with medical informatics systems.

Looking Ahead

For any system, the first and most important step in providing security is understanding the security requirements and deciding which policies to enforce. This step is often ignored, and developers expect available security technologies to ward off attacks. In this chapter, we discussed some important policies for medical informatics systems and some technologies available and under development for enforcing such policies. We believe this information will allow designers of medical informatics systems to write appropriate access policies and enforce them with the available technologies.

References

Blaze M, Feigenbaum J, Ioannidis J, Keromytis A. September 1999. The KeyNote Trust Management System Version 2. Internet Engineering Task Force (IETF) RFC 2704. http://www.rfc-editor.org

Comité Consulatif International Téléphonique et Télégraphique (CCITT). December 1988. Recommendation X.509: The Directory Authentication Framework. http://www.webopedia.internet.com/Standards/Standards_Organizations

Cheswick W, Bellovin S. 1994. Firewalls and Internet Security: Repelling the Wily Hacker. Reading, MA: Addison-Wesley.

Dierks T, Allen C. January 1999. The TLS Protocol Version 1.0. Internet Engineering Task Force (IETF) RFC 2246. http://www.rfc-editor.org

Diffie W, Hellman ME. 1976. New Directions in Cryptogtaphy. IEEE Transaction on Information Theory 22(6):644–654.

Kent S, Atkinson R. November 1998. Security Architecture for the Internet Protocol. Internet Engineering Task Force (IETF) RFC 2401. http://www.rfc-editor.org

Neuman BC, Ts'o T. 1994. Kerberos: An Authentication Service for Computer Networks. IEEE Communications 32(9):33–38.

Proctor PE. 2000. The Practical Intrusion Detection Handbook. Upper Saddle River, NJ: Prentice Hall.

Ryutov T, Neuman C. January 2000. Representation and Evaluation of Security Policies for Distributed System Services. In Proceedings of the DARPA Information Survivability Conference and Exposition. Hilton Head, SC.

Wahl M, Howes T, Kille S. December 1997. Lightweight Directory Access Protocol (v3). Internet Engineering Task Force (IETF) RFC 2251. http://www.rfc-editor.org

For Further Reading

Committee on Maintaining Privacy and Security in Health Care Applications of the National Information Infrastructure, National Research Counsel, Computer Science and Telecommunications Board (CSTB). May 1997. For the Record: Protecting Electronic Health Information. Washington, DC: National Academy Press.

Committee on Enhancing the Internet for Health Applications: Technical Requirements and Implementation Strategies. National Research Council, Computer Science and Telecommunications Board (CSTB). June 2000. Networking Health: Prescriptions for the Internet. Washington, DC: National Academy Press.

6
Digital Libraries and Scholarly Communication

RONALD L. LARSEN and JEAN SCHOLTZ

The rapid advancement of information technology (IT) is transforming the world economy into an information economy. Just as capital and energy replaced land and labor two centuries ago, codified information and knowledge are now replacing capital and energy as the primary wealth-creating assets. This gradual shift has changed the nature of human work. Laborers of the twentieth century who used and transformed physical resources are being replaced by "knowledge workers" skilled in interpreting and transforming information. The emerging information economy is growing two and a half times faster than the goods economy, and although the IT workforce is growing six times faster than the total workforce, the demand for skilled IT professionals far exceeds supply.

The growth of networked information resources, largely through the Internet and the World Wide Web, is both a result and a source of the growing information economy. Digital libraries have emerged within this context as the vehicle for organizing collections of information, much as traditional libraries have done for print and related media. They are becoming a major component of a global information infrastructure.

Because the technology is young, there are still debates about what a digital library is. Under sponsorship of the Defense Advanced Research Projects Agency (DARPA), the DLib Forum (http://www.dlib.org) was organized to address emerging issues in this critical area of IT research. At the kickoff meeting of the DLib Forum's Metrics Working Group, held in January 1998 at Stanford University, a digital library was defined as the collection of services and information objects that support users in dealing with information objects and their organization and presentation, available directly or indirectly via electronic means (http://www.dlib.org/metrics/public/papers/dig-lib-scope.html).

This is a solid working definition; digital libraries allow individuals and organizations to efficiently and effectively identify, assemble, correlate, manipulate, and disseminate information resources, regardless of the medium in which the information exists. Digital libraries make no assumptions about commonality of language or discipline between the problem solver and the information space. Instead, they provide tools to navigate and manipulate a multilingual, multidisciplinary world. Task context, user values, and information provenance are critical elements in the information seeking process.

The Emergence of Online Publication

Skyrocketing serials prices in the 1980s and 1990s, coupled with the dramatic success of the World Wide Web in the 1990s, introduced instability into collection development and optimization in traditional print libraries. While libraries reacted to the cost spiral by cutting serials subscriptions and seeking budget increases, the Web hosted experiments in alternative publishing models like electronic publication. Few libraries took these experiments seriously, arguing that the digital medium was only the most recent in a long series of diverse media that libraries have successfully accommodated. However, since the digital medium is the first one fully capable of subsuming all other media, this one was different. By the close of the 1990s, the full impact of digital publication was still not realized, but few doubted that its ultimate impact would be revolutionary. Libraries, users, publishers, service providers, and sponsors are now beginning to shape the infrastructure supporting our most fundamental intellectual pursuits.

The Development of Networked Information Infrastructure

The growth of the World Wide Web is well documented, but the effects are so far-reaching that the basic data bear repeating. Although estimating the size of the Web is difficult, those who try counted over 200 million Web pages in July 1997. This estimate rose to 800 million in February 1999 (Lawrence & Giles, 1999), and in November 2000, the Google search engine reported 1.2 billion Web pages. On his Web site (http://www.lesk.com/mlesk/ksg97/ksg.html), Michael Lesk suggests that the volume of information available on the Web rivals that of the Library of Congress.

The Web has demonstrated its potential to support serious scholarship, including the publication of scholarly journals. As with other new technologies, this initially meant implementing the older medium within the new medium, i.e., producing print journals to be read on the screen. Soon, however, experiments explored the Web's power to extend publication interactively and dynamically. A publication could now contain audio, video, simulations, models, data sets, and anything else that could be represented digitally.

Economic forces are also driving the movement toward the Web. While the purchasing power of libraries has declined ten-fold over the past 30 years, library collection budgets have remained relatively flat. New construction costs for book stacks typically run between $20 and $100 per book, whereas scanning a book typically costs $10 to $40. Is it any mystery why administrators are less than enthusiastic about large library construction projects?

With the euphoria of the Web, however, came slow recognition of its disorganized, chaotic nature. Finding useful materials is difficult, the "signal-to-noise" ratio is low, and even useful documents often contain no information about origin and authorship. Skilled librarians are increasingly valued for their role in taming the Web and helping it to realize its potential for scholarly communication. The rigor commonplace in research libraries must become commonplace on the Web. The ideal of global collections representing the best and most current information is achievable, but will not come easily. Many of the challenges are not technical, but relate to the complex national and international legal and economic context.

The Pull on Digital Libraries: Timeliness, Accessibility, and Cost

Traditional economic models treat information as a commodity. It is created, packaged, purchased, loaned, copied, and sold, and the containers of information—books, magazines, newspapers—often are equated with the information. The economic model for print is based on a pay-to-read model, and copyright provisions governing fair use and first sale make the model fit the free access and lending requirements of libraries.

Information on the Web is different. By assuming the cost and liability of putting their materials online, authors pay to have their material read, and readers expect information to be free. This pay-to-publish model is feasible because of the low barrier to entry for Web-based publishing. The ease with which authors can do this questions the traditional role of publishers. As the need to manufacture and distribute physical information artifacts diminishes, the publisher's role becomes adding value to the information itself. Although authors can easily put their materials on the Web and make them globally accessible, the user seeking quality information still values vetted sources from a trusted publisher. Besides verifying the legitimacy of information, a publisher also encourages authors to cover particular topics of interest.

The Web reduces barriers to publishing by eliminating printing costs and enabling global distribution at a low cost. Selfpublishing is available and accessible to anyone with modest skills and a personal computer, and roles previously filled by middlemen seem less necessary. Publishers and computer centers are examples of entities that fill these middle-roles, but the effects extend beyond these to secondary information providers (e.g., abstracting and indexing services) and catalogers. Although the functions of these middle-layer providers will still be viable, the question is how the services will be offered in the near future.

The Push for Digital Libraries: Complexity, Collaboration, and Interactivity

Information delivery and use through the Web, although far more interactive than print publication and broadcast media, is still dominated by a mode of operation in which the user accesses material produced by another and reads, displays, or plays it. Although increasingly complex document formats offer information compatible with devices like personal computers, personal digital assistants (PDAs), ebooks, and even cellular telephones, the Web does little to help the user correlate the content of one resource with another. The ability to manipulate materials without compromising intellectual property rights is only beginning to emerge as a possibility. Research on multivalent documents (http://http.cs.berkeley.edu/~phelps/Multivalent) has demonstrated the potential for manipulating, annotating, and sharing marked-up versions of Web resources, but much work remains before these concepts become mainstream.

Web portals like Yahoo, Netscape Netcenter, and AOL function as the user's entry point and enable Web customization. Much more than search engines, these sites provide categories of information that users can access, such as travel information or weather. Portals allow users to customize news and financial information, and they now provide wireless and phone access to vital information. There are two major categories of portals: "horizontal," which offer services for a broad range of users, and "vertical" which, cater to a focused group. As the Web grows, research will focus on how users can automatically monitor specific information.

Early Explorations: The U.S. Digital Library Initiative

The growth of the Web in the 1990s dramatically expanded the amount of accessible and potentially useful information. Identifying, acquiring, and interpreting this volume of information requires much time and diligence, luxuries many users lack. Digital library research makes the information accessible and usable to busy users facing information-intensive activities.

The U.S. Digital Library Initiative (DLI) began in 1994, and a successor (DLI-2) began in 1999. It represents a multi-agency commitment to lead research fundamental to developing digital libraries; to advance the use and usability of globally distributed, networked information resources; and to encourage existing and new communities to focus on innovative applications areas. Led by the National Science Foundation (NSF), which has also partnered with the European Commission, the Deutsche Forschungsgemeinschaft, and the UK Joint Information Systems Committee (http://www.nsf.gov/pubs/1998/nsf9863/nsf9863.htm), the initiative encourages the creation of next-generation operational systems in areas like education, engineering and design, earth and space sciences, biosciences, geography, economics, and the arts and humanities. The entire information life cycle is addressed, from information creation, access, and use to archiving and preservation. Additional research focuses on understanding the long-term social, behavioral, and economic effects that digital libraries will have on education, commerce, defense, health services, and recreation.

Emerging Directions for Modern Digital Libraries

Digital libraries face significant technology challenges that question old assumptions. Three of these are:

- **Real time ingest.** Capturing, interpreting, cataloging, and indexing high rate multimedia data flow in real time.
- **Federation of distributed repositories.** Organizing heterogeneous distributed information sources into comprehensive, discipline-oriented, user-accessible repositories.
- **Translingual interaction.** Automatically accessing and using information across multiple natural languages.

Issues of ingest and federation have attracted attention within the Digital Library Initiative, but translingual interaction is a relatively new direction. Translingual services have received little attention within the Web community and even less attention within digital library research. The TIPSTER Text Program, led by the Defense Advanced Research Projects Agency (DARPA), fostered work in cross-lingual information retrieval, but the effective use of information in different languages presents challenges beyond retrieval.

Although language is an obvious barrier to the broader use of Web resources, it is not the only one. Research is still necessary to infuse digital libraries with the power of the conventional research library, including the basic infrastructure provided by rigorous catalogs, indexes, abstracts, and reference support. Digital libraries can even go far beyond the performance and services traditional libraries offer. The goal is to establish a globally interoperable, open digital library infrastructure that offers multimodal access to multimedia materials in multiple languages. Multimodal access is the ability to combine, substitute for, and smoothly move between various modes of interaction, including keyboard and mouse, voice, gaze, and gesture. The directions and goals are summarized in Table 6.1.

Substantial research is required to:

- Advance the technologies supporting federated repositories so that generic software is readily available and supports thousands of distributed, federated repositories.

Table 6.1. Research directions and goals

Capability	Present	Goal
Federated Repositories	Tens (Customs)	Thousands (Generic)
Items/Repository	Thousands	Millions
Size of "large" item	1 MB	100 MB
Typical response time	10 seconds	100 milliseconds
Mode	Play & Display	Correlate & Manipulate
Interoperability	Syntactic	Semantic
Filters	Bibliographic	Contextual
Language	Multilingual	Translingual
Content extraction	Forms & Tags	Text, image, audio

- Enlarge the collection capacity of a typical repository from thousands to millions of digital objects, including scalable indexing, cataloging, search, and retrieval.
- Support digital objects as large as 100 megabytes and as small as 100 bytes.
- Reduce response times for interaction with digital objects to sub-second levels, striving for a tenth of a second where possible.
- Couple high duplex bandwidth with low response time to explore new modes of interacting with information.
- Expand the user's ability to interact with networked information, from the present "play and display" Web facilities to the correlate and manipulate requirements of network-based research and problem solving.
- Raise the level of interoperability among users and information repositories from a high dependence on syntax, structure, and word choice to greater reliance on semantics, context, and concepts.
- Extend search and filtering beyond bibliographic criteria to include contextual criteria related to the task and user.
- Reduce language as a barrier to identifying and evaluating information resources by providing translingual services for querying and extracting information.
- Advance technology for general-purpose content extraction beyond forms and tagged document structures to include extraction of summary information (e.g., topics) from semi-structured information sources.

Architectural Considerations

A fundamental lesson of the Internet is that open systems based on standards that evolve from collaboration, experience, and best practices yield a highly productive environment for creating globally scalable infrastructure. While nations wrestled with the details of a grand design for Open Systems Interconnection (OSI) in the International Standards Organization (ISO), the Internet thrived under the guidance of the Internet Engineering Task Force (IETF), a volunteer forum open to all. The top down, centrally managed ISO process was ultimately abandoned, in belated recognition that the world community had built a working solution and pioneered new thought about global systems.

Digital library development is incorporating these lessons. The Internet was founded on the concept of free movement of data packets among separately developed, heterogeneous networks that use the Transmission Control Protocol/ Internet Protocol (TCP/IP) suite. Digital library research aspires toward a global information infrastructure in which information is self-describing and organized and can be freely shared among applications in distinct, heterogeneous systems.

Scalable Content and Collections

Scalability and interoperability are fundamental requirements for digital libraries. Scalable repository technology must support the federation of thousands of repositories, present to the user a coherent collection of millions of related items, and do this rigorously across many disciplines. As the size and complexity of information objects increases, so does the bandwidth required to use these objects. Time-critical assessment of complex situations requires real-time interactivity, pushing the bandwidth requirements even higher. As this capability emerges, broadband interoperability becomes feasible. The user's inputs are no longer constrained to a few keystrokes, with the return channel carrying the high volume materials. Further research must explore the nature of such broadband interoperability and the opportunities it can yield.

Ubiquitous Accessibility and Responsiveness

Human performance using online systems and information is strongly correlated with accessibility and system response time. The Web suffers from highly variable response time, and common experience suggests that the size and complexity of Web pages are growing faster than the typical user's available bandwidth. Optimal human performance depends on system performance that is close to human response time. Consistent system response of one to a few tenths of a second matches human performance well, but most users today experience response times of several seconds.

Improving response time is a complex problem with many dimensions. Brute force approaches to expanding the physical availability of bandwidth are necessary and valuable, but not sufficient. Efforts also require careful protocol design, intelligent caching, and ergonomic design of information resources and their delivery.

Persistence, Uniqueness, and Provenance

The Web has not only made vast amounts of information available; it has also raised users' sensitivities to the "brittleness" of networked information. The Uniform Resource Locator (URL) identifies a Web page by specifying its physical location. Search engines index this address, which individuals then use to retrieve the Web page. If the page is moved to a new location or removed from its host system, the retrieval fails with the familiar "Error 404."

Librarians learned long ago that the name of an item differs from its location. To move an item, one need only maintain a common index through which users can determine the item's location. The name remains constant, and the index always contains its current address.

Such a strategy will help ensure persistence of information in the Web. Holdings in a digital library, known as digital objects, attain such persistence by acquiring a unique identity that is unaltered by physical movement and is resolved at retrieval time to a physical address (see the Digital Object Architecture Project, http://www.cnri.reston.va.us/doa.html). Systems that provide these features have been built and are being deployed. An example is the Handle System (http://www.handle.net/index.html), built under DARPA sponsorship by the Corporation for National Research Initiatives (CNRI) and commercialized by the International DOI Foundation (IDF) (http://www.doi.org) as Digital Object Identifiers (DOIs). Persistence and uniqueness are necessary but not sufficient conditions for establishing the provenance of an information object.

Federated Repositories

A federated repository of digital objects is a member of a group of repositories that share a common purpose like a shared topic area or academic discipline. Participants typically share a common interest, expressed as a set of resources that are implemented, managed, and maintained in a distributed fashion but appear to the user as a coherent collection. An example is the Networked Computer Science Technical Reference Library (NCSTRL) (http://www.ncstrl.org), a federated repository of technical reports and other "gray literature" produced by more than 100 computer science departments in universities worldwide. NCSTRL, a federal research project, was intended to test the underlying concepts and develop an operational pilot. While it has achieved these goals, it has also uncovered the need for a scalable, generic, widely deployable set of tools for federated repositories. The goal is to make development of federated repositories as easy as Web site development.

User Considerations

Today, electronic information resides in digital libraries and on the World Wide Web. Michael Lesk (http://www.purl.net/NET/lesk), Director of the

Information and Intelligent Systems Division at NSF, estimates that the Library of Congress, if digitized, would contain about 3 petabytes (3,000 terabytes) of information. He bases this estimate on 13 million photographs (13 terabytes), 4 million maps (200 terabytes), 500,000 movies (500 terabytes), 3.5 million sound recordings (2,000 terabytes), and 20 million books (20 terabytes). The "deep Web" is estimated to contain 7,500 terabytes of information (http://www.completeplanet.com/Tutorials/DeepWeb/index.asp).

The World Wide Web already has more information than the Library of Congress and is growing each year. Lesk also observes that the amount of disk space in the world is increasing, and that soon we may be able to save all the information we generate, including movies, telephone conversations, images, television broadcasts, music, and traditional textual information. This information will be useful only if we can quickly retrieve and use what we need.

The information explosion demands that we view problems with it from the user's perspective, not only the technological aspects. Today's users need to locate information of all types, in any language, from many different sources. The user's task must be easy and fast, and it must provide the needed information in the desired form.

Early evaluations of information retrieval focused on precision and recall; that is, for a given search engine, how many documents were retrieved and how relevant these documents were to the keywords used in the search. The Text Retrieval Conferences (TREC), cosponsored by the National Institute of Standards and Technology (NIST) and DARPA, allow researchers to use the same set of data to compare results, substantially advancing the state of the art in information retrieval (http://trec.nist.gov/).

Begun in 1992 as part of the federal TIPSTER Text program, the purpose of TREC is to support research within the information retrieval community by providing the infrastructure necessary for large-scale evaluation of text retrieval methodologies (http://www.itl.nist.gov/iaui/894.02/related_projects/tipster/). In particular, the TREC workshop series aims to:

- Encourage research in information retrieval based on large test collections
- Increase communication among industry, academia, and government by creating an open forum to exchange research ideas
- Speed technology transfer from research labs to commercial products by demonstrating substantial improvements in retrieval methodologies on real-world problems
- Increase the availability of appropriate evaluation techniques for use by industry and academia, including development of new evaluation techniques for current systems.

In accordance with the last goal, TREC expanded to include multi-lingual retrieval tracks, interactive tracks, and question and answering tracks to focus on the "user experience." The user's attention is the critical resource, and the technological objective is to optimize the user's attention in the least amount of time with a powerful array of tools and automated facilities.

User Interface Design

Growth in networked information infrastructure encourages us to rethink the manner of interaction between the user and the information source and reconsider where mediation is appropriate. Conventional designs still assume a narrowband, text-based user interface. The typical query, for example, is a sequence of 20 to 50 characters and is rooted in dialup technologies capable of delivering a few hundred characters per second. Current and future networks are much faster than this. Broadband, active networks accessed through high performance workstations offer semantically and contextually rich query expression and interaction with information spaces. Low cost infrastructure helps us create new products and services never before envisioned.

Norman (1986) identified seven stages of human-computer interaction that cycle until the user obtains the desired result or gives up in frustration.

1. The user identifies a desired goal.
2. The user forms the intention to carry out the goal.
3. The user formulates what step must be taken toward the goal. This action must be translated into commands the computer can use.
4. The user carries out the action.
5. The user perceives the information given back by the computer.
6. The user evaluates the information with respect to the goal.
7. Evaluation may result in reformulation of the goal and an iteration of the steps.

Within these seven stages, Norman identified two gulfs: the gulf of interaction and the gulf of evaluation. The gulf of interaction occurs when the user knows what he wants to achieve but cannot formulate the correct commands to make the computer perform the task. The gulf of evaluation occurs when the user is unable to assess correctly what the computer has done. These gulfs can be narrowed and possibly eliminated by a system with intuitive commands and well designed feedback that helps the user understand what the system has done with the input.

One pathfinding example of bridging the execution gulf in user interfaces is the Visible Human Project® (http://www.nlm.nih.gov/research/visible/visible_human.html). The longterm goal of this project is to produce a system of knowledge structures that transparently links visual knowledge forms to symbolic knowledge formats like the names of body parts. The Visible Human Explorer (VHE) prototype, created at the Human Computer Interaction Laboratory (HCIL) at the University of Maryland, is an experimental user interface for browsing the National Library of Medicine's

Visible Human data set that demonstrates a general interface for volume exploration. The interface allows users to browse a miniature Visible Human volume, locate images of interest, and automatically retrieve full resolution images over the Internet from the National Library of Medicine archive.

Such user-oriented analysis environments are more than just an interesting attempt to improve search and retrieval capabilities. An analysis environment allows the user to search, refine searches, and explore more of the information space by using analysis tools and combining other sources of information. One compelling example of a user analysis environment is the GeoWorlds project (http://www.isi.edu/GeoWorlds) at The University of Southern California Information Sciences Institute (USC ISI). The GeoWorlds prototype uses a spatially based information management approach, meaning the system can rapidly create customized repositories of maps, images, and documents from spatially distributed sources. Users can move back and forth between text queries and map-based queries. If a user community has existing analysis methods, the prototype allows scripting so that these methods can be carried out automatically. The researchers working on GeoWorlds are also looking at non-spatial domains, such as biological, molecular, and neurological.

Shneiderman's work on dynamic query generation for information retrieval (Ahlberg et al., 1992; Shneiderman, 1994) attempts to eliminate both the gulf of execution and the gulf of evaluation. The prototype interfaces developed here can:

- Represent the query graphically
- Provide visible limits on the query range
- Provide a graphical representation of the database and the query result
- Give immediate feedback after every query adjustment
- Allow novice users to begin working with little training while still providing expert users with powerful features.

Prototype systems for dynamic queries include a graphical representation of the database. The user manipulates a series of sliders corresponding to the values that constitute the query, and the database representation changes to reflect the current query values. This shows in graphical terms the number of database values that satisfy a given query, and the user can select individual data points to obtain detailed information.

Content-Based Multimedia Access

Information retrieval systems rely heavily on indexing the text of documents. Although this is effective in bounded domains in which the usage and definition of words are shared, performance suffers when materials from multiple disciplines are represented in the same collection, or when disparate acquisition or selection policies are active. This is typically the rule, not the exception, especially on the Web. Techniques for mapping between structured vocabularies begin to address this problem for disciplines with a formalized vocabulary (http://www.sims.berkeley.edu/research/metadata/).

Several techniques in development look beyond the words to the meaning and concepts expressed. For example, the University of Illinois Urbana-Champaign (UIUC) and the University of Arizona developed automated techniques for collection categorization in their "Interspace" project, where substantial success is reported using statistical approaches on large collections of documents (http://www.canis.uiuc.edu/interspace/).

Query languages and tools identify materials in a collection that are similar to the characteristics expressed in a query. These characteristics focus on the information artifact and have yet to consider non-bibliographic attributes that might tighten the focus of a search. Examples include identifying the types of individuals who have been reading specific material, the value they associated with it, and the paths they traversed to find it (http://scils.rutgers.edu/baa9709/).

Although the navigational metaphor for information seeking in the network environment has become ubiquitous, tools for visualizing and navigating these complex information spaces are still immature. Incorporating concept spaces and semantic category maps in visualization tools is a promising improvement. Concept spaces and semantic category maps illustrate statistically based techniques to analyze collections, associate vocabulary with topics, suggest bridging terms between clusters of documents, and portray the clusters of related documents in a multidimensional, navigable space, enabling both high-level abstraction and drill-down to specific documents (http://www.canis.uiuc.edu/projects /interspace/).

Increasingly, users want to retrieve multimedia information, much of which is unstructured. Instead of using several different retrieval systems based on the types of media desired, the goal is to develop a multilingual, multimedia information retrieval system. One such project at HNC Software (http://www.hnc.com/innovation_05/projects_0503.cfm) uses LISSOM, a unified neural network learning principle. LISSOM trains on preprocessed data and produces a set of vector representations that the neural networks use to form a content-addressable database. In retrieving data, the representations are ordered according to their similarity to the query representation.

The Informedia Experience-on-Demand (EoD) (http://informedia.cs.cmu.edu) project at Carnegie Mellon University allows users to capture complete records of personal experience and share them in collaborative settings. The project is developing techniques for managing these vast quantities of multimedia data, including searching, summarizing, and visualizing content from multiple perspectives. They have dynamically summarized events recorded in video from different EoD capture units in the same spatial region. They have also incorporated historic, archived video into the system so that a user may view a location as it appeared at an earlier time. The researchers have developed mechanisms that can track one or more individuals in relatively complicated videos.

Mobile Access

Information on the World Wide Web is formatted using HyperText Markup Language (HTML), which defines a predetermined set of "tags" that indicate how information is to be displayed. Because this set of tags is guaranteed to be understood by any Web browser, the information should be uniformly displayed. The eXtensible Markup Language (XML), which is currently used on the Web, is a method for putting structured data like spreadsheets, address books, and technical drawings into text files. A set of conventions for designing text formats, XML produces files that can be easily generated and read by computers, can be internationalized, and are platform independent. XML is more flexible than HTML, as it allows the information designer to create any tags he or she wishes. A Document Type Definition (DTD) is created by grouping the tags into a set of grammar rules.

Access to information today, however, is not limited to the desktop. Users want to access information with their laptops, handheld devices, and even cell phones. The Wireless Markup Language (WML), based on XML, is used to describe data to be displayed on low-bandwidth, small display devices. WML was designed to minimize transactions with remote servers and can download multiple screens in a single transaction. Devices that can use information marked up with WML are called Wireless Application Protocol (WAP) capable, meaning they have the necessary software to translate the WML markups.

The problem with this methodology is that it requires several versions of information—one that supports mobility and another that supports a full desktop-capable browser. This creates versioning and update problems. As content creators develop more devices, they will have to devise other markup languages or develop transducers that translate the information and its display from the capabilities of one markup language to another.

As with federated repositories, it would be preferable to have information marked up so that different devices could be supplied with software to interpret the data in the context of that device's capabilities. Because devices and software change faster than information, the structure of information should be flexible enough to outlast numerous devices and software for interpretation and display. The DARPA Agent Markup Language (http://www.daml.org) adds machine-readable information to information on the Web. This markup language includes semantic tags that help software agents understand the content on a Web page.

Machine Translation and Cross-Lingual Information Retrieval

English is the target language for most tools available today on the Web. As the Web continues to expand, however, its growth rate in non-English speaking countries exceeds its growth rate in the U.S. This is due in part to the earlier and greater penetration of the Web in the U.S. Estimates made early in 1999 suggested that the number of non-English language Web pages would exceed English Web pages by midyear (Frederking R, personal communication, February 1999). The user relying entirely on English language materials risks missing nearly half of the information on the Web and introduces an Anglo-centric bias. A comprehensive approach must include the ability to locate, acquire, and use information resources in unfamiliar languages. This is the focus of DARPA's research program in Translingual Information Detection, Extraction, and Summarization (TIDES) (http://www.darpa.mil/ito/research/tides/index.html). As of 1999, search engines working across select language boundaries performed about half as well as those working within one language.

The Web is already multilingual. Standards like Unicode have addressed multilingual character representation, but if materials in many languages are to provide value, users need the tools to find them, interpret them, and interact with their authors. Constructing this kind of "translingual" Web is a major challenge and the subject of current research through DARPA's TIDES program and the joint National Science Foundation/European Union Multilingual Information Access (MLIA) program (http://www.dli2.nsf.gov/eu_e.html#_Toc432270462).

Multi-Lingual User Interfaces

Besides cross-lingual content, we must also address the presentation of content or Web site design for globalization. Traditional software development has struggled with globalization issues. Typically the English version of a software product is released, and months later, the internationalized versions are released for some larger markets. Multi-lingual Web sites present new challenges because of the rapid change rates of Web sites and the design expressiveness displayed on the Web. Fonts, colors, spatial layouts, icons, content organization, formats for dates, and monetary units must be considered and internationalized.

Guidelines for globalization do exist (Fernandes, 1995), but a rapidly changing environment like the Web needs tools to facilitate globalization. There is little research on the preferences and performance of internationalized Web sites. One study by Barber and Badre (1998) explored and categorized cultural markers for international sites. Further research in this area compared performance and preferences for Web sites containing cultural markers to those of Americanized Web sites (Sheppard & Scholtz, 1999).

Usage Considerations

We can think of the state of the art in information access and use in relatively linear terms. The process begins with a query, the start of an information retrieval process that generates candidate documents. Various document-processing algorithms can be run against this set to understand it without exhaustively studying it. Topic detection algorithms can recognize with reasonable precision the occurrence of stories about specified topics (Wayne, 1998). Named entities (e.g., names of people, places, things, dates, or events) can be extracted with very good recognition accuracy (Message Understanding Conference, TIPSTER Text Program). Automatic summarization of documents has met with modest success, although much work remains (Summarization Evaluation Results, TIPSTER Text Program).

Each of these processes introduces errors, which tend to propagate through the analysis, leaving significant compound errors by the time the process is complete. Relevance feedback improves information retrieval performance by about 50%, but the other analytic steps have received few analogous improvements, and we still have limited understanding of how the processes interact.

Digital library users can opt to leverage the searches of previous users. Packhunter (http://www.packhunter.com), developed at Hughes Research Laboratories, is a collaborative search tool that allows groups of users to traverse the same search paths through a Web site, branching off to individual pages when they discover interesting links. AntWorld (http://aplab.rutgers.edu/ant/), developed at Rutgers, saves the history of searches and users' ratings of the usefulness of visited pages. New users can access the results of an earlier search similar to theirs.

Extraction and Summarization

Information users who rely on large volumes of material with a short period of relevance (e.g., news reports) are increasingly seeking techniques for automated content extraction. The standard approaches to content extraction, derived largely from database technology, rely on structured forms and tagged data fields and do not work for less structured and more dynamic information. Encouraging results have been achieved with automatic extraction of information important to understanding events-based textual reports, such as the names of people, places, things, dates, and fundamental relationships among entities (http://www-nlpir.nist.gov/related_projects/tipster/muc.htm).

Research in this area focuses on four problems of increasing difficulty:

- **Named entity recognition.** Examples of named entities are people, organizations, locations, dates, times, currencies, and other numerical measures, such as percentages.
- **Coreference identification.** This problem concerns identifying all mentions of a given entity, either directly or by indirect reference (e.g., he, she, it).
- **Template element extraction.** Template elements are intended to extract basic information related to a named entity (e.g., George W. Bush is President of the United States).
- **Scenario template completion.** Scenario templates relate event information to named entities (e.g., George W. Bush was elected President of the United States in 2000).

Entity recognition capabilities are being coupled with speech recognition to interpret news broadcasts and automatically identify and track news reports on specific topics, a strategy that has achieved promising results (DARPA Proceedings, 1999). A broad range of content extraction capabilities must cover the full range of media, with the understanding that data of the most interest will be highly dynamic, largely unstructured, and often "noisy."

Search and Retrieval

Information resources on the Web are highly diverse, distributed, and heterogeneous, with varying content and quality. Searching loses effectiveness as information volume grows and source heterogeneity increases. Increased document and information density resists discrimination by traditional search technologies; Lawrence and Giles (1999) estimate that as of February 1999, the largest percentage of the Web covered by any search engine was just over 38%.

Because the overlap in coverage between different search engines is relatively low, combining the results of multiple search engines can improve coverage. A new document on the Web can take several months or longer to be indexed. Lawrence and Giles found that the mean age of a page when indexed by one of the search engines was 186 days; the median age, 57 days. Clearly, research must focus on scaling issues for indexing.

Adaptive Presentation and Interpretation

Digital libraries do little to adapt information presentation to the unique needs, desires, or preferences of a specific user with a particular device. Dynamic Web pages are based on limited knowledge of the user, and transducers are being developed to adapt standard Web pages for display on other devices. Future efforts will continue to help users explore and understand information. Topic-O-Graphy™, developed at Battelle/Pacific

Northwest National Laboratory, produces visualizations of lengthy text documents to promote information exploration. It uses a multi-resolution wavelet-based methodology to decompose a document into thematically coherent and hierarchically related pieces. Further work must explore such alternative presentations that facilitate comprehension, comparison, and synthesis at multiple levels of abstraction.

Looking Ahead

The information user's attention is a critical resource. Digital library research—and by extension, digital publication—must provide the technological capability to maximize value for time- and attention-constrained users. In short, the rigor and organization normally associated with a research library must be virtually rendered and extended in the networked world of distributed information and users.

The digital library research agenda can be broadly structured into context- or task-independent repository-based functions and user- or usage-dependent analysis activities. This is the way traditional libraries have divided their activities. However, it is important to note that digital library research and development is about much more than tasks and users. At its core, it is about developing a global infrastructure that raises information to the level of a first-class object.

References

Ahlberg C, Williamson C, Shneiderman B. 1992. Dynamic Queries for Information Exploration: An Implementation and Evaluation. Proc ACM CHI 92: 619–626.

Barber W, Badre A. 1998. Culturability: The Merger of Culture and Usability, Fourth Conference on Human Factors and the Web. Basking Ridge, NJ.

Corporation for National Research Initiatives. Digital Object Architecture Project. http://www.cnri.reston.va.us/doa.html. Accessed 07/12/01.

Fernandes T. 1995. Global Interface Design. Boston: Academic Press.

Lawrence S, Giles C. 1999. Accessibility of Information on the Web. Nature 400: 107–109. http://www.metrics.com/

Message Understanding Conference. TIPSTER Text Program. http://www-nlpir.nist.gov/related_projects/tipster/muc.htm. Accessed 07/12/01.

Norman D. Cognitive Engineering. 1986. In Norman D, Draper S. (eds). User Centered System Design. Hillsdale, NJ: Lawrence Erlbaum Associates, Inc., 37–61.

Proceedings of the DARPA Broadcast News Workshop. 1999. February 28–March 3. Hilton at Washington Dulles Airport, Herndon, Virginia. http://www.itl.nist.gov/iaui/894.01/proc/darpa99/

Sheppard C, Scholtz J. 1999. The Effects of Cultural Markers on Web Site Use. Fifth Conference on Human Factors and the Web. Gaithersburg, MD. June 5, 1999. http://zing.ncsl.nist.gov/hfweb/. Accessed 07/12/01.

Shneiderman B. 1994. Dynamic Queries for Visual Information Seeking. IEEE Software 11 (6): 70–77.

Summarization Evaluation Results. TIPSTER Text Program. http://www-nlpir.nist.gov/related_projects/tipster_summac. Accessed 07/12/01.

Wayne C. 1998. Topic Detection and Tracking (TDT): Overview and Perspective. http://www.nist.gov/speech/publications/darpa98/html/tdt10.htm. Accessed 07/12/01.

Section 3
Standards and Vocabulary

Christopher G. Chute and Curtis P. Langlotz
Section Editors

Introduction
The Spectrum of Existing and Emerging Health Data Standards: Their Relevance and Application to Cancer Information

Christopher G. Chute and Curtis P. Langlotz

Healthcare practice, policy, and research have all become profoundly information-intensive and intertwined. Perhaps in no discipline is this more true than in cancer. Whether one seeks best practice, rational and compassionate resource allocation, or the application of mouse model genomics to human disease, all these activities increasingly depend upon an underlying body of data, inferences, and knowledge to progress intelligently. How then are we to make sense of the burgeoning mass of information relevant to matters in the cancer community? Furthermore, how can we ensure that basic science breakthroughs have an efficient and timely impact upon improved care practices and appropriate policy decisions?

Progress toward answering the foregoing questions can be leveraged by the development and application of relevant information standards—this is a key message of this entire volume. However, lest we engage in a frenzy of brilliant but isolated standards for cancer information, the universe of related health information standards bears examination and evaluation for adaptation to cancer concerns. The chapters in this section consider many health data standards that are highly relevant to cancer issues. The hope is that putting many of these available and emerging resources into a single work might prevent the redundant and potentially fragmenting emergence of similar but different standards parochial to cancer interests. That the broader health standards and cancer standards needs are more similar than different may be the conclusion of a thoughtful reader.

The section is opened by Chute (Chapter 7), who outlines a brief history of cancer-related standards and the pioneering progress made possible by the foresight of workers in this field toward the comparable, consistent, and analytic representation of cancer patient data. The message is that some inertia might exist in this century-long trend toward ever more precise and interoperable patient data, which may have caused many to overlook what was happening outside the cancer continent in the overall health world. Increasingly the remainder of the health world is becoming interlinked by a sea of standards, which may equally carry the data cargo of the cancer community among the multidisciplinary ports of the larger health community.

Tuttle and colleagues (Chapter 8) commence a suite of chapters on terminology comparing the importance of shared concepts, terms, and codes in the biomedical sciences, and especially cancer-related disciplines, to the profound impact that email and the World Wide Web have had on the world in general. They review, with authoritative detail, the emerging foci of controlled terminology efforts, and explore their relation with and evolution toward shared concepts systems in cancer. Sujansky (Chapter 9) continues some discussion on the importance of controlled terminologies and the classic desiderata that pertain. However, he emphasizes the role of human interface terminology, a sort of vocabulary shorthand, which is of paramount concern to the practical incorporation of vocabularies in electronic medical records (EMRs). The general discussion foreshadows the importance of controlled terminology for the care of cancer patients as a special application of general principles and standards.

Hartel and Coronado (Chapter 10) restate the basic problem of comparable and consistent data representation depending ultimately upon common vocabularies, yet pose this in the broad context of National Cancer Institute (NCI) activities, which range from basic science research on the genome to clinical trials in patients. They overview the enlightened and highly active NCI responses to these problems, providing a comprehensive context for terminology as the basis of many standards used (albeit with continuing needs for development) in the cancer community. Langlotz (Chapter 11) makes these efforts at NCI unambiguously clear by outlining the process by which the CDE (Common Data Elements) for cancer protocols (and a larger body of cancer information), emerged and evolved.

Although content and terminology are important, they are not sufficient. Spackman and Hammond (Chapter 12) review the compelling evidence for templated information, particularly in the domain of cancer pathology. They go on to highlight the evolution of data elements or content for these templates, which logically evolved to become controlled terminologies such as SNOMED. They highlight the close linkage that SNOMED has historically enjoyed with the cancer registry and coding community, most notably in the context of ICD-O (International Classification of Disease for Oncology).

Huff, Hammond, and Williams (Chapter 13) overview the history, evolution, and present status of Health Level 7 (HL7), the dominant health information standard for messaging among connected systems. HL7 has been explicitly adopted by many in the cancer community, particularly in the domain of cancer registries and public health reporting, although its heritage emerged almost exclusively in the patient care arena. The interplay of HL7 message contexts and their embedded contents is highlighted by the examples with ICD-O and SNOMED. Expanding on the theme of embedded context, Shakir (Chapter 14) provides an overview of the HL7 Reference Information Model, which is the overarching architecture for the creation of the new HL7 Version 3 messages. This model is increasingly finding an enthusiastic audience among thoughtful health information leaders who seek a common basis for understanding the context and relationships among health information, a task which may have increasing importance in the overall domain of cancer data.

A short chapter by Braithwaite reviews the Health Information Portability and Accountability Act (HIPAA) and provides insights into its requirements and their implications.

The overview by Greenes, Tu, Boxwala, Peleg, and Shortliffe (Chapter 16) explores the similarity and differences between clinical trial protocols and the structure of clinical guidelines. Fundamentally, protocols outline procedures for hypothesis-driven experiments, upon which guidelines hope to promote a consensus model for best practices in medicine. Despite these tangential differences, the principle of providing a standard template for care practices based on underlying standards offers more similarities between trial protocols and guidelines than not. Finally, Hiatt (Chapter 17) provides the big picture from the public health and information infrastructure perspective as they relate to cancer information. Overviewing many existing information networks—from genetics to early detection to prevention—the role of information standards and interchange is clear.

The scope of these reports is unusual, as is the authoritative association of the authors with the major themes of health information standards and their cancer applications. Although no such work can be exhaustively comprehensive, the treatment in these chapters is substantive and detailed. Together, we hope that they convey an informative picture about existing and emerging health data standards and their relevance to cancer informatics.

7
Cancer Data, Information Standards, and Convergent Efforts

CHRISTOPHER G. CHUTE

The cancer community is no stranger to informatics or data standards. Indeed, within health care, tumor registries and clinical treatment protocols heralded a rigor of data representation and structure that the rest of health care took decades to match. However, once underway, the larger arena of healthcare standards embraced the principles of inter-operability and data sharing at a scale that the early cancer templates, codes, and profiles were not designed to address. The universe of cancer information remains very large, however, and the utility of parochial standards persists. The question is how might the domain specific data standard needs of the cancer community be leveraged by the existing and emerging health information standards that surround it? Furthermore, because the domain of cancer is among the most striking multi-system and multi-organ disciplines in clinical medicine, what advantages might ensue from adoption of larger spectrum health information standards? Few of these questions will be answered in this introductory chapter; suffice that they be raised, cast into historical perspective, and followed by an authoritative suite of chapters that provide depth and insight on the relationship between cancer informatics and the larger world of health information standards.

The Heritage of Cancer Information Standards

Although many accede that the sixteenth-century London Bills of Mortality was the prototype for our modern notion of standardized mortality classifications, it was the systematic study of surgical outcomes at the turn of the 20th century (Mayo, 1905; Codman, Mayo et al., 1914) that prompted attention to morbidity classifications. Because morbidity, by its nature, requires considerably more detail than mortality, these outcome initiatives prompted the advent of standards for patient data abstraction. Arguably, the analytic methods enabled by the advent of mechanical punch cards and relatively high-speed data sorters provided the critical technology that made structured data abstraction, coding, and analysis practical. Although the most dramatic evidence of this technology was the unparalleled success of the 1890 U.S. decennial census by Hollerith's card sorters (U.S. Census Office, 1899) and the subsequent formation of what we know today as the IBM Corporation, the enablement of cancer registries and statistical tabulation are also direct consequences.

Perhaps lost in this early history of computer science and biostatistics is the fact that the primary applications of the newly extended morbidity data were to cancer conditions and outcomes (Mayo, 1921). Indeed, much of the early body of biostatistical methods were also derived to address the analysis of cancer cohorts and treatment variations. From this developed a more formal mechanism to describe patients living with illness, or more pertinently to characterize their disease. Beginning in the 1920s, organized efforts to register patients treated for cancer emerged within the American College of Surgeons (ACS) (Mayo, 1924), a heritage of the ACS that persists to this day (ACS, 1999). The clear intentions of the early cancer registries were to conduct what passed for outcomes research of the period, or at least to compute cancer survival statistics for subsets of cancer patients.

Analysis of cancer outcomes did not proceed very long before the knotty problem of disease severity, or extent of disease, was recognized as a serious confounder. We all know today that advanced stage disease fares more poorly than early stage conditions, yet even that intuition is biased by a modern notion of disease staging. How then did the early pioneers in the cancer domain address a consistent, reproducible mechanism to subset patients for survival analysis? The history of cancer staging is well outlined in the work of Gospodarowicz et al. (1998); suffice it to say our now familiar division of disease description into standard measures of tumor size, nodal extent, and metastatic status (TNM: Tumor, Nodes, Metastasis) began over 50 years ago. Staging in cancer registries today, while still controversial in some of the more sophisticated clinical trials, persists as a direct intellectual descendent of these efforts (American Joint Committee on Cancer, 1997).

Paralleling the allocation of patients into subsets by disease severity was the recognition of the need for standardized classification of histologic cell types. Formalized in 1951 by the Manual of Tumor Nomenclature and Coding (MONTAC) committee (American Cancer Society, 1951), this terminology became the "histology axis" for the modern ICD-O for oncology (ICD-O, 2000). In Chapter 12, Spackman and Hammond outline the interrelationships that MONTAC had and still has on the SNOMED systems in this volume. This is perhaps the first obvious interface between an emergent cancer standards community and the larger health data standards world.

The next evolution beyond cancer registries was the emergence of randomized clinical trials as the backbone for evaluating cancer treatment effectiveness. While the mechanics and theory for trial design had been well established by the 1940s (Gehan & Schneiderman, 1990), drawing heavily upon the statistical basis for agricultural yield optimization, it was perhaps not until President Nixon's War on Cancer undertaken in 1971 that the infrastructure of cancer trials ramped up to industrial scale. The evolution of increasingly sophisticated data collection methods required for those trials, again coupled with the technological advent of modern computing, continued to drive the search for interoperable data interchange and shared infrastructure, the very substance of health data standard. The most recent and well publicized effort in this lineage is the advent of the Common Data Elements (Chute, 2000; also see Chapter 11).

Today, the major cancer clinical trial cooperative groups have highly sophisticated internal data and protocol standards. Increasingly, groups working together have evolved commonly accepted data standards across the standards community, such as the Cancer Therapy and Evaluation Program's Common Toxicity Criteria (CTEP's CTC). The goal, of course, is to broaden the scope and inclusiveness of these groups to extend outside the domain of cancer.

Health Standards Across Biology and Medicine

Although the cancer community has an indisputable claim to being the pioneer of modern health information standards, the rest of the healthcare community has not been idle. Beginning in the late 1980s, a plethora of standards groups formed and, over time, consolidated. The chapter by Huff, Hammond, and Williams in this monograph (Chapter 13) overviews the recent history and status of many of these efforts, focusing attention on the largest and most important—HL7. Internationally, an International Standards Organization (ISO) technical committee was formed in 1998 to begin the coordination and recognition by ISO of health standards around the world (see http://www.astm.org/COMMIT/ISO/tc215.html). All of these activities have become highly relevant as the once distant dream of electronic medical records (EMRs) has become an immediate challenge—a challenge made more difficult by the paucity of mature standards.

The relevance of these standards to the cancer community is obvious from at least two perspectives: (1) cancer as a field involves virtually all body tissues and organs, and thus it overlaps with all other healthcare interests, and (2) consider whether we need special standards for each of these in order: health, cancer, prostate cancer, early stage prostate cancer, and early stage prostate cancer among Medicare beneficiaries. Hopefully, the reduction to absurdity is apparent in the second line of reasoning, though independent standards do exist for each of these nested instances.

The trajectory of our cancer standards legacy, fortunately, is becoming increasingly clear. The cancer community needs to become engaged in the standards development in the larger health information world, a task for which the National Cancer Institute (NCI) has already set a welcome example. The overall health standards community has much it can learn from the near century-long tradition of cancer standardization activities and practical developments. Similarly, it is time for the cancer community to recognize, adapt, and leverage the increasingly elegant and useful work emerging from the health informatics and standards universe.

References

American Cancer Society (ACS). 1951. Manual of Tumor Nomenclature and Coding (MONTAC). New York: American Cancer Society.

American College of Surgeons (ACS). 1999. Commission on Cancer. Standards of the Commission on Cancer. Chicago, IL: American College of Surgeons.

American Joint Committee on Cancer (AJCC), American Cancer Society, American College of Surgeons. 1997. AJCC Cancer Staging Manual/American Joint Committee on Cancer, 5th ed. Philadelphia: Lippincott-Raven.

Chute CG. 2000. And Data for All: The NCI Initiative on Clinical Infrastructure Standards. MD Computing 17(2):19–21.

Codman EA, Mayo WJ, et al. 1914. Report of the Committee Appointed by the Clinical Congress of Surgeons of North America: Standardization of Hospitals. Surgery, Gynecology and Obstetrics 18(Suppl.):9–12.

Gehan EA, Schneiderman MA. 1990. Historical and Methodological Developments in Clinical Trials at the National Cancer Institute. Statistics in Medicine. 9(8): 871–880; discussion 903–906.

Gospodarowicz M, Benedet L, Hutter RV, Fleming I, Henson DE, Sobin LH. 1998. History and International Developments in Cancer Staging. Cancer Prevention & Control 2(6):262–268.

Mayo CH. 1925. Address of the President. Delivered at Convocation of American College of Surgeons, New York, October 24, 1924. Surgery, Gynecology and Obstetrics(3):447–448.

Mayo CH. 1905. Mortality, Disability, and Permancy of Cure in Surgery. Northwestern Lancet 25:179–182.

Mayo WH. 1921. Mortality and End-Results in Surgery. Surgery, Gynecology and Obstetrics 32:97–102.

United States Census Office. 1889. 11th Census, 1890. Report of a Commission Appointed by the Honorable Superintendent of Census. Washington, DC: Judd & Detweiler.

World Health Organization. 2000. International Classification of Diseases for Oncology (ICD-O), 3rd ed. Geneva, Switzerland: World Health Organization.

8
Toward Terminology as Infrastructure*

Mark S. Tuttle, Keith E. Campbell, Kevin D. Keck, and John S. Carter

In the near future, high-level meetings at cancer care and research enterprises may be distracted by discussions of the terminology computers use to support collaborative interactions. Because the productivity of these enterprises will depend on comprehensive and timely terminology, discussions of terminology shortfalls may dominate management discussions until they are overcome and creating and maintaining quality terminology become part of the enterprise infrastructure. Because cancer research and care is necessarily broadly collaborative, this may happen to cancer enterprises before it happens to most other biomedical and healthcare enterprises.

An analogous situation occurred in the computer science department at the University of California Berkeley, where the first author of this chapter was then a lecturer. The Internet had existed for at least a decade, but despite growing use, it was still little appreciated—until the widespread introduction of email. In less than a year, the computer science faculty had embraced email as a way of conducting department business. Because the faculty began to use email to conduct its routine business, committee meetings became less frequent. The committee meetings that were held became more intense because the agenda items that could not be resolved by email were the difficult ones. Email also became a critical part of research, because it permitted teams of graduate students and faculty in different buildings and different academic departments to communicate about common objectives, e.g., the development of the then-novel notion of Reduced Instruction Set Computing (RISC), which joined software and hardware researchers in close collaboration.

When predictable scaling, reliability, and robustness problems emerged with the then-available network, computer, and software resources, email was often the first subject brought to the table at faculty meetings,

*Partially supported by contracts funded by the National Cancer Institute Office of Bioinformatics, and National Library of Medicine Contract #LM-9-3519—"Research Support Services for the UMLS Metathesaurus."

independent of the stated agenda. Although there was laughter and good humor, sometimes heated discussions both began and ended the meetings. (The irony of a computer science faculty arguing about the management of email was not lost on those in attendance.)

In hindsight, email and the network-based applications that followed heralded profound changes in the work processes within academia. Before the widespread use of email, effective group size was limited to that of a wolf pack—no more than 30 members, so that the leader—the alpha wolf—could maintain frequent eye contact with each member. After email achieved widespread use, effective and productive groups could grow larger, amorphous, informal, overlapping, or more geographically dispersed, especially if group members knew one another and maintained occasional face-to-face contact.

Over time, computing resources became more robust. It became crucial to administer and maintain smooth computing environments, a modest but important part of which was support for email. Email digressions from the stated agendas of faculty meetings became rare and eventually disappeared. In short, email and its maintenance became part of the assumed infrastructure of most enterprises. Energy crises might cause the university to cut off heat to some of its buildings during vacations, but many faculty and students kept working anyway; on the other hand, if the email system was down for any appreciable length of time, everyone went home.

The critical nature of email is well known to those who read this chapter. Why, then, will the enterprise use of terminology become even more critical?

Three Scenarios

To communicate the importance of terminology, we pose three scenarios:

- A cancer enterprise director wants to answer the question: "What are we doing related to X?" X could be a phenomenon (cell death), a method (gene therapy), a class of things (endocrine cancers), a population (Gulf War veterans), or any named thing.
- A patient's search for help on a cancer Web site begins with "My doctor tells me I have Y cancer" or "I have Y cancer, and my doctor wants to treat it with Z." Y might be a general category like lung cancer, or it might be specific and include histologic and genetic staging. Similarly, Z could be very general, very specific, or anything in between.
- A cancer researcher asks, "I want to compare my mouse 'clinical trial' outcome data with data from other mouse model researchers. This ought to be easy, but it isn't. Can the enterprise help?"

Cancer enterprises must address these challenges to fulfill their missions, and terminology is a critical part of the solution. The "terminology problem" is one of process; namely, how can terminology be created and managed productively and become part of enterprise infrastructure?

Questions Arising from Terminology-as-Infrastructure

Healthcare enterprises often begin planning for enterprise use of terminology with questions like "Should we use the International Classification of Diseases (ICD) or the Systematic Nomenclature of Medicine (SNOMED)?" Because both are needed but are not sufficient, other more important questions arise. These include:

- What terminology infrastructure do we need?
- Who should pay for its creation and maintenance?
- Who should own the resulting intellectual property?
- What pieces of the infrastructure must cancer enterprises create, because, for example, the pieces are cancer specific?
- To what degree should an enterprise re-use external terminology infrastructure internally?
- To what degree should an enterprise seek to support re-use of its local terminology infrastructure externally?
- To what degree should an enterprise be a terminology infrastructure leader, follower, or collaborator?
- To what degree will sources outside biomedicine supply necessary portions of the infrastructure, e.g., information technology standards?

These questions are not easy, but enterprises can answer them incrementally by fulfilling current, practical terminology infrastructure needs. At the same time, enterprises must implement policies that represent the best answer to every question above and others not yet formulated. (For a list of the qualities of a good terminology, see Cimino, 1998.)

The Email Analogy

Email is often called the "killer app" (killer application) that made the Internet successful. Before the development of the World Wide Web (WWW)—another terminology analogy we address in this chapter—most Internet traffic was email, and before email there was relatively little Internet traffic. For email to become the phenomenon that made the Internet widely available and used, several elements had to converge.

First, the Internet infrastructure had to be well maintained and supported financially. Because this infrastructure existed, uniquely associating an email address with a particular account on a particular computer became a "local" problem. However messy these solutions were in the early days, they were "bounded" because of the predictable handling of a larger problem: maintaining Internet IP addresses, or identifiers for computers or devices on a Transmission Control Protocol/Internet Protocol (TCP/IP) network. The IP creation and maintenance process helped solve the terminology (naming) problem for computers. Because of IP addresses, we can both name and find computers on the Internet. (A detailed explanation of how this works and how those responsible are attempting to meet scalability challenges can be found at www.3com.com/nsc/501302.html.)

Secondly, for email to succeed, receiving computers also had to understand the "username" part of an email address. This was also a local problem. It eased the terminology problem for users and their mailboxes, given a computer reachable from the Internet.

A third email success factor concerns the mailer software, or the programs that support the many functions of email. These had to run on each computer and interact with each another uniformly on the Internet, despite different software environments. Email had to be a standard message that helped leverage solutions to the terminology problem for computers and people. ("Standard message" does not mean that every message is the same; it means that every message can be processed the same way.)

The Web-as-Terminology Analogy

Although we take email for granted as an essential piece of biomedical infrastructure, almost everyone in the field of biomedicine can remember the world without the Web. As with email, the World Wide Web achieved scalable, global adoption by solving certain naming—i.e., terminology—problems.

Uniform Resource Locators (URLs) and HyperText Markup Language (HTML) have both provided solutions to Web-critical naming (terminology) problems. A URL is the global address of a document or other Web-based resource. The first part of the address indicates what protocol to use (e.g., FTP, HTTP), and the second part specifies the IP address or the domain name where the resource is located. HTML is a standard way to tell another computer how to display a page of text, images, and hyperlinks and how to follow hypertext links; it defines structure and layout of a document with various tags and attributes. In parallel with email, URLs uniquely identify resources on a usually remote computer, and HTML "pages" are standard messages that a local Web browser can interpret to produce the intended display.

As Berners-Lee discussed in *Weaving the Web* (1999), the challenge with URLs and HTML was to define just enough functionality to solve the problem and no more. With information technology, too much functionality or complexity impedes success and sometimes prevents it entirely. Regardless, URLs and HTML have fostered unprecedented information technology success, and they have done so by ignoring the "meaning" of anything on Web pages or other Web resources.

Terminology and the Web: Similarities

A term is a unit of formal, technical language (Tuttle, 1995), and a terminology is an explicitly inter-related collection of terms. Every term in a terminology is related to one or more other terms within the terminology using an explicit relationship. For example, in the emerging "Heme" terminology of the National Cancer Institute's Mouse Models of Human Cancers Consortium (MMHCC), formulated by Kogan et al. in the fall of 2000, "myelomonocytic leukemia" IS_A "myeloid leukemia," where the two leukemias are each terms, and the relationship of the former to the latter is "IS_A" (see www.lexical.com/MMHCC). Since it doesn't do much good to create terms and relationships in a single computer, the goal of this kind of terminology exercise is to make it possible for all computers in an enterprise to use key terms, such as "myeloid leukemia," in the same way.

Even if almost every enterprise computer did this, computers would still have to verify a common meaning to interoperate productively. As William T. Hole, who leads the Metathesaurus effort at the NLM, has observed, this will become even more difficult when transgenic models of human diseases are created in diverse species. For example, we refer to "diseases of the breast" in humans, but with mice it is more appropriate to call these "diseases of the mammary gland or the mammary fat pad." This difficulty will continue until a more universal understanding of the "biology of life" and "comparative anatomy" is established and reflected in a suitable terminology.

How does a computer, or a human, verify that a term has the same meaning at two different sites? One way is for each side of the computer-computer, computer-human, or human-human pair to confirm that it is using the same terminology reference model as the other half of the pair. For example, IP addresses all use the same reference model, and URLs use the same reference model. (Although the notion of a reference model for terminology or terminology as a reference model arose in the context of healthcare enterprise information technology, it applies equally well to enterprises needing terminology for biomedical research [Cohn & Chute, 1997; Chute et al. 1999b].)

Terminology and the Web: Differences

Biomedical terminology is profoundly different from IP addresses or URLs, at least to humans. Most of these differences stem from a single distinguishing characteristic: *terms in biomedical terminologies usually name categories of things, while IP addresses and URLs name instances of things.* An IP address, like 204.162.102.101, names a specific computer, and the URL http://www.lexical.com/MMHCC/ names a specific Web page stored on that computer. There is nothing "categorical" about either of these elements; they are not ambiguous, and their identity is not in doubt, given the reference models for IP addresses and URLs. Conversely, the name or term, "murine myelocytic leukemia" (a kind of mouse leukemia) is a category of transgenic mice that have the disorder (Kogan et al., 2001). Because naming and defining categories are both important and difficult, almost all terms in biomedical terminologies name categories. (Some exceptions occur in MeSH [Medical Subject Headings], the terminology the NLM uses to index MEDLINE, in which instance names include federal agencies and other funding sources.) Simply put, the importance of categories to biomedicine and other endeavors merits the trouble of naming and defining them and maintaining the names and definitions in a terminology. As the late Jacob Bronowski observed, the task of science is to draw the dotted lines in the universe; part of the task of terminology is to name and help define the resulting pieces.

This profound difference between naming instances and naming categories has led to the notion of concept representation in terminologies. As part of some distinctions clarified during the early part of the 20th century, a concept is a unit of thought (Richards & Ogden, 1989). Thus, instead of thinking about a category as a group of mice—part of some larger population of mice—that have myelocytic leukemia, we develop a concept, the name of which is myelocytic leukemia. This is related to the contemporary view of probability that opposes the frequency view. Earlier definitions of probability focused on direct connections with a physical reality, which led to an alternate view that probability was a measure of uncertainty. The latter establishes a language of descriptions first, and then a measure is applied to the truth of the descriptions. Both probabilistic descriptions and terminology exist to help describe reality, but details can differ markedly depending on the approach. In our opinion, the study of terminology is the study of descriptions.

To those accustomed to the use of the term "concept" by philosophy and cognitive psychology during the latter half of the 20th century, associating terms with concepts seems hopelessly ambitious. Although everyday notions like "chair" and "cup" (referring to man–made objects), and (phenotypically) "dog" (a natural object) have no required attributes that computers can use to define them, humans find these concepts perfectly serviceable. But when terminologists speak of a concept-oriented terminology, they mean that a single meaning or concept is associated with one or more terms that name the concept. This puts corresponding stress on the need to make terms have "face validity," that is to make them free standing (not context dependent), defining names of concepts. Until recently, most terminologies were not concept-oriented.

This one-to-one association between concepts and their preferred names generalizes to the organization of terms by concept, instead of the other way around. The largest example of such an organization is the UMLS (Unified Medical Language System) Metathesaurus, the latest (2001) edition of which collects 797,359 concepts named by more than 50 biomedical terminologies (see www.nlm.nih.gov/research/umls/).

While a concept is associated with the computer known on the Web as 204.162.102.101, the concept is less important than the physical object, namely the manufactured organization of silicon and copper powered by electricity in a metal box in the machine room down the hall. On the other hand, the concept named "murine myeloid leukemia" brings to mind, among other things, pathological cellular processes occurring in different organs. Our knowledge of and descriptions of these processes are deeply intertwined mixtures of theories and observations.

An example of this intertwining resulted from the Annapolis Meeting, during which terminology for murine breast cancer was created to be more scientifically valid than the terminology for human breast cancer (Cardiff et al., 2000). This difference is a preview of the core terminology maintenance challenge. In biomedicine, concepts may be named using the best technical, scientifically based notions available at the time of their formulation; a simple example might be "ductal carcinoma." As science progresses, however, identification of cells, cell processes, and pathology becomes more precise and reproducible, but the naming often does not keep pace because humans adjust their model of the concept in response to new information without changing the name to keep up.

Therefore, time imposes a more subtle difference between the way IP addresses and URLs are handled on the Web and the way terminology must be handled in biomedicine. Instances rarely have a relationship with time; they either exist or they do not. A computer with a given IP address or a Web page with a given URL is either accessible or not accessible on the Internet. By contrast, a goal of science is to create lasting, useful categories, even if those categories are refined over time (for example, the many refinements of viral hepatitis—hepatitis A, hepatitis B, hepatitis C). Improving the naming of leukemia types in mice and humans does not change the nature of the disease, though it certainly reflects changes in our understanding of it.

As asserted previously, properties of terminologies are properties of descriptions, and while the phenomena addressed by descriptions might change over time, changes in terminology may or may not be related to those changes (Blois, 1984). Regardless, a terminology infrastructure must accommodate change gracefully and allow computers and humans to process pieces of information that straddle changes in terminology. The most visible example of such an infrastructure and associated processes is Medical Subject Headings (MeSH) and MEDLINE. Because annual changes to MeSH are used to "re-index" MEDLINE, we can retrieve citations from more than 30 years ago using the biomedical terminology of today.

Such functionality is not common in health care. Perhaps because most of the categories are simpler, the business world discovered some time ago that preserving enterprise data was more important than preserving enterprise software (Brodie & Stonebraker, 1995), unlike the usual situation in clinical settings, in which changes to software often make information collected before the change unretrievable, and if retrievable then non-comparable (Tuttle, 1999). In clinical settings, systems should preserve data so that important patient information (such as a penicillin allergy) is not lost when a new clinical system is deployed (Safran C, personal conversation).

To a computer, the difference between an instance and a category is not so deep as it is for humans. A computer can define both instances and categories as concepts, with the latter being simply a more complex type of the former because of the role of time. For example, a clinical attribute like "penicillin allergy" often has an associated acuity that a caregiver can determine from context. If the attribute is separated from its context, important information is lost because the term "penicillin allergy" is not precise enough on its own. Still, the scalable methods that have so changed our use of information in computers—namely, the use of IP addresses, URLs, and associated standards—are at least partially applicable to the biomedical terminology problem.

Terminology Servers, Messages, and Operational Semantics

Clearly, computers do not truly "understand" IP addresses, URLs, and HTML, and no program "understands" email. Still, each of these methods helped solve terminology (naming) problems and processes. We can think of how they work in terms of operational semantics. In other words, the meaning of an IP address can be defined through various low-level services on the Internet that correctly handle an IP address. A similar approach defines the physical location (on a disk drive) of the resource named by a URL and specifies how to display the pages. These operational definitions work so well that users do not have to think about them, unless they are performing certain kinds of specialized software development.

How can we reach the point at which terminology works so well that users do not have to think about it, except when the meanings of terms are themselves the subject of scientific research? Part of the burden here is that once terminology uses scale, the associated problems become interdisciplinary. What might be an easy terminology problem for a group with 30 members becomes harder as group size increases to 100, 1000, 10,000, and even 100,000.

Experience has shown that the best response to this challenge is to create operational semantics for important terms and terminologies by creating terminology services and standard messages. NCI has already started this by creating their Enterprise Vocabulary Server (EVS). A Web interface to the EVS that "serves up" terminology for human use is available at ncievs.nci.nih.gov/NCI-Metaphrase.html. Table 8.1 illustrates an example of the contents of the EVS, also known as the NCI Thesaurus (an NCI enhancement of the NLM UMLS Metathesaurus).

In this example, one of the services (operational semantics) the EVS provides is to return a list of concepts, represented by their preferred names, that might be related to the term (concept name) entered. No concept in the EVS corresponds to the term "murine myelocytic leukemia," but an EVS

TABLE 8.1. Matching concepts for murine myelocytic leukemia

Matching concepts	
Term enetered: murine myelocytic leukemia	
Myelocytic leukemia (Myeloid Leukemia)	Neoplastic process
Murine leukemia	
Murines (Muridae)	Mammal
Murine	Pharmacologic Substance; Organic Chemical
Murine (Mouse)	Mammal
Myelocytic	
Leukemial	Neoplastic process
If you did not find the concept you are looking for, and you're sure your spelling is correct, please click.	

service returns a list of concepts with preferred names. Except for a commercial eyedrop preparation named "Murine" all retrieved concepts are relevant and potentially useful. The message at the end of the list, "If you did not find—, please click," prompts the user about another EVS service—namely, to add "murine myelocyctic leukemia" to the terms available in the EVS. (The decision about accepting or rejecting the suggestion is one of editorial policy.)

While the EVS is still developing, the services it provides may be precursors to standard services (Chute, 1999a). The fact that within the EVS "murine myelocytic leukemia inhibitory factor" is related to "growth inhibitors" and "lymphokines" but not to "myelocytic leukemia" is not a shortfall of a service but of the EVS terminology data.

Operational semantics have several immediate practical advantages. They make terminology useful, if imperfect, and that helps users regard it as an organic resource rather than an intellectual or clerical abstraction. Forcing concepts, terms, and inter-concept relationships through the formalization process that enables computers to "serve" them helps reduce and highlight ambiguity. This formalization establishes the foundation for improving terminology and operational semantics. Operational semantics may prove to be the most productive way to define semantics.

Emerging Terminology Reference Models

The unequaled strength of the EVS is that it covers ostensibly all of health care and biomedical research, with special depth in cancer research and care. Its weakness is that, for cost reasons, this breadth prevents it from being organized so that a computer, for instance, can rely on a named relationship between every disease inhibitor and the disease it inhibits. A new generation of biomedical terminology reference models, depicted in Figure 8.1, is attempting to create analogous kinds of predictability; their descriptions follow.

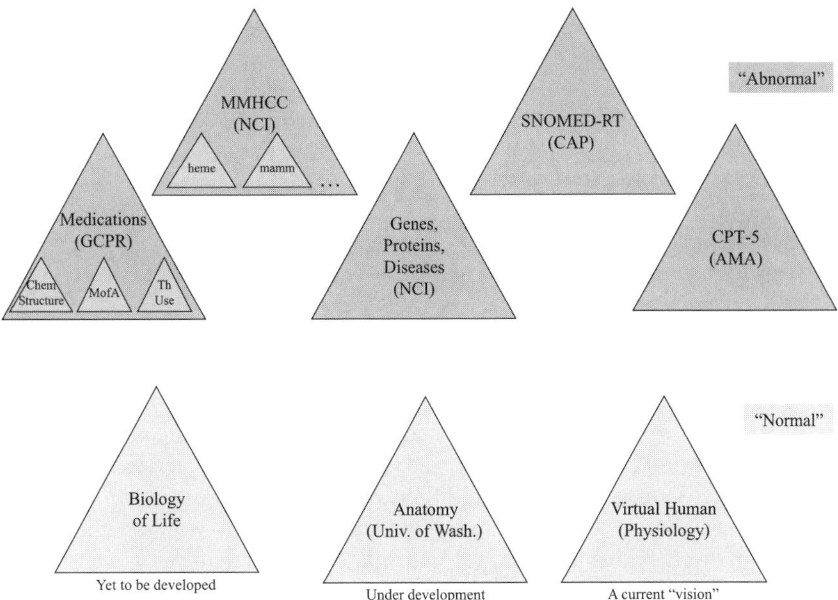

FIGURE 8.1. Emerging biomedical reference terminology models.

• **Medications (GCPR).** The Government Computer-based Patient Record (GCPR), a joint undertaking of the Veterans Administration (VA), Department of Defense (DoD), and Indian Health Service (IHS), will depend on a reference terminology model (RTM)—specifically, a medication RTM (mRTM). The mRTM seeks to define medications by active ingredient, chemical structural class, mechanism of action, kinetics, and therapeutic use, and represent associated attributes (e.g., dose, route, form).

• **MMHCC (NCI).** The Mouse Models of Human Cancers Consortium (MMHCC) is developing micro-terminologies of murine neoplasms and related disorders, beginning with the hematologic, breast, and prostate domains. Using specified reference taxonomies like morphology, genetics, and pathophysiology, these micro-terminologies will define, for a computer, each relevant neoplasm and disorder.

• **Genes, Proteins, and Diseases (NCI).** In this terminology, many genes, proteins, and diseases already named in the NCI EVS are associated more formally with one another to the extent that connections between them are known.

• **SNOMED-RT (CAP).** The College of American Pathologists (CAP) has released a new version of SNOMED that includes "Aristotelian" definitions of diseases. Most diseases are defined through class memberships and anatomic and pathophysiologic references. SNOMED reference terminology (SNOMED-RT) may become a de facto, or even de jure, standard for recording and preserving the meaning of healthcare descriptions. A future version of SNOMED-RT, called SNOMED-CT (for clinical terms), is slated to include British healthcare terminology.

• **CPT-5 (AMA).** The American Medical Association (AMA) is producing a major revision of Current Procedural Terminology version 4 (CPT-4), which will include computer-processible definitions of each coded procedure.

• **LOINC (Regenstreif Institute).** Not shown in Figure 8.1 is Logical Observation, Identifiers, Names, and Codes (LOINC), a terminology used to report and define laboratory testing results. LOINC (www.regenstrief.org/loinc/) receives support from the Hartford Foundation and two federal agencies, Agency for Healthcare Research and Quality (AHRQ) and the National Library of Medicine (NLM).

• **The Biology of Life.** As NCI Director Richard Klausner has observed, one needs to go back to one-celled animals to find divergence from the basic biochemistry shared by humans and their evolutionary predecessors. These shared biochemical processes and other commonalities should be made explicit once—for example, when all mouse model disease definitions are in place. Thereafter, the portion of the definitions common to mice and humans can be "normalized" and maintained in a single reference model. This will highlight the true differences among different species. Although cancer enterprises have a strong interest in developing such a reference model, and thus may want to begin work on its development, it is of sufficiently general interest that its maintenance should be taken over by an umbrella biomedical organization, such as the National Institutes of Health (NIH).

• **Anatomy.** Spurred by the success of the Visible Human projects, the NLM has sponsored the creation of a formal terminology of anatomy being developed by Cornelius Rosse and colleagues, at the University of Washington. They have completed macro-anatomy and begun work on micro-anatomy. Their dramatic achievement is the degree of coverage by IS_A and PART_OF relationships between named parts of the human body.

• **Virtual Human.** Various researchers have postulated the need for a computer-based model of normal physiology, analogous to the Visible Human. This model might, for example, explain the results of certain surgical or medical interventions (Chute, C., personal communication).

The significance of these emerging reference models is that both computers and humans can use them productively. Computers need predictable relationships that result from consistently applied principles, and humans need concept names (terms) that have face validity and do not depend on context for interpretation. The predictability helps software developers build applications that enable computers to interoperate by meaning. The face validity helps us verify that meanings are being used reproducibly. Several reference models have explicit change tracking representations, though no two are alike. One objective of the notion of operational semantics is to develop a universal terminology change transaction.

Because we do not yet know how to create and maintain one, a single biomedical reference model will not exist in the foreseeable future. Still, for obvious practical reasons, we must avoid needless proliferation of reference models. Determining the right number of reference models remains an empirical question.

Creating Operational Semantics

The operational semantics for IP addresses, email, URLs, and HTML were the result of an extraordinary set of circumstances. A large amount of benign neglect allowed otherwise immature ideas to mature sufficiently for widespread use (Segaller, 1998). We may not have the luxury of relying on benign neglect for the development of terminology operational semantics; in fact, after years of the terminology technology speeding ahead of the market, the reverse may now be true.

Experience indicates that narrow operational semantics—how one computer interoperates with another using shared meanings defined in a reference terminology—should be the result of market forces and appropriate consensus (standards) processes. Once the U.S. market decides it wants a standard, one is usually developed or anointed, although the process and result may not be ideal. The terminology definitions in the reference terminology, the broader operational semantics, pose another challenge. Healthcare informatics as a field has now accumulated more than 100 person-years of experience trying to create, maintain, and deploy concept-based terminologies and terminologies with formal semantic definitions (i.e., those that specify the meaning of a term for a computer, as SNOMED-RT and several Emerging Reference Terminologies shown in Figure 8.1 have done).

One key to this emergence is the notion of configuration management developed by Campbell (1997). Combined with earlier work by Mays et al. (1996) that supported scalable editing of formal terminologies, this notion overcame a formidable terminology infrastructure impediment and enabled SNOMED-RT development. The key was to equip each terminology creator/editor with an advanced, free-standing, client interface and to combine the work of multiple editors into a single configuration of a terminology.

This proved to be a valuable contribution. In large terminology development efforts, workflow—the management of geographically and professionally diverse domain experts on units of terminology work—quickly begins limiting development. The impact of this observation, now repeated in different contexts, cannot be overestimated. In addition, convening unstructured face-to-face terminology consensus groups works only under unusual circumstances. Because experts are used to knowing nearly everything there is to know about a particular subject, focusing them on the less well defined parts of their domains makes them uncomfortable and less productive. The tools developed by Mays and Campbell solve this problem by assigning multiple editors the same unit of work. They can quickly dismiss agreements without further review and then return disagreements directly to the disagreeing parties, allowing each to see the work of the other. Once editors see the opposing work, they often quickly agree on a resolution without communicating with one another, except through the workflow software.

One important lesson learned is that when editors still disagree on definitions, the best solution is to send them to a higher authority, e.g., a specialist, with sub-specialists held in the wings for extreme cases. In this way, terminology development units-of-work are spent most productively, with minimal time wasted and maximum confidence achieved in the validity of the result. While the field is still learning to do this reproducibly and scalably, the currently available tools represent a breakthrough in achievable quality and productivity.

Cancer research and care are by definition multidisciplinary and interdisciplinary. Because terminology development will have to be similarly multi- and interdisciplinary, the challenge is achieving this without draining resources devoted to care and cure. As with the Internet and the Web, a small number of curators will probably have to sustain the creation and maintenance of the underlying semantic definitions and face-valid term names in a cancer enterprise terminology infrastructure. Any stakeholder will be encouraged to complain about perceived terminology shortcomings, but a small minority of caregivers and researchers will do the actual maintenance. How to drive a new terminology into existence is still a pressing question, because it is so much less expensive to start with the terms already used in a domain. This strategy stresses the development process because large changes may be needed, but overcoming these stresses is usually worth the time and effort. As Betsy Humphreys at the NLM has observed, with terminology development it matters less where we start than where we go (personal communication).

Mixing Terminologies for Research and for Clinical Care

While deep qualitative differences exist between most research terms and most clinical terms, they are too subtle for formal semantics to capture (Blois, 1986). We understand that qualitative differences exist, but we are unable to explain them to a computer in a useful way. Still, we can make practical engineering adjustments for the differences in volatility in the Emerging Reference Models. If we know that terms will change often because the domain they describe is immature, then we can undertake formalization less aggressively than we would with stable clinical concepts, where reproducible interpretation is the primary goal. At our current level of sophistication, it makes sense to build an infrastructure that knows only that term A has a different definition from that of term B, not that term A is a "research" term, and term B is a "clinical" term.

Operational Semantics and the Three Scenarios

At the beginning of this chapter, we posed three scenarios:

- A cancer enterprise director wants to answer the question: "What are we doing related to X?"
- A patient's search for help on a cancer Web site begins with "My doctor tells me I have Y cancer" or "I have Y cancer, and my doctor wants to treat it with Z."
- A cancer researcher asks, "How can I compare my mouse 'clinical trial' outcome data with data from other mouse model researchers?"

Whatever the operational semantics do, they should begin by helping to accomplish the objectives laid out in the scenarios. Once we can operationally handle these and related scenarios, we can consider more esoteric functions. The problem is that as simple as the scenarios may sound, we are not yet able to directly reuse the solution to one to solve other problems. Medical centers, research centers, and software companies are making good progress to change that.

The challenge with operational semantics is to ensure that necessary and useful aspects are working in a way that allows all to learn from the experience and does not impede future enhancements. This is not impossible, but it cannot be done casually.

Looking Ahead

Successful terminology will eventually pass into the background, just as IP addresses, email, URLs, and HTML are taken for granted by most cancer caregivers and researchers. For this to happen, we will have to focus on deploying and using operational semantics to solve enterprise-wide problems. These operational semantics pose interdisciplinary challenges because they must involve information technology developers, management, content (terminology) developers, and others throughout the enterprise. The reward for overcoming these challenges is multi- and interdisciplinary empowerment of the targeted caregivers and researchers.

Despite the drama "working" examples can produce, too much effort in narrow domains—whether the focus is on technical or content issues—can be difficult to sustain. Planning for breadth-first approaches to terminology objectives, even if narrow demonstration projects are necessary, is the most productive way to proceed. Email did not achieve global use overnight, but it could not succeed until everyone on the Internet, regardless of computing environment, could receive it. The availability of the Web has removed many of the technical barriers to interoperation by meaning. What remains are the functional barriers and content hurdles that are the targets of operational semantics.

Disclosure. Apelon, Inc. (www.apelon.com) sells terminology software components and services.

Acknowledgments. Stuart Nelson, William T. Hole, Betsy Humphreys, John Silva, Scott Kogan, Cheryl Marks, Robert Cardiff, Sherri De Coronado, Frank Hartel, Cornelius Rosse, Christopher G. Chute, Steven Brown, Michael Lincoln, and David Sherertz each made important contributions to the ideas presented here, though, as is customary, they should not be held responsible for statements made in this chapter. Related material was presented at Pharmacology Grand Rounds, Vanderbilt University, Nashville, TN, October 2000. Portions of this chapter were presented at a colloquium and a seminar hosted by Reed Gardner, Chairman, Medical Informatics, University of Utah, October 2000.

References

Berners-Lee T. 1999. Weaving the Web: The Original Design and Ultimate Destiny of the World Wide Web by Its Inventor. Harper: San Francisco.

Blois MS. 1984. Information and Medicine: The Nature of Medical Descriptions. Berkeley: University of California Press.

Blois MS. 1986. Medicine and the Nature of Vertical Reasoning. New England Journal of Medicine 315:740–744.

Brodie ML, Stonebraker M. 1995. Migrating Legacy Systems: Gateways, Interfaces and the Incremental Approach. Palo Alto: Morgan Kaufman.

Campbell KE. 1997. Distributed Development of a Logic-Based Controlled Medical Terminology (CS-TR-97-1596). Dissertation, Stanford University. Available at http://elib.stanford.edu

Cardiff, et al. 2000. The Mammary Pathology of Genetically Engineered Mice: The Consensus Report and Recommendations from the Annapolis Meeting. Oncogene 19(8):968–988.

Chute CG, et al. 1999a. Desiderata for a Clinical Server. Proceedings of AMIA Symposium 42–46.

Chute CG, et al. 1999b. National Conference on Terminology for Clinical Patient Description: Terminology II: Establishing the Consensus, Lessons from Experience. April 27–29, Tysons Corner, VA. Also at www.amia.org/cpri/terminology2/overview.html.

Cimino JJ. 1998. Desiderata for Controlled Medical Terminologies in the Twenty-First Century. Methods of Information in Medicine 37:394–403.

Cohn SP, Chute CG. 1997. Clinical Terminologies and Computer-based Patient Records. Journal of AHIMA, 68(2):41–43.

Kogan SC, et al. NCI/MMHCC Proposals for the Classification of Murine Non-Lymphoid Hematopoietic Neoplasms and Related Disorders. In preparation, 2001.

Mays EK, et al. 1996. Scalable and Expressive Medical Terminologies. In Cimino J, ed. Proceedings of AMIA Symposium. Philadelphia: Hanley & Belfus. 259–263.

Richards IA, Ogden CK. 1989. The Meaning of Meaning: A Study of the Influence of Language upon Thought and of the Science of Symbolism, reissue ed., New York: Harcourt Brace.

Segaller S. 1998. Nerds 2.0.1: A Brief History of the Internet. New York: TV Books.

Tuttle MS. 1995. Concept, Code, Term, and Word: Preserving the Distinctions. In Masys D, ed. Proceedings of Fall AMIA Symposium. Philadelphia: Hanley & Belfus, 956.

Tuttle MS. 1999. Information Technology Outside Health Care: What Does It Matter to Us? Journal of the American Medical Informatics Association 6(5): 354–360.

9
Clinical Terminologies for Data Analysis and Structured Data Entry

Walter Sujansky

Electronic medical record (EMR) systems, once considered esoteric technologies confined to research settings, are now entering the mainstream of healthcare computing. In 2000, 64% of providers who responded to the HIMSS Leadership Survey were at some stage of EMR implementation, whether developing a plan (23%), beginning installation (29%), or implementing a fully operational EMR (12%) (HIMSS Leadership Survey, 2000). Increasingly, provider organizations believe EMRs can help address operational challenges, such as increasing clinical staff productivity, billing accurately, monitoring and reporting on care quality, and offering patients access to their medical data. Some organizations are also looking to EMRs to improve the efficiency of retrospective clinical research.

To meet these challenges, an EMR system must do more than store medical records as electronic renditions of paper-based charts. It also must provide an internal model of the stored medical data so that computers can automatically process the data, "understand" them to some extent, and perform valuable analysis (Sujansky, 1998b). An EMR system that includes such a model is called a structured EMR.

A cardinal element of a structured EMR is a *controlled medical terminology* (Cimino 2000). An entire subfield of medical informatics studies and develops terminologies to enable the analysis of data in structured EMRs. However, equally important are terminologies that enable clinicians to *enter* data into structured EMRs. Although terminologies for data entry have generally received less attention, data analysis is impossible without prior data entry, and data entry is difficult without appropriate terminologies. Figure 9.1 illustrates the flow of clinical data in a structured EMR and highlights the roles of terminologies for data entry and analysis.

In this chapter, we discuss the requirements and desired attributes of terminologies for data analysis (reference terminologies) and data entry (interface terminologies), and consider the differences between them. We also describe a strategy for reconciling the differences to create a structured EMR system, one that supports both entry and analysis of clinical data.

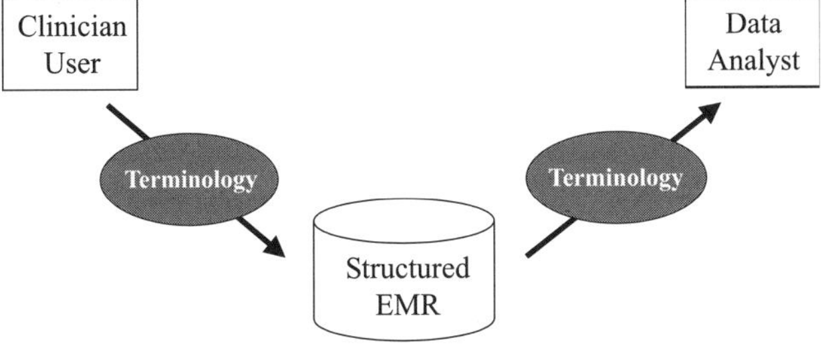

FIGURE 9.1. II

Requirements and Desired Attributes

The terminology model used for data analysis, now called reference terminology (Spackman et al., 1997), supports aggregation and analysis of clinical data. Aggregation is pooling data from multiple observers for multiple patients, and analysis is correctly answering queries based on data. Researchers and developers have done much work to develop medical terminologies that support these two tasks.

For users to effectively enter data into an EMR, the terminology must complement their workflow. Because clinicians generate approximately 80% of the information in patient records, any structured EMR that does not allow direct data entry will have limited analysis capabilities, and it will not address the wide variety of operational challenges healthcare organizations face. Direct data entry, also called structured data entry, requires no transcription and coding staff or intermediate processing of natural language into a structured format. Terminologies designed for structured data entry are called interface terminologies or user terminologies.

Interface terminologies must support convenient, complete, and useful capture of structured clinical data. Convenient data capture is rapid and consistent with normal workflow; complete data capture satisfies all clinical documentation needs; and useful capture means that the stored information can support data analysis or be mapped to a reference terminology that supports data analysis. All three requirements are equally important. For example, free-text data entry meets the convenience and completeness requirements, but since it cannot be reliably mapped to a reference terminology, it fails to satisfy the usefulness criterion.

Because reference terminologies and interface terminologies must support different activities, they have different requirements. Specific requirements of reference terminologies include:

- **Completeness with respect to the domain of interest.** The terminology must include the terms and phrases representing the real-world phenomena to be aggregated and analyzed.
- **Non-redundancy of representation.** The terminology cannot allow multiple terms or combinations of terms to represent the same observation. The

exception is an allowance for synonyms, which must be explicitly represented as such.

- **Non-ambiguity of representation.** The terminology cannot include single terms or combinations of terms that represent different observations.
- **A rich multiple classification hierarchy.** The terminology must organize terms into a hierarchy with useful aggregating concepts and allow terms to be classified beneath multiple concepts.
- **Formal logical definitions for the concepts.** The terminology must define concepts so that a computer can automatically detect unintended additions of redundant terms and discover valid relationships among terms.

Others have described these criteria extensively (Cimino, 1998).

Although interface terminologies share many characteristics with reference terminologies, such as domain completeness and explicit synonymy, they also have several distinguishing characteristics. Some of the most important are:

- Compositional construction
- Redundancy when necessary
- Modifier-based grouping of observations
- Shallow hierarchies
- Non-definitional modifiers
- Negation and temporal attributes.

To illustrate these requirements in practice, we use a specific EMR tool, shown in Figure 9.2, to describe structured data entry (Sujansky, 1998a).

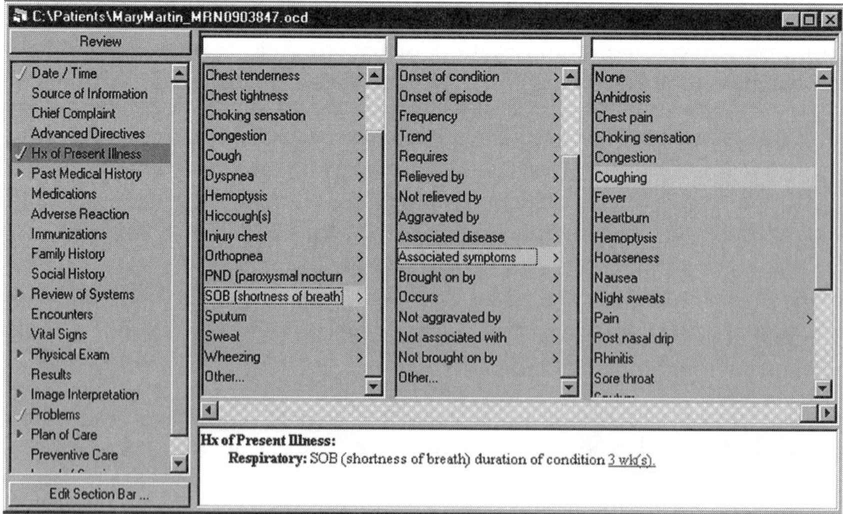

FIGURE 9.2.

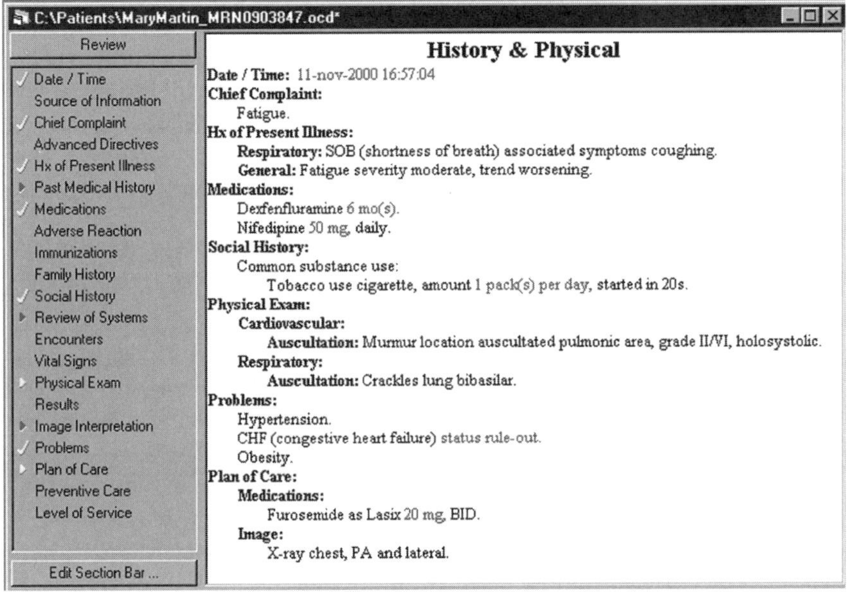

FIGURE 9.3.

The tool and its interface terminology allow clinical users to specify a context for clinical observations ("history of present illness"), a primary concept or subject to be documented ("SOB"), a set of relevant modifiers ("associated symptoms"), and appropriate values for each of those modifiers ("cough"). A formal interface terminology underlies the user interface of this tool. By interacting with the interface terminology, users can generate sentences that form the components of a clinical note. Data underlying the sentences are structured and conform to the interface terminology. As shown in Figure 9.3, a user can complete an entire document in this way.

Compositional Construction

As Kirby and Rector (1996) observe, clinical care "requires that patients be described rather than labeled." To this end, interface terminologies must allow clinicians to compose complex patient observations, not just choose from pre-enumerated, pre-defined patient classifications. Figures 9.4 and 9.5 illustrate this contrast. Figure 9.4 shows a compositional model for documenting the findings of a physical examination. The structure of the terminology allows users to select from diverse findings, modifiers, and values to construct a complete description of each finding.

By contrast, Figure 9.5 shows a hypothetical data entry tool that uses pre-enumerated, pre-coordinated terminology to represent physical findings. Because of the pre-combined findings, modifiers, and values, it is difficult to

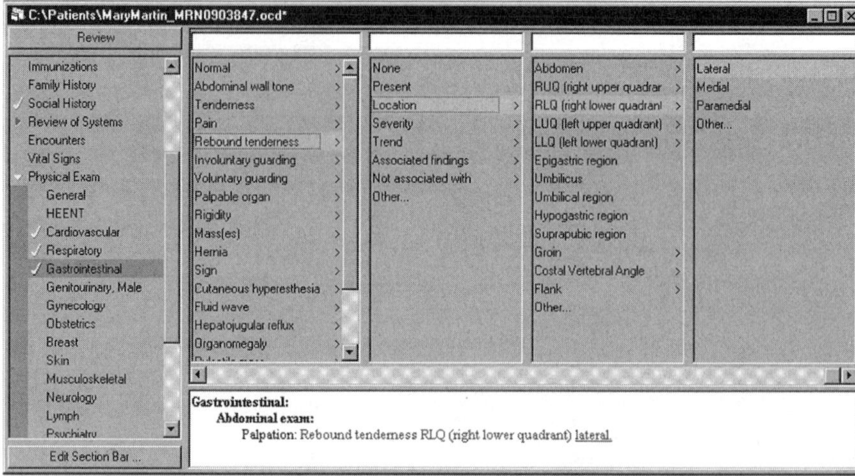

FIGURE 9.4.

identify the correct combination from a lengthy list of choices and impractical to include all the clinically possible combinations.

Compositional terminology models promote complete and convenient structured data entry: complete because they allow clinicians to combine a

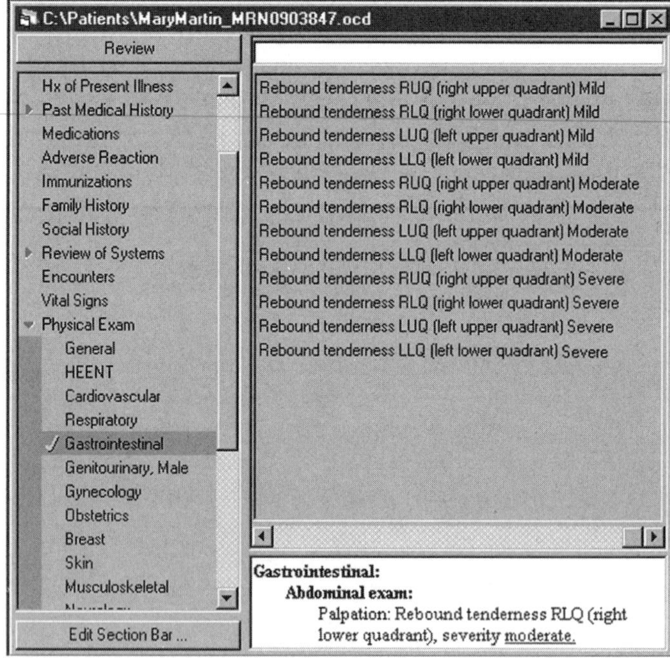

FIGURE 9.5.

large set of descriptors to characterize a patient, and convenient because they eliminate the need to search long lists of similar observations.

Redundancy

Although redundancy is anathema to reference terminology development, it is actually desirable in interface terminologies. Representing the same concept in multiple ways is useful, because optimal representation may vary depending on the clinical context and user style. Allowing users to appropriately enter information fulfills the convenience requirement for structured data entry. For example, the structured data entry tool offers two ways of entering family history information. With the first option (shown in Figure 9.6), the user can first specify a disorder in the family and then enter information about relatives that have it. This approach is often useful when a physician is working up a particular problem, such as a breast mass. With the second option (shown in Figure 9.7), a user can specify individual relatives first and then list the disorders they have, a process typical for a general history and physical. Interface terminologies should offer both options.

Modifier-Based Grouping of Observations

With modifier-based grouping, clinicians specify a modifier value for an entire set of observations. This method of documentation, common in clinical records, requires modifiers to precede concepts in the terminology hierarchy. For example, clinicians documenting physical exam findings will

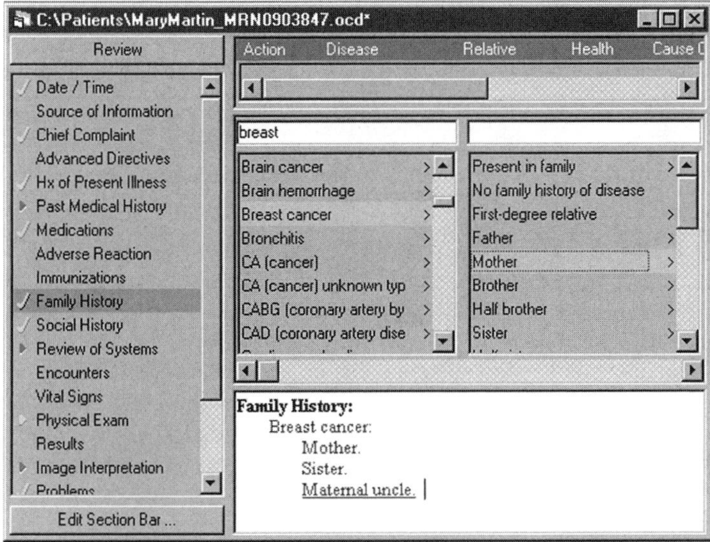

FIGURE 9.6.

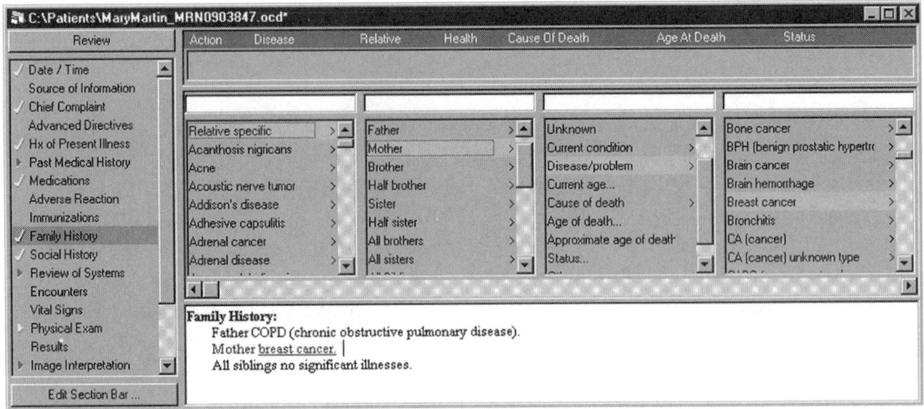

FIGURE 9.7.

specify an anatomical location (such as "neck") and all the positive and negative findings at that location (such as "tenderness," "swelling," and "bruit"). Figure 9.8 illustrates the use of this technique in the data entry tool and the generated text that results.

Users depending on reference terminologies, which typically nest modifiers below their concepts, would have to repeatedly specify the "neck" location for each of the negative findings in the example, a tedious process contrary to normal documentation habits. Modifier-based grouping supports fast, convenient data entry, especially when users must record several negative findings in the same anatomical context.

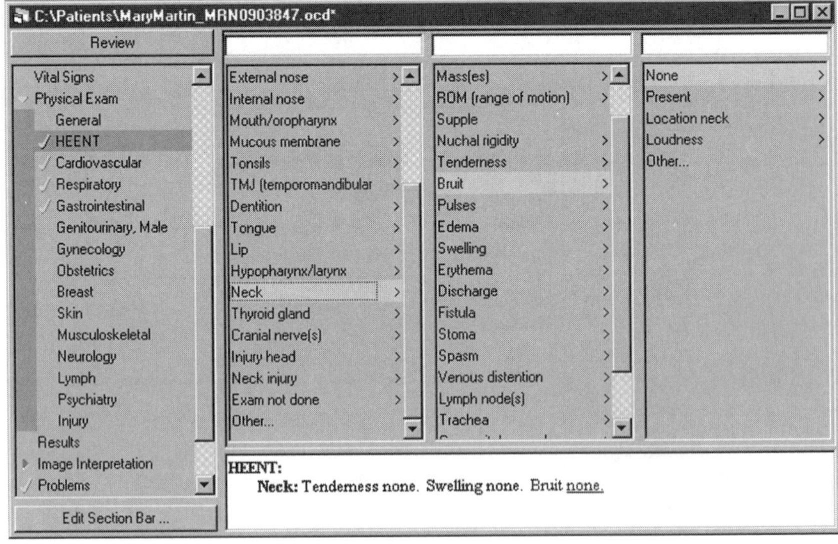

FIGURE 9.8.

Shallow Hierarchies

Reference terminologies benefit from deep, rich hierarchies of clinical terms that provide many levels of data aggregation. For example, the SNOMED reference terminology (College of American Pathologists, 2000) provides six levels of aggregation above the term "atrial fibrillation," as illustrated in Figure 9.9. This feature allows reporting and other data analysis programs to identify groups of patients who manifest any cardiovascular disease, any disease of the heart, or any conduction disorder of the heart.

However, multiple hierarchical levels above the clinical terms can also impede data entry. Studies have shown that users of structured data entry tools prefer shallow hierarchies, which reduce path uncertainty and the number of navigational clicks, to deeper and more complex hierarchies that support data analysis. Furthermore, physicians do not require aggregating terms when entering clinical data. Instead of documenting diagnoses at non-specific levels of abstraction, such as "conduction disorder of the heart" or "cardiovascular disease," they document specific signs, symptoms, and diagnoses, such as "atrial fibrillation" or "second degree heart block."

For example, in the "problems-list" section of the structured data entry tool, shown in Figure 9.9, there is only one level of abstraction above the specific problems. The problem "atrial fibrillation," hence, appears directly below the heading "cardiovascular system." Because the data entry tool has

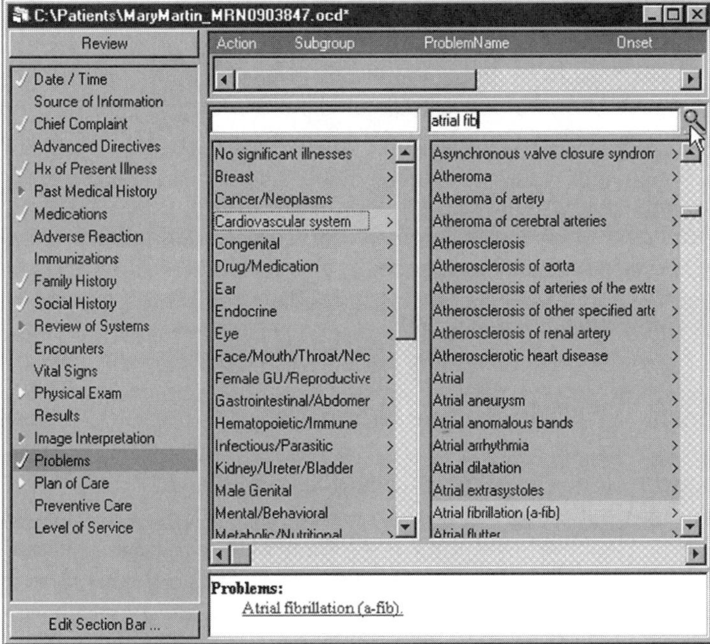

FIGURE 9.9.

rapid text search capabilities, the interface terminology can contain a long, "flat" list of problems under very general headings. In practice, users find it faster to search a long list of varied observations than to navigate many levels to arrive at a short list of specific observations. Therefore, shallow hierarchies help interface terminologies meet the convenience criterion.

Non-Definitional Modifiers

Another distinction between reference terminologies and interface terminologies is the usefulness of definitional modifiers, also called definitional attributes. Definitional attributes, supported by reference terminologies like SNOMED-RT, are modifier/value pairs that unambiguously define the concepts to which they are assigned. For example, the concept "breast cancer" may be formally defined as a disorder with the anatomical location "breast" and the morphological characteristic "carcinoma." Such definitions help maintain large and complex terminologies by averting accidental introductions of redundant terms.

In terminology systems with definitional modifiers, redundant terms can be automatically detected by advanced terminology-editing environments because the redundant terms, although textually distinct, carry the same definitional modifiers. However, definitional modifiers for concepts like breast cancer usually are not relevant for documenting the diagnosis of breast cancer in a specific patient. More useful is a list of the possible but not necessary values for the topography, morphology, and other characteristics of the disease. For example, lists of the possible topography values such as "axillary tail," "subareolar region," and "upper inner quadrant" and the possible morphology values such as "ductal Ca in situ," "infiltrating ductal Ca," and "comedocarcinoma" are much more useful for documenting breast cancer using a structured data entry tool.

Some reference terminologies represent the appropriate sets of modifier values for clinical documentation as "sanctions" (Solomon et al., 2000). Terminologies with such "sanctioned" sets of modifiers allow users to fully describe the details of diagnoses and other clinical observations, thus meeting the completeness criterion.

Temporal Attribution and Negation

To support realistic clinical documentation, terminologies must also include temporal attribution of clinical observations. Although the onset and duration of a clinical symptom is fundamental to decision making and record keeping, reference terminologies rarely include explicit terms for temporal attribution. Interface terminologies must include such temporal modifiers as "onset" to meet the completeness criterion, and the values of the modifiers, such as "one year ago," must be contextually appropriate to meet the convenience criterion. The latter element relieves users from searching through a long list of values for temporal modifiers.

Explicit negation of symptoms, findings, and other concepts is also a necessary part of clinical documentation and must appear in interface terminologies. Reference terminologies rarely include negating terms. In the clinical data entry tool, various terms explicitly negate clinical concepts, and the negating terms are related to concepts in a contextually appropriate manner that is consistent with the clinical vernacular. For example, in the documentation of the symptoms review, symptoms reported by the patient are typically negated by the modifier "denied," (as in "shortness of breath denied"). In the documentation of physical findings, however, phenomena the physician directly observes are typically negated by the modifiers "no," "none," or "absent" (as in "no rebound tenderness").

Reconciling Reference and Interface Terminologies

Given the differences between interface terminologies and reference terminologies, how can organizations combine the benefits of both in an EMR that effectively captures clinical data and supports data analysis? Options include:

- **Using a reference terminology for capturing clinical data.** Although this approach enables immediate data analysis, it also impedes data entry. Many reference terminologies are excessively precoordinated, lack modifier-based grouping capabilities, force users to navigate deep hierarchies to enter clinical observations, and include only definitional modifiers.
- **Using an interface terminology for analyzing clinical data.** Although this approach promotes complete and convenient data entry, it impedes effective aggregation and analysis. Interface terminologies lack useful aggregating concepts in their shallow hierarchies, include redundant representations of clinical concepts, and provide minimal semantics for making inferences from collected data.
- **Mapping the interface terminology to the reference terminology.** This approach uses an interface terminology to capture clinical data and transform and normalize it so it conforms to the requirements of a reference terminology. This hybrid strategy promotes complete and convenient data entry and supports effective aggregation and analysis of captured data.

The last option merits expansion. Data normalization and transformation involve several steps, as follow.

- **Normalizing redundancies.** When the interface terminology includes several ways of entering the same information, the data must be transformed so that only one structure can represent each type of observation. For example, the data entry tool shown in Figures 9.6 and 9.7 offers two ways to enter family history information: specifying the family member as the primary observation and the disorder as the modifier(s), or vice-versa.

TABLE 9.1. Data normalization in a single structure

	Primary Observation	Modifier(s)
Interface Terminology	Breast Ca	Relative = Mother, Sister
	Father	Disorder = COPD
Reference Terminology	Mother	Disorder = Breast Ca
	Sister	Disorder = Breast Ca
	Father	Disorder = COPD

However, this flexibility violates the non-redundancy requirement for reference terminologies.

To consistently represent family history information, data must be normalized to a single structure, in this case one in which the family member is always the primary observation and the disorder is the modifier. This normalization step, illustrated in Table 9.1, depends on simple data-transformation rules invoked when exporting data from the production database into a reporting database or data warehouse.

• **Distributing modifier-based groupings.** Although clinicians may find it convenient to group multiple observations by a common modifier, such as an anatomical location ("neck") or a method of examination ("auscultation"), the resulting data are structured inversely to the model of most reference terminologies. Reference terminologies define primary clinical concepts like "swelling" or "bruit" and associate modifiers like location, severity, and duration with these concepts. To map data captured with the interface terminology to a reference terminology, the modifier-based groupings must be distributed across the observations. This normalization step (illustrated in Table 9.2) also uses simple data-transformation rules.

• **Precoordinating composed terms.** Most reference terminologies have limited ability to represent complex clinical observations as constellations of linked features, such as a primary observation and a set of related modifier-value pairs. Reference terminologies more often represent complex concepts as single precoordinated entities, while interface terminologies must allow clinical observers to construct more complex observations. As shown in Table 9.3, a transformation must occur to map primary observations and their modifier-value pairs to the appropriate precoordinated concepts in the reference terminology.

TABLE 9.2. Data normalization through modifier-based groupings

	Modifier-Based Grouping	Primary Observation
Interface Terminology	Neck	Tenderness, swelling, bruit
	Primary Observation	Modifier
Reference Terminology	Tenderness	Location = Neck
	Swelling	Location = Neck
	Bruit	Location = Neck

TABLE 9.3. Precoordinating composed terms

	Primary Observation	Modifier(s)
Interface Terminology	Diabetes mellitus	Type = 2 Complications = Absent
Reference Terminology	Type 2 diabetes mellitus without complications	

Looking Ahead

As increasing numbers of healthcare organizations express interest in developing and implementing EMRs, they must educate themselves about the features that will satisfy their complex needs. To manage data effectively, advanced EMRs must support both structured data entry and automated data analysis. Because different features of controlled medical terminologies are suited to each of these tasks, no single terminology can meet all the needs of an EMR. Based on experience with a structured data entry tool, we believe successful EMRs will require separate terminologies for data entry and analysis. By using a flexible interface terminology to transform collected data into data that reflects the rigorous features of a reference terminology, we can reconcile the distinctions between reference and interface terminologies.

References

Cimino JJ. 1998. Desiderata for Controlled Medical Vocabularies in the Twenty-First Century. Meth Inf in Med 37:394–403.

Cimino JJ. 2000. From Data to Knowledge Through Concept-Oriented Terminologies: Experience with the Medical Entities Dictionary. Journal of the American Medical Informatics Association 7(3):288–97.

College of American Pathologists. 2000. SNOMED®-RT (Systematized Nomenclature of Medicine Reference Terminology). Northfield, IL: College of American Pathologists. Available at http://www.snomed.org

11th Annual HIMSS Leadership Survey. 2000. Sponsored by IBM. Available at http://www.himss.org

Kirby J, Rector AL. 1996. The PEN&PAD Data Entry System: From Prototype to Practical System. Proceedings of the 1996 AMIA Fall Symposium. Philadelphia: Hanley & Belfus. 709–713.

Solomon WD, Roberts A, Rogers JE, Wroe CJ, Rector AL. 2000. Having Our Cake and Eating It Too: How the GALEN Intermediate Representation Reconciles Internal Complexity with Users' Requirements for Appropriateness and Simplicity. Proceedings of the 2000 AMIA Fall Symposium. American Medical Informatics Association. 819–823.

Spackman KA, Campbell KE, Cote RA. 1997. SNOMED RT: A Reference Terminology for Health Care. Proceedings of the 1997 AMIA Fall Symposium. Philadelphia: Hanley & Belfus. 640–644.

Sujansky W. 1998a. A Document-Centric Electronic Medical Record System with Database-Centric Reporting Capabilities. Toward An Electronic Patient Record. Proceedings Manual. San Antonio, TX.

Sujansky WV. 1998b. The Benefits and Challenges of an Electronic Medical Record: Much More than a "Word-Processed" Patient Chart. Western Journal of Medicine 169:176–183.

10
Information Standards Within the National Cancer Institute

FRANCIS W. HARTEL and SHERRI DE CORONADO

As a federal research institution, the National Cancer Institute (NCI) both funds a large portfolio of external research and conducts scientific research in its own laboratories. It creates, maintains, and analyzes data related to funding grants and contracts; manages a large science portfolio; conducts and shares research; and manages its internal operations. The science supported both internally and externally ranges from the most basic research to large-scale clinical trials conducted by national cooperative clinical trials groups. Now more than ever, with "business to business" interoperation and data sharing among the members of the cancer community, NCI must meet the challenge of managing millions of data points.

Data sharing and process integration are cornerstones of clinical trials processes and critical to other diverse fields, such as genetics, molecular biology, and development of human cancer models. The data systems at NCI grew over time; each was designed to meet a specific need or serve a segment of the overall organization. Because aggregation of information from these systems was not a priority, both the vocabulary they used for keywords and coding and the communications and data standards they supported were sub-optimal. Only in recent years has the lack of Institute-wide data standards and vocabularies come to be recognized as a strategic problem.

In fiscal year 1999, the NCI Deputy Director for Extramural Research established what would come to be called the Institute Information Systems Advisory Group (IISAG). Recognizing that inconsistent terminology and usage caused serious information search and sharing problems, the IISAG studied how to standardize coding across the Institute. In the resulting report (Gray & Spaholtz, 2000), the IISAG recommended that the NCI establish a central repository for NCI vocabulary, centralize coding activities, develop software to support consistent use of vocabulary to store and retrieve data in NCI systems, and establish an Institute-wide oversight group for guidance. The NCI Executive Committee adopted the recommendations and has authorized an implementation group that will begin work in FY 2002.

Written from the perspective of vocabulary service developers, this chapter further examines the role of information standards at NCI. It describes the NCI's current use of vocabulary, the governance structure needed to address challenges, and the technology infrastructure that NCI has built to date to support vocabulary services. Included are synopses of major near-term and longer- term initiatives and a brief discussion of the importance of intellectual property issues.

Terms Versus Concepts: A Vital Distinction

Throughout this chapter we refer to concepts and terms. These are related but not synonymous. It is vital the distinction be kept clearly in mind. We use the word "term" to mean a lexical unit, such as an acronym, word, or phrase. We use "concept" to refer to semantic units, that is, the meaning of a term. An example makes the distinction clear. The term "mole" is ambiguous. It can refer to at least three different concepts: a small mammal, a unit of measure, or a skin nevus.

Much of our work has centered on enabling NCI staff to work with terms in automated systems without running afoul of this sort of semantic ambiguity. The vocabulary systems that we build are concept based, because concepts possess attributes like semantic type, which we can use to make their meaning clear.

The Need for Vocabulary Standards

At the NCI, the broad range of research and supporting activities creates many different settings for data creation, maintenance, sharing, and analysis, and therefore many different needs for vocabulary. Since the NCI is first and foremost a research institution, it generates and uses vast quantities of data from basic research laboratories, clinical trials, and epidemiologic studies. Given that NCI supports a large research portfolio, it has an obvious need for information to analyze the science portfolio, from basic research through clinical standard practice. Such information is used to identify gaps and opportunities for new research or initiatives and for planning, goal setting, and evaluation. These activities can occur only through synthesis of information sources across the Institute, which has been laborious and time-consuming in the past.

Another major use for data and information at NCI is reporting, which ranges from budget to clinical trials summary data. A few examples are:

- Reporting expenditures and describing progress in areas of high interest to Congress
- Developing ad hoc summaries of research funded in disease areas like breast or prostate cancer, or science areas like potential antiangiogenesis treatments

- Summarizing gender and minority accruals to clinical trials
- Reporting to the Food and Drug Administration (FDA) adverse events that occur during clinical trials
- Answering Freedom of Information Requests about specific grants or contracts
- Disseminating cancer incidence and mortality statistics.

The sources of information for reporting are generally databases: for example, grant databases, clinical trial databases, databases that collect incidence and mortality data from cancer registries, and science databases on such topics as genetics. Most of the data in them are "coded" with vocabulary terms to enable retrieval for reporting.

The NCI also uses data and information for its publications, many of which appear on the Web. A broad range of information is contained in these sources, for instance:

- Clinical trials information includes eligibility criteria, protocols, treatment statements, and other related documents
- The NCI Web site contains a variety of information about research programs, funding opportunities, cancer trials, and other resources for scientists and the public
- Annual research and budget documents are frequently accessed by the public.

Much of the data for publication originate from the same databases described previously, plus several others. Information made available through the Internet is ripe for "coding"* or indexing to facilitate retrieval, and NCI staff recognize the potential value in providing links to definitions of the cancer concepts in these documents, as well as broader and more specific terms users may not understand.

Several issues emerge from this need to create, use, synthesize, and share information—issues that drive the need for a shared vocabulary:

- **Consistency and completeness.** For financial reporting, as well as for other published data and statistics accessible by the public or scientists, consistency and completeness of retrievals is paramount.
- **Data sharing.** Science does not operate within well-defined boundaries; it is multi-disciplinary and advances through the sharing and synthesis of multiple sources of data. For example, data from genetic, pathology, and clinical trials databases need to be combined and shared to clarify the molecular basis of cancer.
- **Storing and communicating information.** Where and how to store information that will be used for analysis is also an issue. Should users create data in their own databases using a common vocabulary, should they

*Assigning alphanumeric strings to a data base record to facilitate retrieval.

enter their data into large shared repositories, or should they do post-facto mapping of their data to the standards of a "group" database?

Nearly every time a database is developed at NCI, the developer needs to adopt or create a "coding" system that will represent the content of the database and facilitate retrieval and analysis. The database owner would need to "interpret" the results of a search and retrieval report for a data consumer. Over the years, databases have adopted their own idiosyncratic ways of representing content; however, as the need to share and synthesize data across databases has grown exponentially, it has become clear that a shared (standard) vocabulary is needed. The science is driving the need for vocabulary standards that will ensure consistency and completeness of retrieval and enable data from multiple retrievals to be combined in a meaningful way.

Vocabulary Challenges at NCI

The challenges facing NCI with respect to controlled vocabulary and related standards reflect the diverse nature of the Institute's activities. Because of its clinical trial activities, NCI has many of the vocabulary and data interchange requirements familiar to hospitals and clinicians. NCI is engaged in basic biological research and applied biological and biomedical research, and these activities generate extensive vocabulary and data interchange requirements. Administrative activities, too, have their own distinct vocabulary and data interchange requirements.

Even within the context of clinical trials however, significant differences exist between the NCI environment and that of typical clinical medicine. For example, reimbursement—a major focus of reporting and data interchange in the typical hospital setting—has been of small consequence for NCI. On the other hand, regulatory reporting and correlation of detailed, voluminous data from multiple institutions looms large in NCI clinical trials. Commercially available medical information systems meet some but not all NCI clinical needs, and no single standard vocabulary or set of vocabularies is adequate.

Biology and biomedicine present the greatest vocabulary challenges. These areas generate a high volume of new knowledge, and the coverage of research concepts in standard vocabularies is relatively shallow. Mechanisms are needed to rapidly model new concepts in controlled vocabulary as they surface in sources like Entrez (http://www.ncbi.nlm.nih.gov/entrez/) and to provide the vocabulary to NCI for operational use.

To meet its administrative needs, NCI has developed a highly specialized vocabulary. The administrative vocabulary is used principally for Congressional and management reporting, as well as financial accounting and oversight of grants and contracts. NCI administrative activities require a tightly controlled vocabulary, so that reports and analyses are consistent and comprehensive.

These three vocabulary areas—clinical, biological, and administrative—are interdependent. As new concepts enter the research vocabulary, they quickly begin to be used in the NCI clinical trials and grants administration applications. This requires that the vertical and the horizontal relationships among NCI concepts are simultaneously valid in the ontological sense and navigable by members of many disciplines.

The Problem of Hierarchy

Ideally, in formal hierarchies, vertical relationships are "is_a relationships," in which everything true of the "parent" is true of the "child." In practice organizing principles such as "part_of" are needed, for example, in anatomy hierarchies. The organizing principle, notwithstanding, when vocabulary is used for keywords or retrieval codes in a database, the hierarchical relationship of the concepts must be valid.

For instance, queries against NCI enterprise databases will depend on vocabulary servers for query "explosion" and aggregation. When a query is exploded, the database user specifies a search term. The database passes it to the vocabulary system. The vocabulary system identifies the retrieval concept referred to by the search term, and then walks the vocabulary tree downward, starting with the specified concept, and returns all the "children," or results, to the user's database. The user's database system then constructs a query consisting of the original concept and all its children. Conversely, in an aggregation, the user starts with a concept, is shown all its parents, and selects among the broader concepts for one at the desired level of generality. If NCI enterprise systems are to generate search results that are consistent and comprehensive, NCI concept trees must correctly embody the parent-child relationships as the communities within NCI have defined them.

The Problem of Semantic Relationships

Horizontal relationships among concepts specify how a concept is semantically related to another. Given the need for navigability by a diverse population of users, the NCI vocabulary systems use semantic relationships among concepts to provide links between the clinical, research, and administrative areas. For example, the administrative vocabulary possesses a number of reporting categories that are generally broad and may have no valid clinical or scientific meaning. However, they do have important social, political, or other meaning, and are related in some sense to sets of scientific or clinical concepts. "Head and neck" may not be a meaningful anatomical term, but it is recognizable as a token for a set of anatomical sites where specific oncology diseases occur. In this case, no valid "is_a" relationship may exist, but valid semantic relationships of some sort most likely do. By modeling the semantic relationship explicitly (Campbell, 1997), the NCI vocabulary system can help the clinician understand if a specific disease site is considered "head and neck" for reporting purposes. There is danger that the burden of modeling and maintaining such semantic relationships will become overwhelming. For this reason, modeling must be limited to relationships of clear value to NCI operations.

The Problem of Representing Molecular Biology and Medicine

Arguably the greatest challenge facing NCI's vocabulary and standards work is dealing with the explosion of molecular biology and its accelerating impact on cancer medicine. Cytogenetic notation has begun to appear in standard vocabularies like ICD-Oncology(O)-3 (Harris et al., 1999), as prognostic indicators and as diagnostic criteria. A standard way of representing this and other molecular biology information in the context of controlled medical vocabulary must be developed. NCI may be forced to address this issue for cancer-related vocabulary sooner than others (Klausner, 1999).

More and more novel therapeutic interventions are being developed, like ONYX-015, a genetically engineered adenovirus that, in preclinical and clinical studies, has been shown to replicate in and kill tumor cells deficient in p53 tumor suppressor gene activity (Makower et al., 2000). As the mechanisms of action for these new interventions are understood, and as they are proven useful and enter the clinic, NCI will have to develop principles governing how to place them in a hierarchy (or "tree" them) and semantically relate them. A major goal of these principles will be to avoid continuously reworking the fundamental vocabulary model as scientific and clinical details emerge.

Collaborations with the Cancer Community

NCI currently has a large number of home-grown vocabularies in use; however, standard vocabularies are used in several areas of the Institute, most notably in the clinical area. In these areas, NCI participates in vocabulary development with the cancer community.

The Surveillance, Epidemiology and End-Results Program (SEER), for example, uses the ICD-O-2 vocabulary for collecting and coding data on incidence and survival from cancer data registries around the country and is now converting to the newer ICD-O-3 vocabulary (http://www-seer.ims.nci.nih.gov/). The ICD-O-2 was developed by the World Health Organization with substantial NCI participation. NCI also participated in the development of the ICD-O-3 that was released by the WHO in early 2001.

Other areas of NCI that have not previously used the ICD-O are beginning to use the new version, because it is the first vocabulary to include relevant cytopathology information as part of the disease classification.

The Cancer Therapy and Evaluation Program (CTEP), which manages a large portfolio of funded clinical trials, is required to report adverse event information to the FDA. The vocabulary used to code these adverse events is the Medical Dictionary for Regulatory Activities (MedDRA) vocabulary, formerly International Medical Terminology (IMT). The researchers responsible for these clinical trials report the adverse events to the NCI using this vocabulary, and NCI transmits the data to FDA. MedDRA is another internationally developed vocabulary in which NCI participated, contributing heavily to the Neoplasms, Benign and Malignant System Organ Class (SOC), a major part of MedDRA (http://www.msso.org/default2.htm).

The Physician Data Query System (PDQ), a part of the NCI Office of Cancer Communications (formerly the International Cancer Information Center), incorporates a vocabulary used extensively in the cancer community and by the public to retrieve information from that system. Although not a nationally or internationally developed vocabulary, it has been submitted to the Unified Medical Language System (UMLS) for several years, and is therefore made available to the community to use as it wishes. The vocabulary is currently undergoing extensive revision and review, and the new version will be used by the PDQ database and other CancerNet databases and submitted to the UMLS in the future. The PDQ staff currently also provides a glossary of lay cancer terms for use with PDQ and NCI Web documents (http://cancernet.nci.nih.gov/pdq.html).

Development of Basic Science Vocabulary

Although the clinical side of the Institute has a history of working with the community in developing and using standard vocabularies, basic cancer researchers and science managers have only recently begun to interact with the cancer and biomedical communities in vocabulary development and use. In the past, the basic science vocabularies used by NCI have been mostly small and home-grown, sufficient for program managers to answer individual questions about the relatively small portfolios they manage, and for a central indexing organization to produce information for NCI budget reports. Although this satisfied the need to answer questions like "How much did the Institute spend in a particular disease area or special interest area in a particular year?," it did not help answer questions about the science itself or facilitate collaboration with other agencies or interdisciplinary research programs.

The need to answer science questions across multiple data sources requires standard vocabularies that are detailed enough to describe the science precisely, especially since the distinction has blurred between information about the science and the science data itself. Consequently, the Institute has engaged in several basic science vocabulary related activities that address both the science and the science information aspects.

One such activity is NCI's ongoing effort to "model" the vocabulary for cancer-related genes and proteins and provide that information to the UMLS as it becomes available. This will benefit the entire biomedical community and spur further development. Another activity, the Mouse Models of Human Cancer Consortium (MMHCC), is beginning to build a vocabulary that will help clarify the differences and similarities among mouse and human cancers so that better models can be built. A completely different type of activity is the NCI's Common Scientific Outline of cancer research, developed jointly with the Defense Department to enable exchange of information about the NCI and Defense Department cancer research portfolios.

An NCI database that contains spectral karyotyping and comparative genomic hybridation data for the high-profile Cancer Chromosome Aberration Project is being designed for international use. The scientists and database designers, working with an external group of scientists who will also contribute data to the database, have decided to use the ICD-O-3 as the standard for assigning topography (site) and morphology (e.g., cell type) coding to their sample data. This will be one of the enablers for combining data from many different research projects. By providing access to the NCI Enterprise Vocabulary System (discussed later) to potential users and contributors of the data, those who choose to use a different standard vocabulary like SNOMED International in their own systems can map to the ICD-O-3 vocabulary for placing data in the "shared" database.

A relatively new effort to create and maintain standard vocabularies for NCI clinical trials is discussed in Chapter 11. Called the Common Data Elements (CDE) project, it heavily involves the cancer community in developing vocabulary relevant to particular clinical forms, like case reports, along with values for these data elements in the context of the appropriate form. Other CDE projects are expanding the scope of the vocabulary under development to pathology, radiology, epidemiology, and other information relevant to the clinical trials.

Increased Recognition of the Need for Vocabulary Standards

Over the past year, a wide variety of players at NCI—scientists, administrators, planners, systems developers, program managers—have recognized that vocabulary standards are crucial to the continuing progress of cancer research. It is a strategic issue, because it provides the only way to share data meaningfully, and it will be vital to linking the basic and clinical research that will lead to new treatments.

Willingness to participate and engage in discussions and planning has increased markedly. Top NCI leadership has recognized the need for an Institute-wide vocabulary review board. We believe there ought to be an advisory component staffed with leading experts from outside NCI to provide external input into NCI vocabulary activities. Further, many NCI components have realized that it is easy to create a vocabulary but difficult to maintain it. Thus, a major implication of the recognized needs will be additional use of standard vocabularies that are maintained by the scientific and medical communities.

Emerging Trends

Several trends within and outside of NCI have underscored the importance of vocabulary development and standards. These trends provide a focus to NCI's initiatives.

Migration from Isolated Systems to Integration

Several years ago, the NCI director and other senior managers envisioned a system that would answer questions about the science NCI supports, clarify the gaps and opportunities in the portfolio, and synthesize information from many different systems that historically have been isolated. This vision has driven NCI to move towards integration. As the size of the NCI program, the pace of discovery, and operational requirements for greater integration all increased, NCI undertook major investments to create enterprise systems that shared a data model and adhered to defined standards. These systems aimed to help NCI develop integrated applications supporting all critical internal activities and share data with business partners in government and the research sector. Many applications that access this database are integrated in an internal NCI Web site called the NOW (NCI Online Workplace).

The availability of enterprise systems means that given a robust vocabulary and business rules about how to do "coding," the NCI now has the means to store the various sets of coding that exist for a given grant or contract. Coding from various programs can be combined in a single database to enable single queries about a topic across the portfolio using a common language. This moves the Institute considerably closer to its vision.

An exemplar of this integration model is The Science Place, a knowledge management application that may be used to support the work of the Mouse Models of Human Cancer Consortium or other specific NCI activities. This application provides a place for scientists, analysts, and managers to retrieve information from many sources, organize that information according to their own preferences, and share information about topics in which they are experts. The Science Place depends on the rich synonymy provided by the

NCI Enterprise Vocabulary System, which enables search, retrieval, and organization of information from bibliographic databases, genetics databases, the Internet, its internal database, and NCI science data warehouse. (The Science Place is a NCI version of the now commercially available software, The Research Place, from LGA, Inc.)

The Coming of Governance

Although NCI systems like The Science Place can retrieve comparable information in several databases even if the information is coded with different keywords, it is better to avoid inconsistent vocabulary to begin with. Avoiding them is a major goal of governance. Governance is the best way to sidestep the "Tower of Babel" effect in databases.

Recently, the Long Range Planning Committee (LRPC) advised the NCI that establishing new processes to speed development, approval, conduct, and reporting of clinical trials would require considerable investment in governance (Chapter 1). Because of NCI's central role in funding and conducting cancer-related research and in translating findings into cancer care, decisions the NCI makes about vocabulary, messaging, and metadata standards affect the operations of others. For this reason that we advocate that NCI establish an external advisory group. We feel the NCI's governance procedures must reflect the needs of both its business partners and the whole cancer community.

The Long Range Planning Committee recommended that NCI establish a standing advisory group composed of leaders from across the cancer community and various standards development organizations. The group would provide strategic advice to NCI regarding vocabulary and health-related standards and critique NCI's decisions and activities in these areas. The committee also recommended that NCI become the focal point for representing the cancer community in the standards development organizations.

Laying the Groundwork: NCI EVS

Well before consensus was reached that vocabulary standards and governance were needed, NCI began to lay the infrastructure to support them. The NCI Enterprise Vocabulary System, or NCI EVS, provides a variety of vocabulary-related services to NCI. Among them is the NCI Metathesaurus, which is a core infrastructure component. Created to neutralize the Tower of Babel effect that had grown among legacy NCI systems, the NCI Metathesaurus is a technology-based stopgap that has enabled NCI, for the first time, to:

- Identify gaps and inconsistencies among the informal terminologies being used by the Institute

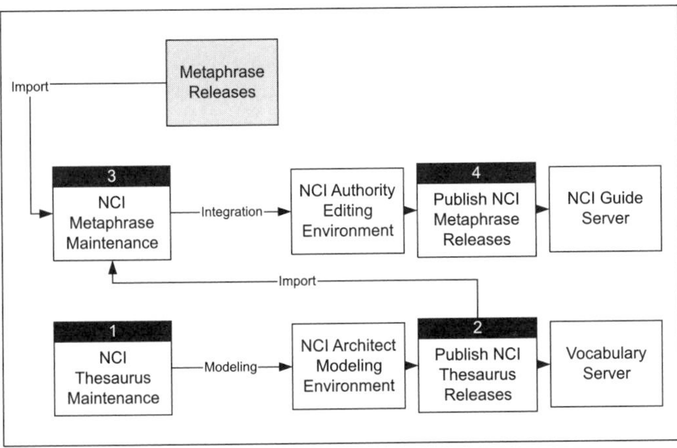

FIGURE **10.1.** Overview of NCI EVS processess and components.

- Provide a central point for maintenance of these terminologies
- Provide a single resource from which all NCI systems could obtain vocabulary
- Place the NCI terminology into trees and map it to standard vocabularies.

The NCI EVS infrastructure consists of technology and human resources. The technology includes server hardware, database, editing and management software, and applications programming interface software. The human resources include operations staff to care for the servers, vocabulary databases and software, curators who edit and maintain the content of the vocabulary databases and applications support staff who interface the NCI EVS to other NCI systems. Figure 10.1 provides an overview of NCI EVS processes and components.

Licensed Software

NCI has attempted to construct the NCI EVS from commercial products that appear to be emerging de facto or formal standards. The Apelon Incorporated TDE™, (Technology Development Environment) Authority™, Concept-based Retrieval™ System, and Metaphrase™ products are being used operationally, and the Mayo Vocabulary System, the FDA's Autocoder and Apelon DTS Metaphrase™ (Distributed Terminology System) products are being actively evaluated. These products are attractive to NCI because, except for Autocoder, they support "open" Java Application Program Interfaces (APIs). In the case of the TDE™ and Mayo products, they are also compatible with the description logic vocabulary representation (Campbell, 1997) that is becoming widely used in private sector entities like the College of American Pathologists (Hochhalter, 2000; College of American Pathologists, 2000a) and in government initiatives like the

Government Computerized Patient Record consortia, the National Library of Medicine government-wide SNOMED-RT acquisition, and National Health Service of the United Kingdom (College of American Pathology, 2000b).

Vocabulary Services to NCI

Two distinct vocabulary service offerings are needed to meet NCI's needs. The NCI Thesaurus is a description logic-based vocabulary that contains only NCI terminology. The NCI Metathesaurus contains many of the sources contained in the UMLS Metathesaurus, plus the NCI vocabulary. Tailored to the needs of NCI database systems, the NCI Thesaurus ensures formally correct concept modeling, which in turn provides reliable navigation among NCI concepts and correct explosion and aggregation of search terms. These properties are vital to consistent and comprehensive retrieval from NCI databases. The NCI Metathesaurus provides rich synonymy, English language definitions, and mappings between NCI terminology and sources like SNOMED, ICD, and MeSH, which are used within NCI or by NCI business partners. The NCI Metathesaurus is especially useful to NCI Web masters for indexing documents and helping users navigate to the biomedical concepts in which they are interested.

EVS Editing, Review, and Change Management

In fiscal year 1999, NCI decided to employ contractors to edit the NCI EVS content. Review would be provided by NCI staff and by outside reviewers. NCI EVS editors use the Authority™ and TDE™ editing environments for content creation, and new releases of the NCI Thesaurus and NCI Metathesaurus are periodically produced and made available for testing. These activities are governed by a configuration management and change management plan. Change requests and dispositions and configuration control activities are tracked and analyzed. These practices bring the NCI EVS close to compliance with the ASTM E2087 Standard Specification of Quality Indicators for Controlled Health Vocabularies. Plans to achieve full compliance with this standard and a variety of others are discussed elsewhere in this chapter.

Vocabulary Update Processes

The NCI Thesaurus is continually updated. Each month, new NCI Thesaurus releases are issued for use by NCI databases and other systems and imported into the NCI Metathesaurus using the Authority™ tool. These minor monthly releases of the NCI Metathesaurus ensure that the rapid evolution of biomedical terminology, especially in the areas of cancer genetics, cellular and molecular biology, and other fast-moving research areas, is available to NCI Metathesaurus users. Once a year, the NCI issues a major release of the NCI Metathesaurus, which keeps the NCI Metathesaurus current with new releases of the National Library of Medicine's UMLS Metathesaurus.

Because NCI concepts "inherit" synonyms and other relationships from Metathesaurus sources, "false" synonymy, definitions, and other relationships to NCI concepts occasionally crop up. NCI editors use the Authority™ tool to delete many of these, but some cannot be eliminated without editing non-NCI sources. Remaining false relationships are the unavoidable price paid for the rich synonymy and other benefits of embedding the NCI Thesaurus in the Metathesaurus-like environment of the Metaphrase Metathesaurus.™ Because of this relative lack of control, most configuration management and quality review effort is directed at the NCI Thesaurus, not the NCI Metathesaurus.

Near-Term Initiatives

To realize the benefits of internal information sharing and business to business operations that an investment in infrastructure can provide, the NCI must implement the governance structure alluded to earlier. In 2002, much of the governance structure envisioned by the Long Range Planning Committee and the IISAG Coding Report should be in place.

External Experts and Internal Stakeholders

The NCI's vocabulary initiatives must deliver appropriate products and well-managed services to clients within the NCI and, where appropriate, to those in the broader cancer community. As recommended by the LRPC, an external advisory group will be needed; as recommended by the IISAG Coding Committee Report, an internal oversight group will be needed. We advocate that these groups be called the NCI Vocabulary and Standards Advisory Committee and the NCI Vocabulary Executive Group. Their combined goals ought to be to:

- Guide the NCI's efforts in vocabulary use and development
- Set expectations for how vocabulary will be used within the NCI and how the vocabulary resources can assist the cancer community
- Oversee the provision of quality vocabulary services to the NCI and to the cancer community
- Maximize the coherence and interoperability between NCI's vocabulary efforts and those taking place outside the Institute.

Figure 10.2 shows how we envision the relationship of these two groups to each other and to the components that have operational responsibility for vocabulary service and implementation of information-related standards.

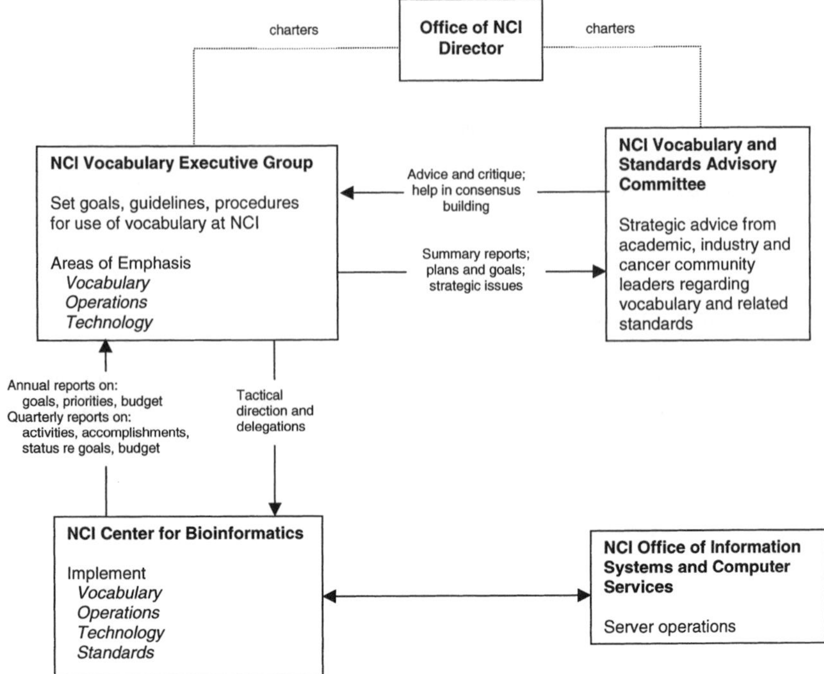

FIGURE 10.2. Governance diagram.

External Advice and Communication

The NCI Vocabulary and Standards Advisory Committee could be created under the aegis of the NCI director's Advisory Group. The individual roles of the NCI Vocabulary and Standards Advisory Committee should be to:

- Maintain a high level of awareness regarding the directions of vocabulary-related products, services, and standards in external communities of interest to the NCI
- Convey this information to the NCI Vocabulary Executive Group for further dissemination within the NCI
- Maintain awareness of NCI initiatives and needs regarding vocabularies and related standards and ensure that they are clearly presented to relevant parties outside the NCI
- Provide advice to the NCI director
- Serve as liaison to the cancer community, the standards-setting community, and the publishers of vocabularies, ensuring an effective bi-directional flow of information, concerns, and plans.

Members of this advisory committee should be prominent and influential within the communities in which they are active. They should be chosen to represent relevant standards development organizations, cancer researchers and clinicians, advocacy groups, industry, and other influential stakeholders in the cancer community. Advisory committee meetings should take place two or three times per year.

Internal Oversight and Direction

The responsibilities of the NCI Vocabulary Executive Group should consist of an overall mission and three more specialized roles. Overall, the group should:

- Ensure that NCI's vocabulary efforts maintain maximum coherence with the direction of industry technology, methods, content, and standards
- Ensure that software and vocabularies acquired and developed by NCI will have lasting value by maximizing interoperability with those outside the Institute
- Ensure that NCI develops clear and persuasive presentations of its needs for vocabularies and related products, services, and standards
- Convey these needs through participation in external activities and through the efforts of the NCI Vocabulary and Standards Advisory Committee.

The three more specialized roles concern vocabulary, operational issues, and technology-oriented factors. For vocabulary, the executive group's responsibilities should be to set goals, guidelines, and procedures for the use of vocabulary at NCI, select commercial vocabularies for integration with the NCI EVS, and oversee editing of the NCI vocabulary. Responsibilities for operational issues include monitoring delivery of vocabulary-related services, acting as advocate for NCI organizations where service falls short of needs, and serving as the NCI EVS Configuration Control Board. Finally, for technology-oriented factors, the group should act as a liaison with publishers of vocabularies and represent the NCI on selected standards groups.

The NCI director or deputy director should charter this executive group, the membership of which should be NCI staff members. Senior staff representing the entire NCI organization at the division level should be included, and other NCI staff will be nominated as appropriate to supply specialized knowledge or to meet specific responsibilities. The group should meet quarterly.

In connection with vocabulary services and information standards related to medical or biological requirements, NCI's Center for Bioinformatics should have a range of responsibilities:

- Assessment and selection of commercial technology and methods for vocabulary services
- Development and testing of new technology for vocabulary services
- Advice and assistance in using vocabulary resources

- Vocabulary editing and other operational responsibilities
- Operation and maintenance of vocabulary-related software
- Representation of the NCI on IT-related standards groups.
- Operation of servers for vocabulary and software.

Standards Relevant to Cancer

We envision the NCI becoming the focal point of the cancer community with respect to information standards and vocabulary. Within this vision, more fully described in the Long Range Plan, the NCI Vocabulary and Standards Advisory Committee would serve as an ongoing forum for dialog between the standards development community and the cancer community. Determining which standards are relevant to cancer would be one result of this dialogue. Table 10.1 contains a summary of several standards with clear relevance. Others will emerge in time.

NCI has been an informal—or, in several cases, formal—participant in some Standards Development Organization (SDO) activities, and it should become a formal participant in all SDO activities judged relevant to its information needs. Through the Vocabulary and Standards Advisory Committee and other outreach activities, NCI representatives should become aware of the needs and opinions of the broader cancer community. They should represent NCI and the larger community to the SDO and inform the NCI and the community of important plans and decisions.

Table 10.1. Standard development activities with clear relevance to NCI and the cancer community

Standard Development Organization	Relevant Standard	Status of NCI Participation	Relevance to Cancer Community/NCI
W3C	XML,DOM		Sharable biomedical document design, creation, use
ISO JTC 1/SC32	ISO/IEC 11179		Sharable database contents
ISO TC 37	ISO 1087:1990		Priniciples and coordination of terminology
ANSI HISB USHIK	ANSI X3.285	Member	Information needed to interpret, use shared data
HL7	MDF, RIM, PRA		Information exchange techniques, interpretation of shared data
ISO TC 215	ASTM E2087		Vocabulary quality
ANSI X 12	ASC X12N		Reimbursement
G-CPR		Ongoing liaison	Secure patient-focused information technology architecture

During 2001, the NCI will likely commence formal membership in each of the SDO activities listed in Table 10.1. The Center for Bioinformatics is developing a Web site devoted to standards and vocabulary, which will be used to foster communication among the NCI representatives to the SDO and between the cancer community and the NCI representatives. The NCI representatives to SDO activities will largely be drawn from the NCI Center for Bioinformatics, since these activities principally involve information technology.

Table 10.2 lists vocabulary products known to be relevant to NCI. During 2001, as with SDO participation, NCI should seek formal representation on editorial boards or similar entities for each of these vocabularies. Because the focus will be on issues of biomedical terminology, most NCI liaisons to these vocabulary developers should be members of the NCI Vocabulary Executive Group.

Each vocabulary in Table 10.2, except SNOMED, is needed for NCI operations. SNOMED is included because of ongoing efforts by a consortium of federal agencies to license SNOMED-RT for use across the federal government. In anticipation of this license, the NCI is investigating formal collaborative arrangements to facilitate rapid migration of new cancer-related concepts, especially cytogenetic and molecular concepts, from NCI Thesaurus to SNOMED-RT. The technical infrastructure to do this is largely in place, because the NCI Thesaurus is being developed using tools

Table 10.2. Controlled vocabularies with clear relevance to NCI and the cancer community

Publisher	Vocabulary Product	Status of NCI Participation	Impact on Cancer Community/NCI
World Health Organization	MedDRA	Subscriber	WHO data set required for adverse event reporting
World Health Organization	ICD-0-3	Coauthor	WHO data set required for cancer incidence reporting, epidemiology
Department of Health and Human Services	ICD-9-CM	Subscriber	HIPAA required data set
Department of Health and Human Services	HCPCS	Subscriber	HIPAA required data set
College of American Pathologists	SNOMED, SNOMED-RT	Subscriber	Commonly used medical records data set
American Mediacal Association	CPT-4		HIPAA required data set
NCI	NCI Thesarus	Publisher	Source of newest cancer-related terminology, internal NCI data set
NCI	Common Data Elements	Publisher	Data set developed for transactions related to clinical trials protocols

and description logic similar to those used by the College of American Pathologists (College of American Pathologists, 2000) in developing SNOMED-RT (http://snowmed.org).

The NCI Vocabulary Executive Group should make decisions about which standard vocabularies to license and how NCI should use them. The direction of NCI Thesaurus development and usage within NCI should also fall to the Executive Board. As mentioned previously, an extensive configuration management process has been developed. It will enable the Executive Board to develop policies and practices to ensure that all users depending on the NCI Thesaurus are made aware of changes to its content, especially changes to the concept hierarchy that could directly affect query performance of databases.

The NCI Thesaurus and NCI Metathesaurus are largely compliant with ASTM E2087 quality indicators, and work continues to make both fully compliant in 2001. Efforts to register the NCI Common Data Elements with the Health Informatics Standards Board (HISB) are ongoing, and the NCI will begin making its systems Health Level 7 (HL7)-compliant, especially any enterprise systems that must interact with clinical grantees and other clinical partners.

The NCI Vocabulary Executive Group should work with the NCI Vocabulary and Standards Advisory Committee to determine priorities for achieving standards compliance within NCI. They should also consider establishing measures for assisting business partners or other members of the cancer community to achieve compliance.

Business Case for Coding

At a minimum, NCI has two business goals for its use of controlled vocabulary and standards: operational efficiency and improved scientific productivity. Operational efficiencies between NCI and external entities—the ability both to share information and to integrate systems—will result in cost savings. For example, clinical trials management procedures using the CDE data set and business-to-business techniques promise to save both NCI and trialists money. More importantly, it will provide much better clinical management; for example, adverse event information would be rapidly disseminated to all relevant protocol directors.

Within the NCI, controlled vocabulary and information standards will enhance research productivity. It will be much easier to find and interpret information relevant to a scientific issue from the multiple systems that contain grant, contract, internal project, and other scientific information. This will benefit both the NCI researcher and NCI research management. It will also greatly reduce the burden of generating routine and ad hoc reports for Congress, the Department, oversight and advocacy organizations, and the press.

Uniform Coding and Keyword Practices

The NCI Vocabulary Executive Group should determine how the licensed and NCI-specific vocabulary is used, both for coding and key wording artifacts in data systems and as aids for search and retrieval in Web sites and other information resources. The IISAG Coding Committee's recommendation that coding and keyword assignment be done by a dedicated, centralized group of experts will be the point of departure. Whatever the Executive Group decides to do with respect to code and keyword assignment, uniformity of practice across the NCI is vital.

The criteria to determine if the NCI's code and keyword strategy is satisfactory should be empirical, and results-based vocabulary assessment should be adopted. This would depart from historical practice at NCI, where code and keyword practices were often driven by the limitations of technology, available staff, or organizational culture. If vocabulary or code/keyword decisions do not result in measurable improvement in the comprehensiveness or consistency of NCI information systems, they should be considered unsuccessful.

Coherence Across NCI Involvement with SDO Activities

Because the NCI is so large and diverse, it is not surprising that many of its components are involved with various vocabulary developers and SDO activities. The NCI Vocabulary Executive Group must ensure that the Institute presents a consistent face across these interactions. In many cases, the NCI is engaged in informal interactions with clearly important vocabulary and standards groups, and the Vocabulary Executive Group should formalize these, with NCI becoming a formal member of important development efforts. These steps are the *sine qua non* of any NCI effort to become the focal point for cancer community interaction with the SDO and vocabulary developers.

Investment in Standards as Community Resource

To become formally involved in development efforts and establish reliable means to ensure that NCI and the cancer community agree about standards and vocabulary, the NCI will have to undertake significant financial investment. More is needed if the cancer community is to benefit fully from NCI investments in standards development and compliance.

The ongoing effort to license SNOMED-RT across the government aims to cover use of the vocabulary by external entities in their interactions with government agencies. In effect, such a SNOMED-RT license would shelter these entities from the cost of licensing vocabulary so they can do business with the government. This license procurement, then, can be seen as the government "buying down" the cost of adopting a standard for business-to-business communications. The NCI may need to establish other ways of encouraging business partners to consider early adoption of standards-compliant systems or vocabulary. In the absence of such inducement, the pace of replacing old, noncompliant technology may well be too slow to meet the country's need to translate rapid cancer research advances into prevention and care improvement.

As mentioned previously, NCI is discussing a cooperative research and development agreement with the College of American Pathologists to help migrate new terminology from the NCI Thesaurus to SNOMED-RT. The Institute is also contributing portions of the NCI Thesaurus to the National Library of Medicine for inclusion in the UMLS. The NCI Director's Advisory Group and the Vocabulary Executive Group should determine other opportunities that the Institute should explore to get new cancer-related concepts and terminology into use across the full range of medical vocabulary and clinical practice.

Long-Term Goals

When the NCI governance structure is mature and its involvement in standards and vocabulary development and utilization is well established, emphasis should shift to helping the cancer community benefit from these activities. It will take several years to develop adequate communication about information exchange opportunities and requirements and the standards and vocabulary needed to support them.

NCI is working on improvements to its public Web sites like PDQ, hoping to make it easier for individual patients to find appropriate clinical trials. These improvements are possible because of improved information sharing among NCI systems, supporting both protocol development and information sites. Adoption of standards and vocabulary conventions underpin such improved services to the community. However, many in the cancer community are uninformed (or are inadequately informed) about the role of standards and controlled vocabulary in facilitating modern information sharing and utilization. The NCI must help increase understanding of these issues, and the NCI Director's Advisory Group could play an important role in identifying ways to spread the word.

Much of the progress being made today in understanding cancer, its treatment, and its prevention comes from molecular and genetic research and from moving basic science insights rapidly into clinical intervention or recommendations for prevention. The terminology used by molecular and genetic science is unfamiliar to many in the cancer community. Some of these terms will be available in the NCI Thesaurus before they are modeled in vocabularies with a more general focus, and arrangements are underway to make them available to the larger community. In the long term, however, the NCI may have to go beyond vocabulary modeling into ontology development.

The key to making clear the relevance of molecular or genetic concepts to clinical practice or to cancer prevention is through semantic relationships that link them. The description logic used in the NCI Thesaurus appears to be capable of representing a useful amount of such semantic information. Still, workable rules to use the capability while avoiding the well-known pitfalls of modeling are yet to be developed. Developing satisfactory rules for such semantic modeling is a difficult long-term challenge for NCI to address.

Looking Ahead

Shared information can enable new science through collaboration, clinical excellence, lowered costs, better programmatic analyses, and research efficiency. This vision depends on sharing vocabulary and other intellectual property that costs a great deal to create. When the government does not defray the cost of development, the producer must charge for use of the property to cover the costs of development. Commercial considerations, combined with the highly unsettled state of intellectual property law in the digital arena, may delay or derail some of the information sharing that would most benefit the community.

The cancer community needs to find a voice in the ongoing political and legal dialogue about intellectual property. Organizations wishing to merge public domain content into proprietary offerings have concerns about losing control of their intellectual property, while organizations wishing to use intellectual property are uncertain of the boundaries of fair use. Across the biomedical marketplace, the pricing of such intangible products as sequences and vocabulary is so inconsistent and confusing that it is impeding adoption of useful products and techniques.

The investment in standards and vocabulary described in this chapter will undoubtedly prove beneficial to the NCI and to the larger community, making accurate information available where it can do the most good. To reap the potential benefits, the Institute must rise to the challenge of addressing difficult technical and process issues. At the same time, it must pay special attention to legal and economic issues, which will determine the scope of the benefits cancer care can realize.

References

Campbell KE. 1997. Distributed Development of a Logic-Based Controlled Medical Terminology. Stanford: Stanford University. Dissertation Abstracts International 01 599 569.

Gray P, Spaholtz B, Chairs. 2000. Goals and Principles for Establishing an Integrated NCI-Wide Coding System. Report of the Institute Information Systems Advisory Group Subcommittee on Coding, National Cancer Institute. (Draft document available only on the NCI Intranet.)

Harris NL, Jaffe ES, Diebold J, Flandrin G, Muller-Hermelink HK, Vardiman J, Lister TA, Bloomfield CD. 1999. World Health Organization Classification of Neoplastic Diseases of the Hematopoietic and Lymphoid Tissues: Report of the Clinical Advisory Committee Meeting—Airlie House, Virginia, November 1997. Journal of Clinical Oncology 17:3835–3849.

Hochhalter B. 2000. Putting Terminology in the Business Plan: Using SNOMED-RT in Kaiser Permanente Information System. Paper presented at Towards an Electronic Patient Record (TEPR 2000). San Francisco, CA.

Klausner R. 1999. The Nation's Investment in Cancer Research, a Budget Proposal for Fiscal Year 2001. Bethesda, MD: National Cancer Institute. 52. (http://2001.cancer.gov). Accessed 07/12/01.

Makower D, Rozenblit A, Edelman M, Augenlicht L, Kaufman H, Haynes H, Zwiebel J, Wadler S. 2000. Oncolytic Viral Therapy in Hepatobiliary Tumors. Cancer Investigation 18(Suppl. 1):111–112.

Gilfillan L, Haddock G, Borek S. 2001. Knowledge Management Across Domains. SPIE, in press. (http://www.theresearchplace.com/SPIEPaper.htm)

Readings

For more information on the new commercial version of The Science Place, see http://www.TheResearchPlace.com

For more information on SNOMED, see http://www.snomed.org

11
CDE Development Model for Chest CT Screening for Lung Cancer

Curtis P. Langlotz

Background

Several years ago, the National Cancer Institute (NCI) embarked on an effort to standardize data collection methods across the cooperative trials groups it funds. These data collection methods included common toxicity criteria (CTC) and common data elements (CDEs). To date, CDEs have been developed for phase III therapeutic trials related to breast, prostate, lung, and colon cancer. Recently, the NCI funded the American College of Radiology Imaging Network (ACRIN, http://www.acrin.org), a cooperative group dedicated to imaging trials. Simultaneously, new imaging tests have shown promise in screening for lung cancer. Thus, several groups within the NCI became keenly interested in developing CDEs for imaging trials. What follows is a description of the development of CDEs for chest CT screening for lung cancer that was undertaken in the last half of 1999.

Motivations

Because there are a large number of existing medical terminological resources and standards, our first step was to determine whether others have already accomplished the same task or a related one. Terminological resources such as the Unified Medical Language System (UMLS, http://www.nlm.nih.gov/research/umls/) (National Library of Medicine, 1999) and SNOMED International (http://www.snomed.org) already provide a rich vocabulary for encoding clinical data. In many cases, these resources can be adopted directly for use in data collection for clinical trials. A number of imaging-specific classification systems are also available. For example, we considered the American College of Radiology's Index for Radiological Diagnoses (American College of Radiology, 1992), a bi-axial classification that was originally developed for the organization of teaching files according to anatomical and pathological information. We also evaluated an extensive classification system for the indexing of scientific literature developed by the

Radiological Society of North America (RSNA, 1999) and a glossary of chest imaging published by the Fleischner Society (Tuddenham, 1984).

Unfortunately, the results of our tests were in accord with the results of previous studies of existing terminological resources, which suggest that existing terminologies are lacking in many of the types of terms used in imaging. For example, while these terminologies contain a rich anatomic and pathological vocabulary, they rarely contain the descriptive visual features that radiologists use to describe findings on imaging studies or the technical terms that describe how images were acquired and viewed. One study of the UMLS, SNOMED, and the ACR Index found that they contained less than half of terms used in ultrasound reporting (Bell & Greenes, 1994). Because we found similar results in a pilot study of chest CT terms (unpublished data), we embarked on the development of a comprehensive set of common data elements for chest CT screening, while relying on the UMLS and SNOMED to guide our use of anatomic and pathological terms.

Attributes of a Common Data Element (CDE)

The goal of the CDE development process was to produce CDEs that could be made available in a Web-accessible database on the NCI's Web site (http://cii.nci.nih.gov/cde). The database contains a searchable list of terms and their definitions, following a dictionary format. In this section we provide definitions of CDE attributes used in that database, and describe the hierarchy of CDE categories that was developed for chest CT screening CDEs. The following attributes are typically specified for each CDE:

1. *Category* is a grouping or classification into which a CDE falls. For example, the Imaging CDE category is broken down into sub-categories, such as anatomic locations and imaging findings.
2. *Short CDE Term* lists a brief unique name for the CDE. For example "Exam Quality" is an imaging CDE that allows a radiologist or other imaging professional to rate the quality of the images being interpreted.
3. *Long CDE Term* indicates how a CDE might be listed on a data collection form. For example, "The overall diagnostic quality of the imaging study" is the Long CDE Term for the "Exam Quality" CDE.
4. *CDE Values* itemize the list of possible values that a CDE can take on. For example, the Exam Quality CDE can take on values of Optimal, Diagnostic, Limited, Non-diagnostic, and Uninterpretable.
5. *Definition* is a text description of a CDE Term or CDE Value. For example, the definition of the "Uninterpretable" CDE Value is "No useful diagnostic information. The study should be repeated."

Because our CDE development effort was the first to focus on imaging trials, no groupings of imaging CDEs had been developed. We also found that no

TABLE 11.1. CDE categories developed for CT imaging to screen lung cancer

Study Technique
- Equipment
- Acquisition
- Protocol
- Contrast Agent
- Display

Exam Quality

Image Location

Anatomic Location
- Lung Lobes
- Right Lung
- Left Lung
- Mediastinum
- Thoracic Lymph
- Pleura
- Metastases

Findings
- Nodules
- Other Findings

Conclusion

Recommendation

detailed imaging data model was available from other terminologies or standards. Therefore, we drafted a hierarchy containing several new imaging CDE sub-categories, which served as a simple data model (see Table 11.1). This hierarchy will be refined and augmented as additional imaging CDEs are developed.

The CDE Development Process

The CDE development process resulted in a comprehensive set of approximately 120 data elements over a period of 2–3 months. The process was conducted in cooperation with professional organizations (e.g., the Radiological Society of North America), standards development organizations (e.g., DICOM—Digital Imaging and Communications in Medicine), and interested scientific groups within the NCI. We followed the technical desiderata defined by Cimino et al. (1994) and the conceptual framework outlined by Campbell et al. (1998). Because the technical and philosophical issues have been reviewed in this prior literature, we will focus here on the social, political, and administrative issues we faced. The steps we took in developing the CDEs for chest CT screening are detailed below.

CDE Development Steps

1. *Assemble pertinent resources.* The first step was to assemble a comprehensive set of resources from which proposed CDEs could be extracted. Even when some terminological resources are available in a given domain, there often are additional resources that can be helpful in generating a more comprehensive set of CDEs. These resources include schemas for clinical trial databases, data collection forms from ongoing clinical trials, publications of related preliminary scientific research (e.g., Henschke, McCauley, Yankelvitz et al., 1999), and portions of relevant standards and terminologies.
2. *Involve relevant stakeholders.* As investigators in ongoing clinical trials were contacted to obtain the preceding resources, they were asked to participate in the CDE development process, either by attending panel meetings, participating in electronic mail discussions, or both. Our panel included predominantly clinical researchers and clinical experts—especially those with an interest in informatics and medical terminology. But we also tried to include other relevant stakeholders, including members of cooperative groups, biostatisticians, epidemiologists, and data coordinators. Leaders from professional organizations and standards development organizations nominated additional members to the panel. This resulted in a productive mix of expertise, interest, institutional support, and opinion leadership.
3. *Create initial CDEs and CDE categories.* We convened a small working group of 3–5 people, consisting primarily of informatics and clinical experts to sort through the pertinent resources and create a preliminary list of data elements. In some cases, multiple sources provided similar or duplicate data elements. The working group organized the list of proposed elements into categories and subcategories, and created a reduced list of candidate CDEs to be considered by the CDE panel. When there appeared to be more than one appropriate method to represent a given data element, both possibilities were presented to the panel.
4. *Link proposed CDEs to existing standards and terminologies.* Prior to the panel's deliberations, consistency between the proposed CDEs and existing standards and vocabularies was assessed. We felt that there might be important reasons for any differences between newer data collection methods and existing terminologies and standards. Consequently, prior to the panel meeting we weeded out potential conflicts only when we could identify clearly preferable existing approaches, rather than enforcing rigid consistency to existing terminologies in every case.
5. *Distribute draft CDEs to the full panel.* Prior to the panel meeting, each panelist was sent a list of these draft CDEs in the form of a spreadsheet. Panelists were encouraged to review the spreadsheet to formulate questions and comments that they felt should be discussed by the group.

6. *Convene CDE panel.* Although a face-to-face panel meeting might not be necessary for every terminological development effort, we felt that the relative paucity of existing terminological efforts in imaging, together with the diverse backgrounds of the panelists, made in-person meetings beneficial. The meeting allowed each member of the panel to be oriented to the concerns, needs, and skills of the others. A brief presentation of the results of a recent trial, with special emphasis on data collection methods, highlighted the clinical needs. A presentation of a tentative protocol design for an upcoming trial highlighted the potential near-term utility of CDEs. A demonstration of the CDE Web site provided an informatics emphasis and a focus on the overall goal of the process. Following this brief orientation, the panel deliberated for about five hours.
7. *Finalize CDEs.* Following the panel's deliberations, the CDEs were revised by the informatics working group to reflect the discussion. Additional comments on the revised version were sought via electronic mail. The relationship to other terminologies and standards were rechecked using the UMLS knowledge sources (National Library of Medicine, 1999) and the published DICOM standard (Digital Imaging and Communications in Medicine, 1999).
8. *Publish CDEs in Web-accessible database.* After the panel finalized the new CDEs, the list was provided in spreadsheet form to the NCI's Office of Informatics for inclusion in the Web-accessible CDE database. We then sought to publicize the availability of the new CDEs among the communities of clinical researchers that would find them useful.

Avoiding Pitfalls of CDE Deliberations

To prevent unnecessarily lengthy discussions of side issues, we laid out several principles to guide the panel's deliberations. All of us naturally become attached to the terms we use in our daily work. Likewise, cooperative groups and other large research organizations typically invest considerable resources in their data collection methods. These attachments, together with the heterogeneity of existing data collection systems, create the potential for lengthy discussions regarding the choice between forms of a common data element. We therefore outlined the following principles for the panel prior to its deliberations:

1. *Clinical research, not clinical practice.* The discussion should focus on common data collection methods for cancer research, not for clinical practice. For example, we focused on standard methods to collect data about how chest CT screening studies were performed. Any discussion of standards for how chest CT screening studies *should* be performed clinically was considered outside our purview, since attempts to formulate such standards by the NCI would be viewed with skepticism by professional organizations, who view the creation of such standards one of their key roles.

2. *Data collection, not experimental design.* The panel should address how data should be collected for clinical trials, rather than how those trials should be designed and conducted. For example, the group did not discuss the merits of whether a particular data item should be used as an eligibility criterion or a stratification variable. Instead, the panel focused on how that data item should be collected and encoded if trial designers elect to collect it as part of a clinical trial.
3. *Adoption rather than reinvention.* The panel should be strongly predisposed toward adopting previous terminological standards when possible, rather than "reinventing the wheel." This principle applies not only to existing standards and terminologies, but also to commonly used anatomic classification and staging systems. For example, rather than reinventing a staging system for classifying mediastinal lymph nodes, a standard, widely used classification system (Mountain & Dresler, 1997) was adopted.
4. *Synonyms, not competitors.* Occasionally, two groups use two different terms to describe essentially the same phenomenon. In that case, informatics systems can consider these two terms as synonyms (Cimino, Clayton, Hripcsak et al., 1994), so that each group can use the familiar term to describe the same concept. If each synonym has the same definition, the two synonyms will be used consistently. Thus, terminological "synonym wars" can be avoided. On the other hand, there are occasional semantic differences between similar terms that should be discussed openly and resolved. If the differences cannot be resolved, the two terms should both be retained, each with a detailed definition and specification of the difference between the similar terms.
5. *Expertise, not turf.* The interdisciplinary panel generally should defer to the individual with the training and experience most specific to the term under consideration. For example, most imaging trials collect extensive information about gross pathologic specimens, in order to maintain a reference standard. Although most of the panel members may be radiologists, a pathologist or surgeon is probably best able to resolve terminological issues related to gross pathologic specimens.

Discussion

Using the procedures described above, we created a set of about 120 common data elements (CDEs) over a period of approximately three months. The CDEs were created in cooperation with the several groups within the National Cancer Institute, including the Biomedical Imaging Program, the Lung and Aerodigestive Cancer Research Group, the Office of Informatics, and the SPORE Program. Other cooperating organizations included the American College of Radiology Imaging Network (ACRIN), the Radiological Society of North America (RSNA), and the Digital Imaging and Communication (DICOM) Working Group 18 on Clinical

Trials and Education. Since ongoing CDE development has ongoing importance to NCI's mission, we will now consider several issues related to NCI's continuing role in developing terminology.

It may be beneficial for NCI to strengthen its relationship to other standards-development organizations, such as HL7 (Health Level 7), SNOMED, and DICOM. For example, the NCI could actively monitor and contribute to these ongoing standards activities. This will contribute to the NCI's ability to rapidly develop CDEs that contribute to a convergent and comprehensive medical terminology.

As clinical trial sites adopt the CDEs, the NCI's role will naturally shift from the process of developing CDEs and the methods for their use to the process of encouraging ongoing use and managing change. NCI's role at that point will shift to measuring CDE usage, providing technical assistance to support adoption and implementation, and supporting a change-management process that involves all stakeholders.

There are also several technical enhancements for NCI to consider. For example, the CDEs have been viewed essentially as dictionaries, consisting of a linear list of terms, each with its own definition. However, most successful terminologies have developed a rich set of knowledge about each term that not only provides linkages between terms and a logical context for terms, but also specifies how a term should be instantiated and used in a variety of contexts. The NCI's CDE "Categories" can be viewed as a nascent information model for CDEs. With time, the CDE Categories must evolve into a richer representation of the relationships among terms and term groups. Ultimately, sophisticated knowledge representation techniques, such as semantic networks and description logic, will be required to express adequately the relationships among terms and to facilitate convergence with existing information models. Likewise, more detailed data dictionary entries for new data elements will minimize variation in term meaning and usage according to context and user. In some cases, imaging information or other non-textual data should augment simple text descriptions.

The current Web-enabled interface to the CDE database is designed to encourage consistent data collection not only from the cooperative groups, but also from oncology trials being conducted in other settings. The ability to perform boolean keyword searches in a transparent user interface, and the ability to display and download terms in forms other than HTML will likely enhance its usability to the disparate constituencies that it is intended to serve. For example, users without a great deal of research infrastructure may wish to download CDEs as draft data-collection forms or draft database specifications.

Conclusion

We have described how a well-defined set of common data elements can be created in a relatively short period of time. We have focused primarily on the social, political, and administrative issues, since others have comprehensively discussed the technical and conceptual issues (Cimino et al., 1994; Campbell, Oliver, Spackman, et al., 1998). The resulting CDEs are currently available on the NCI's Web site, and likely will become a part of both SNOMED and the UMLS. The results have been officially sanctioned by the board of directors of the Radiological Society of North America, and will be employed in the design of an upcoming chest CT screening trial to be supported by the National Cancer Institute. We have described this process in detail to allow others to learn from our experience and avoid some of the pitfalls we identified, thereby resulting in more efficient terminological development efforts. We also hope our efforts will identify key informatics research issues that will be the underpinnings of a rich set of informatics resources for clinical research and clinical care.

Acknowledgments. I would like to thank a number of people whose efforts were vital to this chapter and to the CDE development process it describes. Dan Sullivan, who directs the Biomedical Imaging Program at the National Cancer Institute, supported efforts to develop imaging CDEs from the beginning. John Silva provided the leadership that made CDEs a reality. Jeff Abrams and Beverly Meadows shared their valuable experience with CDE development for therapeutic trials. Christine Berg and Jorge Gomez from the Division of Cancer Prevention of the National Cancer Institute provided support for the CDE panel meetings. Denise Warzel and Carolyn Pifer were close collaborators on the creation of draft CDE documents. Marie Zinninger from the American College of Radiology and Dana Davis from the Radiological Society of North America facilitated the involvement of professional societies. This chapter began as an appendix to the report of the NCI's Informatics Long Range Planning Committee. I am grateful to the members of that committee, who provided comments on earlier drafts. Finally, I would like to thank Marion Ball and Judy Douglas, whose able leadership and gentle encouragement made this chapter (and this book) a reality.

References

American College of Radiology. 1992. Index for Radiological Diagnoses. 4th ed. Reston, VA: American College of Radiology.

Bell D, Greenes R. 1994. Evaluation of UltraSTAR: Performance of a Collaborative Structured Data Entry System. JAMIA Symposium Supplement:216–222.

Campbell K, Oliver D, Spackman K, et al. 1998. Representing Thoughts, Words, and Things in the UMLS. Journal of the American Medical Informatics Association 5(5):421–431.

Cimino J, Clayton P, Hripcsak G, et al. 1994. Knowledge-based Approaches to the Maintenance of a Large Controlled Medical Terminology. Journal of the American Medical Informatics Association 1(1):35–50.

Digital Imaging and Communications in Medicine. 1999. DICOM Information Object Definitions. Rosslyn, VA: National Electrical Manufacturers Association.

Henschke C, McCauley DI, Yankelevitz D, et al. 1999. Early Lung Cancer Action Project: Overall Design and Findings from Baseline Screening. Lancet 54(1973):99–105.

Mountain CF, Dresler C. 1997. Regional Lymph Node Classification for Lung Cancer Staging. Chest 111(6):1718–1723.

National Library of Medicine. 1999. Unified Medical Language System Knowledge Sources. 10th ed. Bethesda, MD: U.S. Department of Health and Human Services. p. 147.

Radiological Society of North America. 1999. RSNA Index to Imaging Literature. Oak Brook, IL: Radiological Society of North America.

Tuddenham W. 1984. Glossary of Terms for Thoracic Radiology: Recommendations of the Nomenclature Committee of the Fleischner Society. AJR 143:509–517.

12
Pathology Standards in Cancer Informatics

Kent A. Spackman and M. Elizabeth Hammond

The surgical pathology report has always contained vital information for managing oncology patients. In the past decade, we have come to realize that the value of this information depends on how it is communicated. Synoptic reporting, based on a simplified standard report format, is one efficient communication method (Markel & Hirsch, 1991). In 1992, a landmark study demonstrated that the use of a standard report form or checklist was "the one practice significantly associated with increased likelihood of providing complete oncologic pathology information" (Zarbo, 1992). As a result, individuals and organizations began recognizing the need to standardize the surgical pathology report, particularly for cancer reporting (Kempson, 1992; Association of Directors of Anatomic and Surgical Pathology, 1992; Kempson, 1993; Rosai J et al., 1993; Leslie & Rosai, 1994; Robboy et al., 1994).

The College of American Pathologists Cancer Protocols

The Cancer Committee of the College of American Pathologists (CAP) designed protocols to guide pathologists in examining cancerous pathologic specimens. These protocols specify information the referring physician needs to select primary or adjuvant treatment, estimate prognosis, and analyze outcome. Designed for patient care in all types of practice settings—including community hospitals, urban centers, and universities—the protocols provide common reporting formats to help tumor registrars and others uniformly collect pathology data.

The process of protocol development is multidisciplinary. For common malignant sites like the prostate, breast, and colon, protocols followed the Cancer Committee recommendations on site-specific task forces. These task forces, composed of surgeons, medical oncologists, radiation oncologists, diagnostic radiologists, and pathologists, met as a group and provided guidance based on a review of the literature, personal experience, and consultation with colleagues.

The task forces created provisional protocols that the Cancer Committee and other consultants reviewed. Members of the Cancer Committee or other pathologists developed protocols for less common cancers with the guidance of other medical specialists, listed in the acknowledgments for each protocol. The approval process for all protocols was identical. After gaining approval from the Cancer Committee, each provisional protocol moved to a formal review process with multiple pathologists serving on resource and other governing or review bodies within the organization (Commission on Anatomic Pathology, the Council on Scientific Affairs, the House of Delegates, and the Board of Governors of the College of American Pathologists). Five hundred practicing pathologists received all the early protocols for reality testing and their comments were also incorporated. The primary author, with guidance from other members of the Cancer Committee and the protocol manual editor—Carolyn Compton, MD, PhD—made the modifications suggested by the pathology consultants.

Each protocol contains a general outline for specimen accessioning, evaluation explanatory notes, a list of specific references cited in the notes, and a general bibliography. The explanatory notes contain TNM classifications for extent of disease, site-specific histologic classifications of tumors, and specific information about macroscopic specimens, microscopic features, and diagnostic considerations.

All protocols are divided into three sections: clinical information, macroscopic examination, and microscopic evaluation. For each site, protocols are stratified according to the procedure used to obtain specimens, including cytologic evaluation, biopsy, and resection. Each protocol is identified by the date of publication. Revisions are also dated and names of revising authors are provided. A short form of each protocol (synoptic format or checklist) lists all the elements for easy use. These checklists contain nomograms to ease selection of appropriate pathologic TNM staging information. Figure 12.1 illustrates the checklist from the most recent version of the breast cancer protocol.

Cancer protocols recommend simple, practical ways to provide information clinicians need to treat patients effectively. When a report is long, confusing, or missing key elements, the clinician must interrupt a pathologist or have the slides reviewed, possibly generating rework. Clear and predictable reports will not confuse clinicians, resulting in fewer pathologist interruptions and better, faster patient care. Standardized formats may also lessen interobserver variation among pathologists in a group, ensuring greater clinician satisfaction and fewer errors from misinterpreting pathology information. Because such standardized reports are easier for transcriptionists to produce, the results are also available much faster.

The American College of Surgeons has endorsed the CAP cancer protocols, in their synoptic format, as review criteria for accepting hospitals into their cancer hospital accreditation program. Clearly, the College recognizes that synoptic formats help determine the completeness of an

BREAST: Cytology/Biopsy

Patient name:
Cytology/Surgical pathology number:

MACROSCOPIC (check all that apply)

SPECIMEN TYPE
___ Cytology
___ Biopsy
  ___ Percutaneous core biopsy (e.g. Tru-Cut™)
  ___ Image-guided core biospy
  ___ Incisional biopsy
  ___ Other (e.g. ABBI procedure)

TUMOR SITE
___ Right breast
___ Left breast
___ Unknown

SPECIMEN SIZE: ___ x ___ x ___ cm

TUMOR SIZE (largest dimension), if appropriate: ___ cm

MICROSCOPIC (check all that apply)

HISTOLOGIC TYPE
___ Cannot be determined
___ Noninvasive carcinoma (NOS)
  ___ Ductal carcinoma in situ
  ___ Lobular carcinoma in situ
___ Invasive carcinoma (NOS)
  ___ Invasive ductal
  ___ Invasive ductal carcinoma with an extensive intraductal component
  ___ Invasive lobular
  ___ Mucinous
  ___ Medullary
  ___ Papillary
  ___ Tubular
  ___ Adenoid cystic
  ___ Secretory (juvenile)
  ___ Apocrine
  ___ Cribriform
  ___ Paget's disease of the nipple
    ___ With invasive carcinoma
    ___ Without invasive carcinoma
  ___ Carcinoma with metaplasia
    ___ Squamous type
    ___ Spindle cell type
    ___ Cartilaginous and osseous type
    ___ Mixed type
  ___ Inflammatory
  ___ Other(s) (specify: ________________)

HISTOLOGIC GRADE
___ Cannot be determined

Tubule formation:
___ Majority of tumor >75% (score = 1)
___ Moderate 10% to 75% (score = 2)
___ Minimal <10% (score = 3)

Nuclear pleomorphism:
___ Small regular nuclei (score = 1)
___ Moderate increase in size, etc. (score = 2)
___ Marked variation in size, nucleoli, chromatin clumping, etc. (score = 3)

Mitotic count:
For a 25x objective with a field area of 0.274 mm^2
___ <10 mitoses per 10 HPF (score = 1)
___ 10-20 mitoses per 10 HPF (score = 2)
___ >20 mitoses per 10 HPF (score = 3)
or
For a 40x objective with a field area of 0.152 mm^2
___ 0-5 mitoses per 10 HPF (score = 1)
___ 6-10 mitoses per 10 HPF (score = 2)
___ >10 mitoses per 10 HPF (score = 3)

Total score:
___ Grade I: 3-5 points
___ Grade II: 6-7 points
___ Grade III: 8-9 points

MICROSCOPIC, CONTINUED (check all that apply)

ADDITIONAL PATHOLOGIC FINDINGS
___ None identified
___ Microcalcifications
___ Fibrocystic changes
___ Atypical hyperplasia
___ Other (specify: ________________)

COMMENT
____
____
____
____

FIGURE 12.1. Surgical pathology cancer case summary. (Reprinted with permission from Fitzgibbons PL, Connolly JL, Page DL. Breast chapter (pp 15–18). In: Compton, CC. Ed. *Reporting on Cancer Specimens: Protocols and Case Summaries*. 2000. College of American Pathologists, 325 Waukegan Road, Northfield, Illinois 60093–2750)

BREAST: Complete excision less than total mastectomy (includes wire-guided localization excisions), total mastectomy, modified radical mastectomy, radical mastectomy

Patient name:
Surgical pathology number:

MACROSCOPIC (check all that apply)

SPECIMEN TYPE
___ Complete excision, less than total mastectomy
    ___ Without axillary contents
    ___ With axillary contents
___ Total mastectomy
___ Modified radical mastectomy
___ Radical mastectomy

SPECIMEN SIZE (for excisions less than total masectomy): ___ x ___ x ___ cm

TUMOR SITE
___ Right breast
    ___ Upper outer quadrant
    ___ Lower outer quadrant
    ___ Upper inner quadrant
    ___ Lower inner quadrant
    ___ Central

___ Left breast
    ___ Upper outer quadrant
    ___ Lower outer quadrant
    ___ Upper inner quadrant
    ___ Lower inner quadrant
    ___ Central

TUMOR SIZE (largest dimension): ___ cm

MICROSCOPIC (check all that apply)

HISTOLOGIC TYPE
___ Noninvasive carcinoma (NOS)
    ___ Ductal carcinoma in situ
    ___ Lobular carcinoma in situ
___ Invasive carcinoma (NOS)
    ___ Invasive ductal
    ___ Invasive ductal carcinoma with an extensive intraductal component
    ___ Invasive lobular
    ___ Mucinous
    ___ Medullary
    ___ Papillary
    ___ Tubular
    ___ Adenoid cystic
    ___ Secretory (juvenile)
    ___ Apocrine
    ___ Cribriform
    ___ Paget's disease of the nipple
        ___ With invasive carcinoma
        ___ Without invasive carcinoma
    ___ Carcinoma with metaplasia
        ___ Squamous type
        ___ Spindle cell type
        ___ Cartilaginous and osseous type
        ___ Mixed type
    ___ Inflammatory
    ___ Other(s) (specify: ________________)

HISTOLOGIC GRADE
Tubule formation:
___ Majority of tumor >75% (score = 1)
___ Moderate 10% to 75% (score = 2)
___ Minimal <10% (score = 3)

Nuclear pleomorphism:
___ Small regular nuclei (score = 1)
___ Moderate increase in size, etc. (score = 2)
___ Marked variation in size, nucleoli, chromatin clumping, etc. (score = 3)

Mitotic count:
For a 25x objective with a field area of 0.274 mm^2
___ <10 mitoses per 10 HPF (score = 1)
___ 10-20 mitoses per 10 HPF (score = 2)
___ >20 mitoses per 10 HPF (score = 3)
or
For a 40x objective with a field area of 0.152 mm^2
___ 0-5 mitoses per 10 HPF (score = 1)
___ 6-10 mitoses per 10 HPF (score = 2)
___ >10 mitoses per 10 HPF (score = 3)

Total score:
___ Grade I: 3-5 points
___ Grade II: 6-7 points
___ Grade III: 8-9 points

FIGURE **12.1.** (*Continued*).

institution's cancer pathology reports. Their endorsement will likely encourage more pathologists to use these protocols.

Synoptic Cancer Reporting: Experience with Breast Cancer

In 1990, a review of breast cancer reports provided to clinicians at LDS Hospital in Salt Lake City, Utah illustrated the utility of synoptic reporting

MICROSCOPIC, CONTINUED (check all that apply)

EXTENT OF INVASION

___ TX: Cannot be assessed

___ T0: No evidence of primary tumor

___ Tis: Carcinoma in situ: Intraductal carcinoma, lobular carcinoma in situ, or Paget's disease of the nipple with no tumor

___ T1: Tumor ≤ 2 cm in greatest dimension

 ___ T1mic: Microinvasion ≤ 0.1 cm in greatest dimension

 ___ T1a: > 0.1 cm but ≤ 0.5 cm in greatest dimension

 ___ T1b: > 0.5 cm but ≤ 1 cm in greatest dimension

 ___ T1c: > 1 cm but ≤ 2 cm in greatest dimension

___ T2: Tumor > 2 cm but ≤ 5 cm in greatest dimension

___ T3: Tumor > 5 cm in greatest dimension

___ T4: Tumor of any size with direct extension to chest wall or skin

 ___ T4a: Extension to chest wall

 ___ T4b: Edema (including peau d'orange) or ulceration of the skin of the breast or satellite skin nodules confined to the same breast

 ___ T4c: Both T4a and T4b

 ___ T4d: Inflammatory carcinoma

MARGINS

___ Margins uninvolved by tumor

 Distance of tumor from closest margin: ___ cm

___ Margin(s) involved by tumor

 Specify which margin(s): ______________

MICROCALCIFICATIONS

___ Absent

___ Present

VASCULAR INVASION

___ Absent

___ Present

___ Indeterminate

REGIONAL LYMPH NODES

___ NX: Cannot be assessed (previously removed or not removed for pathologic study)

___ N0: No regional lymph node metastasis

___ N1: Metastasis to movable ipsilateral axillary lymph node(s)

 ___ N1a: Only micrometastasis, none > 0.2 cm in greatest dimension

 ___ N1b: Metastasis to lymph node(s), any > 0.2 cm in greatest dimension

 ___ N1bi: Metastasis in 1 to 3 lymph nodes, any > 0.2 cm and all < 2 cm in greatest dimension

 ___ N1bii: Metastasis to 4 or more lymph nodes, any > 0.2 cm and all < 2 cm in greatest dimension

 ___ N1biii: Extension of tumor beyond the capsule of a lymph node, metastasis < 2 cm in greatest dimension

 ___ N1biv: Metastasis to a lymph node ≥ 2 cm in greatest dimension

___ N2: Metastasis to ipsilateral axillary lymph node(s) fixed to one another or to other structures

___ N3: Metastasis to ipsilateral internal mammary lymph node(s)

DISTANT METASTASIS

___ MX: Cannot be assessed

___ M0: No distant metastasis

___ M1: Distant metastasis [includes metastasis to ipsilateral supraclavicular lymph node(s)]

ADDITIONAL PATHOLOGIC FINDINGS

___ None identified

___ Microcalcifications

___ Fibrocystic changes

___ Atypical hyperplasia

___ Other (specify: ______________)

COMMENT

____

____

____

____

FIGURE 12.1. (*Continued*).

for breast cancer. A significant number of reports (9% of 356) were missing information necessary for patient care, and another 7% were judged confusing in their narrative form. As mentioned before, clinicians must disrupt the pathologist's workflow when reports are confusing or incomplete. A phone log of calls concerning breast cancer reports at LDS indicated significant pathologist disruption to find and review slides and

TABLE 12.1. Breast cancer report review

Category	Reports from 1990	Reports from 1993	Reports from 1995
Total reports reviewed	356	250	190
Total complete reports	299	242	188
Total incomplete reports	32	8	1
Incomplete gross description	10	8	1
Incomplete microscopic description	22	0	0
Confusing narrative	25	0	0

recontact the clinician. In a specific 14-day period, 80% of phone calls about breast cancer reports involved queries about missing information.

To improve the quality of breast cancer reports, Hammond and her colleagues implemented synoptic formats for them. They queried clinicians about the information needed, created a form, and ensured pathologist training. After a 30-day test period, they implemented the new report format. Clinicians were satisfied with the new formats and pathologists readily adopted them. Surveys of breast cancer pathology reports in 1993 and 1995 confirmed that the synoptic reports had eliminated the problem of missing information (Table 12.1), and in a 1996 survey, oncologists reported strong satisfaction with the new formats (Hammond & Flinner, 1997). Synoptic formats for breast cancer were so successful that synoptic report formats for other tumors soon followed.

Subsequent reports have been modified to conform to CAP breast cancer protocol synoptic formats and changed to pick list formats pathologists can use to quickly create and reproduce reports. Synoptic reporting for all cancer types has been adopted throughout Intermountain Health Care, the system of which LDS is a part. Implementing this schema of reporting has enabled other advancements, like voice-activated recording for cancer reports and data acquisition of cancer pathology elements. Collecting data as standardized choices also makes it easier to transmit it to the enterprise data warehouse.

Coded Terminology for Cancer Reporting

Checklists and standard report formats ensure greater consistency and completeness in reporting data on individual cases within a single institution. Still, variation across institutions or even across different recipients of reports in a single institution is in many ways both inevitable and desirable. Some report recipients need additional data for specific clinical trials; some have experimental investigational techniques that need to be accommodated; and variation across institutions and over time will influence reports' size, shape, page placement, formatting, and other characteristics.

These variations present a problem for those who use pathology reports not for their primary purpose—communicating a particular set of results on a single patient—but for secondary purposes. Such secondary uses, such as calculating cancer incidence statistics, usually require aggregating information from many patients. Secondary uses also include intra-institutional or intra-departmental activities like quality assurance, case finding for educational purposes, and automated alerts and reminders.

Paper-based pathology reports inhibit secondary uses because of the time and expense of manually extracting information. Pathology departments have a long history of encoding the final diagnoses electronically, and today it is highly unusual for reports not to pass through some electronic form, at least during word processing. This presents the opportunity to capture and use the information in coded form for secondary purposes. Checklists and standard report formats increase this capability. Connecting the checklists to standard codes facilitates intra- and inter-institutional aggregation and analysis.

SNOMED/ICD-O Encoding of Tumor Morphology and Topography

The Systematized Nomenclature of Medicine (SNOMED) was first published in 1976 as an expanded and revised version of the Systematized Nomenclature of Pathology (SNOP). SNOP, published in 1965, provided a coding scheme for pathologic findings that separated the code for the location of a disorder (the topography code, a number preceded with a "T") from the code for its morphologic characteristics (the morphology code, a number preceded with an "M"). For example, adenocarcinoma of the breast had two codes, M-8143 (adenocarcinoma), and T-0400 (breast).

The morphology sections of SNOP were adopted in 1968 by the Manual of Tumor Nomenclature and Classification (MOTNAC), widely adopted by tumor registrars, and used as the basis for the International Classification of Diseases for Oncology (ICD-O). ICD-O was originally published in 1976 and revised in 1990 and 2001. The morphology codes in ICD-O were a one-digit extension of the SNOP codes. Thus adenocarcinoma became M-81403 (the extra digit was inserted in the fourth position, leaving the "3" as an indicator of malignancy). The neoplasm codes in SNOMED (M-8.... and M-9....) are identical to those in ICD-O, allowing tumor registries using ICD-O morphology codes to use the SNOMED codes in surgical pathology reports. This has continued in the most recent version of SNOMED, called SNOMED Reference Terminology (RT) (Spackman, 2000).

In their most recent revisions, ICD-O-3 and the corresponding tumor morphology section of SNOMED-RT have extensive additions and changes that reflect the ongoing changes in the nomenclature of malignant morphology. To represent new morphologies, 220 codes were added. The most extensively revised sections are those dealing with lymphomas and leukemias (Fritz & Percy, 2000).

SNOMED's topography codes are not the same as those used in ICD-O, because they allow for far more anatomical detail. They can be translated directly to the ICD-O topography codes using a many-to-one mapping table available from CAP.

Additional SNOMED-RT Support of Cancer Data Reporting

SNOMED-RT contains several other enhancements to facilitate cancer data reporting and analysis. These include specific code additions to support cancer checklists, codes for cytology, improved linkage to ICD-9-CM cancer codes, and improved structures for data aggregation and analysis.

The SNOMED "M" and "T" codes are sufficient for encoding the histologic tumor type and the organ of origin, but checklists contain much more information. For example, they encode the type of specimen (including the procedure used to obtain it), the extent of invasion, tumor configuration, histologic grade, involvement of specific margins, distant metastases, and involvement of blood vessels, lymph nodes, or perineural structures. The SNOMED team has added codes for all these data elements by systematically examining every data element in each CAP Cancer Protocol. They also added codes to support use of the revised Bethesda System, widely used as a standard for the narrative portion of cervical cytology reports.

In addition to coding cancer morphology and topography, many organizations also need to use a single diagnosis code from ICD-9-CM. SNOMED provides an ICD mapping file that can be used to automatically identify the ICD-9-CM code corresponding to a given pair of topography and morphology codes. This is a two-step process. The first step is identifying the SNOMED disease/disorder code that corresponds to the pair of topography and morphology codes. This involves examining the definitions of the disease/disorder codes and searching for one that matches, either as directly identical codes or as subtypes. For example, if adenocarcinoma of the female breast has the topography code T-04050 and the morphology code M-81403, a search of disease/disorder codes can match these to the definition of "malignant neoplasm of female breast," D7-F0803. This definition includes associated-topography T-04050 (a direct match) and associated-morphology M-80003 (a supertype of M-81403). The second step in the process is a simple look-up in the ICD mapping table, which lists D7-F0803 and its corresponding ICD code, 174.9.

The definitions available in SNOMED-RT enable easier recording, more flexible and reliable retrieval, and data aggregation along multiple axes. For example, a table lists the larynx as part of the upper aerodigestive tract, the respiratory tract, and the neck, enabling automated retrieval and analysis by tumor site according to any of these categories.

Benefits of Combining Protocols and Standardized Coding

A consideration of the requirements of different groups illuminates the value of combining cancer reporting protocols like checklists and synoptic reports with standardized encoding. To accurately interpret the material and use it in patient care, pathologists who produce the reports need correctness, completeness, efficiency, and flexibility. Users of information in pathology reports have similar requirements that still may not be satisfied by reports optimized for pathologists. Users who need to retrieve and aggregate information require recall, precision, automation, and flexibility. They must be able to retrieve (recall) all cases of a particular kind of cancer for statistical reporting and analysis, and they must be able to exclude irrelevant cases (precision). These activities must be done in a way that permits automation, avoids costly and error-prone manual methods, and can change to meet various data needs.

The traditional narrative pathology report, while efficient and flexible, can become more correct and complete through the use of checklists and protocols. Although some pathologists have justifiably resisted using synoptic reports by themselves, combining checklists and synoptic reports with additional narrative meets pathologist requirements. Using encoded checklists can also meet user needs while not adversely affecting pathologists. Flexibly customized checklists, whether paper, electronic, or a combination, help ensure completeness of information. Electronic approaches to "coding templates in the background" can be readily created from word processor macros or Web-browser scripts or integrated in anatomic pathology information systems. As narrative reports are transmitted for clinicians, coded data can be transmitted for inclusion in databases and incorporation, transmission, and aggregation by other systems. This approach enables retrieval, aggregation, and maximum comparability of data collected at different sites by different people.

Looking Ahead

As the primary source of crucial information about cancer patients, the pathology report merits ongoing and extensive examination. New protocols, checklists, and codes can improve the completeness, accuracy, and usability of this information. Widespread adoption and implementation of these technologies promise significant benefits to pathologists, clinicians, and their patients.

References

Association of Directors of Anatomic and Surgical Pathology. 1992. Standardization of the Surgical Pathology Report. American Journal of Surgical Pathology 16(1):84–86.

Association of Directors of Anatomic and Surgical Pathology. 2000. Recommendations for the Reporting of Surgical Specimens Containing Uterine Cervical Neoplasms. American Journal of Clinical Pathology 114(6):847–851.

Fritz A, Percy C. 2000. Introducing ICD-O-3: Impact of the New Edition. Journal of Registry Management 27(4):125–131.

Hammond EH, Flinner RL. 1997. Clinically Relevant Breast Cancer Reporting: Using Process Measures to Improve Anatomic Pathology Reporting. Archives of Pathology and Laboratory Medicine 121(11):1171–1175.

Kempson RL. 1992. The Time is Now: Checklists for Surgical Pathology Reports. Archives of Pathology and Laboratory Medicine 116:1107–1108.

Kempson RL. 1993. Checklists for Surgical Pathology Reports: An Important Step Forward. American Journal of Clinical Pathology 100(3):196–197.

Leslie KO, Rosai J. 1994. Standardization of the Surgical Pathology Report: Formats, Templates, and Synoptic Reports. Seminars in Diagnostic Pathology 11(4):253–257.

Markel SF, Hirsch SD. 1991. Synoptic Surgical Pathology Reporting. Human Pathology 22(8):807–810.

Robboy SJ, Bentley RC, Krigman H, et al. 1994. Synoptic Reports in Gynecologic Pathology. International Journal of Gynecologic Pathology 13:161–174.

Rosai J, et al. 1993. Standardized Reporting of Surgical Pathology Diagnoses for the Major Tumor Types: A Proposal. American Journal of Clinical Pathology 100(3):240–255.

Spackman KA, et al. (eds). 2000. SNOMED Reference Terminology. Northfield, IL: College of American Pathologists.

Zarbo RJ. 1992. Interinstitutional Assessment of Colorectal Carcinoma Surgical Pathology Report Accuracy: A College of American Pathologists Q-probes Study of Practice Patterns from 532 Laboratories and 15,940 Reports. Archives of Pathology and Laboratory Medicine 116:1113–1119.

13 Clinical Information Interchange with Health Level Seven

Stanley M. Huff, W. Ed Hammond, and Warren G. Williams

The name Health Level Seven (HL7) refers to both an organization and the set of data exchange standards produced by the organization. Data exchange standards are specifications for the syntax (format) and contents (identifiers, codes, and values) of messages sent between computer systems to meet a particular business need. The purpose of this chapter is to:

- describe why messaging standards were created
- provide a brief history of HL7
- illustrate how the HL7 Standard is used to transmit data between computer systems
- show examples of how the HL7 Standard can be used to transmit cancer related data and information

Motivation for Creating Data Exchange Standards

Twenty or more years ago, the typical architecture for hospital information systems was based on a single large computer that serviced all the information needs of a hospital and its associated clinics. These "main-frame" systems had applications for entering and reviewing many kinds of clinical data, including medication orders, laboratory results, nursing observations, radiology reports, blood bank findings, and emergency room evaluations. The systems usually had a consistent look and feel, and the applications shared information between modules in an integrated way. The downside of the monolithic systems was that a given module—for example, pharmacy—might not be optimal. Organizations selected systems for the overall benefits they offered, which did not guarantee that all modules were equally good.

Beginning in the early to mid-1980s, local area networks became generally available and people began to propose systems composed of network modules (McDonald, 1984; McDonald & Hammond, 1989; Hammond, 1988; Simborg, 1984a; Simborg, 1984b). The idea was that experts in a given area could create special-purpose systems that were optimal for a given clinical department. Using this strategy, sometimes called a "best of breed" system, purchasers could buy the best system for a given purpose. These ideas led to the introduction of modular, stand-alone computer systems to serve the clinical laboratory, the radiology department, and the pharmacy.

These new modular systems had a potential drawback. For the systems to work together as an integrated whole, information needed to pass between the independent modules. For example, when a patient was admitted using the hospital registration system, the demographic information would also have to be sent to the laboratory system so that the proper patient name and visit number could be attached to all laboratory tests for that patient. Likewise, the results from laboratory testing had to be sent back to the clinical system so physicians and nurses could use them to direct patient care.

In systems today, interfaces serve several purposes. Data exchange within an enterprise reduces redundant data entry. Optimally, data is entered once, as close to the original source as possible, and then shared with other computers on the network via interfaces. For example, demographic data should be entered as part of patient registration, and then shared with the pharmacy, radiology, and laboratory systems as needed. Laboratory results are entered in the laboratory and immediately shared with the hospital information system or the intensive care unit system. The result is that patients receive better clinical care because data is available when and where it is needed.

Data can also be shared between different enterprises or entities. Standardized interfaces can be used for reporting public health data between a clinical laboratory and a local, state, or federal public health facility. For example, standards have been set for sharing infectious disease data (serologic studies, cultures, and antimicrobial susceptibilities) between clinical laboratories and state or local health departments (Centers for Disease Control, 1997). Reports have shown that using standardized electronic interfaces improves the accuracy and completeness of data and allows reports to reach the health departments faster (Effler et al., 1999; Health Insurance Portability and Accountability Act, 1996).

Data associated with clinical studies (outcomes research and clinical trials) can also be sent using data exchange standards. Using a standard allows reuse of software and knowledge that already exists within the enterprise, and it obviates the need to create special-purpose software for each new clinical study. Standardized interfaces also can be used to exchange administrative and financial data related to patient care. For example, the Health Information Portability and Accountability Act (HIPAA) of 1996 mandates the use of electronic data exchange standards for communication between healthcare providers and payers. The kinds of transactions supported include insurance enrollment, claims submission, payment transactions, and authorization of care. Figure 13.1 summarizes some of the purposes for interface creation.

- ***Intra-enterprise data sharing***
  - reduce redundant data entry
  - better clinical care
- ***Inter-enterprise data sharing***
  - public health reporting
  - clinical studies
  - outcomes
  - clinical trials
  - patient administration
  - enrollment, claims, payments

FIGURE 13.1. Summary of purposes for which interfaces have been created.

A Brief History of Interfaces

The first interfaces were one-of-a-kind programs. Interface designers decided what kind of plugs and wiring to use for the physical connection, whether to use ASCII or EBCDIC character encoding, what convention to use to identify unique instances of messages, and what the data contents would be. Creating special-purpose interface programs was a costly and time-consuming proposition. Software companies often charged $50,000 or more to create an interface, and programming and testing could take a year or more. These high costs and long development times were the main drivers for standardizing the way interfaces were created. If created in a standard way, interface programs could be reused, which would substantially reduce the time and cost of creating and implementing a new system module.

In the mid-1980s, the desire to decrease the time and cost of implementing interfaces led to the creation of organizations interested in standardizing medical data exchange standards. For example, the Digital Imaging and Communications Standards Committee (DICOM) was established in 1983 as a joint effort between the American College of Radiology (ACR) and the National Electrical Manufacturers Association (NEMA) (Bidgood & Horii, 1992; NEMA, 1997). The first version of the DICOM standard was published in 1985. American Standards for Testing and Materials (ASTM) Committee E-31 on Healthcare Informatics was established in 1970, but the first ASTM medical data exchange standard was published in 1988 (ASTM, 1988). The Health Level Seven (HL7) organization was established in 1987, and the first version of the HL7 Standard was published later that year (Health Level Seven, 1987). Accredited Standards Committee (ASC) X12N, which deals with administrative data exchange standards using UN/EDIFACT encoding, was created in February 1991.

A Brief History of HL7

In 1987, a group of healthcare providers established the not-for-profit HL7 organization. As initially organized, HL7 was an *ad hoc* standards development organization. Version 2 of the standard was produced in 1988, a year after the first version, and was the first to be implemented in production systems. Between 1990 and 2000, HL7 produced five additional versions of the standard.

In 1994, HL7 became an accredited American National Standards Institute (ANSI) Standards Developing Organization (SDO). This means that HL7 follows the ANSI guidelines for developing open consensus standards. Following an open consensus process means that any interested party is free to join HL7 and participate in the creation of standards, and that specific rules are followed to ensure balanced participation between software vendors, software users, and academicians. Version 2.2 of the HL7 standard and all subsequent versions of the standard have been approved as ANSI standards.

Today, the HL7 organization has over 500 organizational members, over 2000 individual members, and 15 international affiliates. Current affiliates include Argentina, Australia, Canada, the United Kingdom, Germany, Japan, the Netherlands, New Zealand, Finland, South Africa, India, China, Taiwan, South Korea, and Switzerland. The HL7 Standard has been officially adopted by the governments of New Zealand, Australia, and the Netherlands. The organization holds working group meetings three times a year to create new standards and to revise existing ones; typically, 400 to 500 members attend.

HL7 has become the most widely used clinical data exchange standard in the world. In a survey of 153 chief information officers in 1998, 80% used HL7 within their institutions and 13.5% were planning to implement HL7 in the future. In hospitals with over 400 beds, more than 95% use HL7 (College of Healthcare Information Management Executives, 1998).

Basic Interfacing Principles

To communicate in any language, people need common words and a common understanding of the meaning and rules for putting those words together. When we write a letter, we have rules that define how we address the envelope and how we structure the inside address, date, heading, body, and closure of the letter. The same must be true for the successful interchange of clinical information.

Most integrated delivery systems include many heterogeneous information systems that use neither a common data model nor a common vocabulary. Data often is entered independently into each system, and only in recent years has a standard existed for data exchange among these systems. Despite the existence of a working data interchange standard—HL7—from the early 1990s, much negotiation is still required among heterogeneous systems to determine what items will be sent and to establish vocabulary mapping from one system to another. The growing demand for seamless and cost effective interfacing of two or more heterogeneous systems is driving the move toward interoperable systems.

The IEEE Standard Computer Dictionary: A Compilation of IEEE Standard Computer Glossaries (Institute of Electrical and Electronics Engineers, 1990) defines interoperability as "the ability of two or more systems or components to exchange information and to use the information that has been exchanged." The ability to exchange information is a functional interoperability met largely by standards like HL7 Messaging and Communication Standard. Using that information is more complex and requires, at minimum, an enterprise model that includes a common terminology.

The ISO standard known as ISO/IEC TR9007:1987—Concepts and Technology for the Conceptual Schema and the Information Base—defines the basis for communication in this way: "Any meaningful exchange or utterance depends upon the prior existence of an agreed upon set of semantic and syntactic rules." This standard, which resulted from the Conceptual Schema Modeling Facilities (CSMF) project begun in 1991, introduced the notion of a conceptual schema (enterprise model) and provided a tool to deal with the scope and complexity of enterprise modeling. The two primary objectives for the CSMF standard were to enhance interoperability between enterprise models and to improve the quality (e.g., accuracy, completeness, semantic depth) of enterprise models and the information systems developed from them. Semantic rules were used to define the content of the communication using words with a common, understandable meaning. The syntactic rules define how the content is put together to have meaning.

Successful communication among disparate systems requires interoperability at many levels. Computers communicate with each other using a set of rules or a protocol. Multiple levels of communication protocols are required to support messaging between a sending application on one system and a receiving application on another. The International Standards Organization (ISO) has defined a suite of protocols to facilitate this type of messaging between computers. This suite, known as the Open Systems Interconnection (OSI) Standard, provides the basis for full interoperability. The seven-layer protocol deals with the stacking of communication levels, from the applications level down to the physical level of a sending system, and across to the physical level and up to the applications level of the receiving system. The HL7 standard deals with the application level (what needs to be sent to fulfill business need) and partially with the presentation level (the syntax of the data sent) of the OSI model. HL7 actually derives its name from the seventh (application) level of the OSI stack. Figure 13.2 illustrates the OSI model.

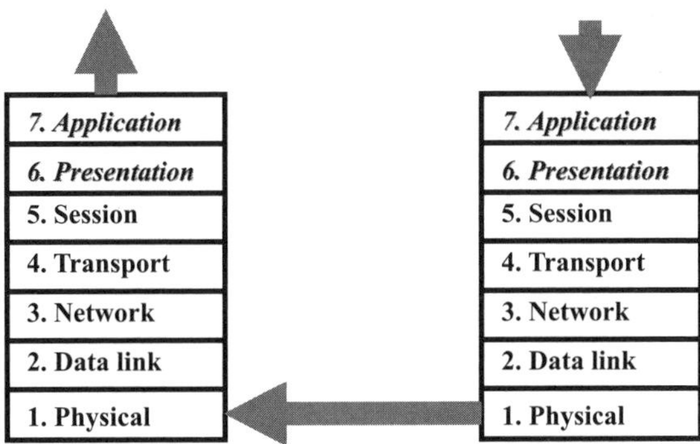

FIGURE 13.2. Seven-level Open Systems Interface model. The International Standards Organization (ISO) has defined a seven-level Open Systems Interface (OSI) model for exchange of data between heterogeneous computer systems. The model provides standardized information exchange between each level of the model so that interfaces can be implemented in a modular fashion.

Vocabulary and Messaging

In one biblical story, the people of the world come together to build a tower to heaven. God decided he did not want the tower built, and caused the people to speak different languages so that Chaos would result. Not surprisingly, some standards developers point to the Tower of Babel as a symbol of standardization efforts.

One unsolved challenge for interoperability is the lack of a single, universal clinical terminology. While significant progress has been made, much time and energy is still required to meet the understanding and usability requirement for interoperability.

Perhaps the most common way to deal with vocabularies at an institutional level is to create local terminologies. A single institution has several vocabularies, often addressing the same subject matter. Whenever a communication is required from one unit to another, local mappings are made. Each time a change is made in either system, however, the mapping is in error and must be corrected. The number of system-to-system mappings that must be made is represented by the following equation: $(n^2 - n)/2$ (Simborg, 1984a). This is the most common method of dealing with vocabulary differences, but because a typical institution has many different systems, the method is also time- and cost-intensive.

A second approach builds on national or international sets of controlled vocabularies. In this approach, a publicly available mapping is created (although perhaps at a cost) among sets of these publicly available vocabularies. The National Library of Medicine Unified Medical Language System (UMLS) is such a public mapping (Lindberg, Humphrey, McCray, 1993; National Library of Medicine, 1993).

Neither of these two options for overcoming vocabulary differences is ideal. If it is possible to map every concept in one vocabulary to one and only one concept in a second vocabulary, no logical reason exists for two separate vocabularies. Still, if the two vocabularies cannot be mapped exactly, it means that information will be lost when data is translated.

The best approach may be to create a standard, public, no-fee or low-fee set of terms and codes that an appropriate authority would continuously maintain. Such a vocabulary set does not exist today, although mergers of key controlled vocabularies may move the community in that direction. The goal is to create a universal vocabulary. Initially, each system would map to the universal vocabulary, which would allow any two systems to communicate via the standard. This is the same principle as Esperanto. If each system knows the universal language, it can talk to any other system through that medium. Over time, the universal vocabulary should replace most or all of the local vocabularies and obviate the need for any translations.

HL7 Messages

All HL7 Version 2 standards are based on some common assumptions and principles. One principle is that all data exchange is motivated by a business need and that a particular instance of data exchange is triggered by some event in the real world. For example, the business need may be sharing order information between a system that allows orders to be placed for laboratory tests and a laboratory information system (LIS) that can fill the order. A particular instance of data exchange is triggered when someone places a laboratory order on the ordering system, an action that causes an order message to be created and sent to the LIS. After a specimen has been obtained from the patient and the testing is complete, the test results are entered into the laboratory information system, which causes a result message to be created and sent to the ordering system. Figure 13.3 illustrates this series of interactions.

All HL7 Version 2 messages have some similar characteristics. As shown in Figure 13.4, each message is composed of segments. Each segment starts with a specific label, which is followed by the contents of fields that have been defined for that segment. Each segment is terminated by a carriage return "<CR>" character. The various fields within a segment are delimited by the vertical bar character ("|"). For example, in Figure 13.4, the first segment in the message is a MSH or message header segment. The first field in the MSH segment shows the set of field delimiters allowed in the message. Subsequent fields indicate the name of the sending facility, the name of the sending application, the name of the receiving facility, the name of the receiving application, the date and time of the message, security information (left blank in the example), and the message type. These fields

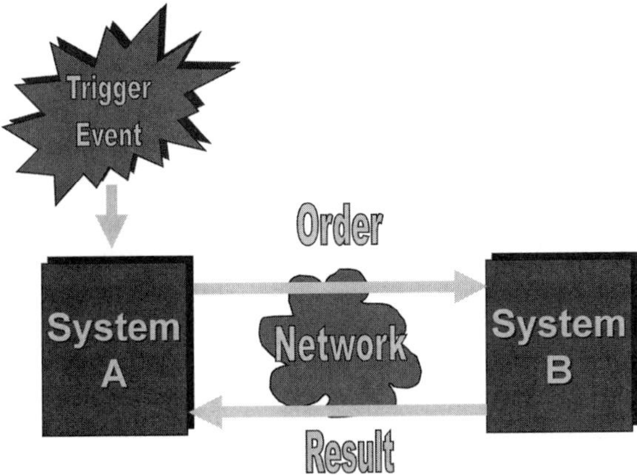

FIGURE 13.3. Trigger events. Trigger events are things that happen in the real world that cause information to be exchanged between systems. In this example, a particular instance of data exchange was triggered by someone placing an order in the ordering system (System A). This action causes an order message to be created and sent to the laboratory system (System B). Entry of the test result into the laboratory information system causes a result message to be created and sent to the ordering system.

direct the message to the correct destination and indicate to the receiving system what kind of message it is.

In the example, the message type has been set to "ORU^M01." A message type of ORU means that this is an unsolicited result message; that is, a message that can be sent whenever results are available. Each field in a message is defined in the standard as a particular data type. Commonly used data types include strings, formatted text, numbers, time stamps, codes, addresses, and person names.

The second segment in Figure 13.4 is a person identification segment (PID), which contains identifying information on the patient that the message is about. The next segment shown is an observation request segment (OBR), which contains information about the context in which the reported data was collected. An ORU message can contain one or more OBR segments, and each OBR segment is followed by one or more OBX (observation) segments. Each OBX segment contains the details of a clinical observation or measurement. In the example, the first OBR segment indicates that the observations to follow are stage/prognostic factors. The subsequent OBX segments contain the T, N, and M stages of the tumor. Subsequent OBR segments and their associated OBX segments provide details of the first treatment and primary site of the tumor.

Fields within an HL7 message are divided into sub-fields using a sub-field delimiter, usually the caret character ("^"). For example, coded fields in HL7 messages are typically represented as triplets consisting of a code, a brief description of the meaning of the code, and the code system from

```
MSH|^~\&|Hospital ABC|Pathology|Tumor Registry QRS|Tumor
Database|20011122100053||ORU^M01|<CR>
PID|||123456789|00000|DOE JOHN||19230306|M||W|123 MAIN STREET ANYTOWN US||S|<CR>
OBR|||XYZ^Registry/22051-7^Stage/prognostic
factors^LN|198703281530|||||||||||||||F<CR>
OBX|1|CE|21899-0^TNM PATH T^LN||T1^T1 STAGE^AJCC||||||F|<CR>
OBX|2|CE|21900-6^TNM PATH N^LN||N0^N0 STAGE^AJCC||||||F|<CR>
OBX|3|CE|21901-4^TNM PATH M^LN||M0^M0 STAGE^AJCC||||||F|<CR>

OBR|||XYZ^SURG|22052-5^Treatment first course^LN|198703281530|||||||||||<CR>
OBX|2|DT|21926-1^DATE RAD^LN||19860628|<CR>

OBR|||XYZ^Lab|22049-1^Cancer Identification^LN|198703281530||||||||||||||||F<CR>
OBX|1|CE|21899-0^Primary Site^LN||C50.4^Upper-outer quad of Breast^ICDO2^T-
4004^Upper-outer quad of Breast^SNM||||||F|<CR>
OBX|2|CE|21900-6^Histology^LN||M8500^Ductal carcinoma^ICDO2||||||F| <CR>
OBX|3|CE|20228-3^Laterality^LN||1^Left^CR410^G-A101^Left^SNM||||||F| <CR>
```

Figure 13.4. Using the HL7 reporting structure to transmit cancer-specific data. As illustrated in italics, this sample message used LOINC codes for the observation and battery identifiers. Various codes are submitted in the observation value location. A comprehensive vocabulary, such as SNOMED, can be supported and reported along with the local values as typically reported in current cancer registration systems. The shaded text illustrates the capability of sending ICD-O codes while including the corresponding but more specific SNOMED codes. The ability to connect the value of a classification to a clinically defined data concept allows integration with clinical decision making and supporting systems. Transmitting both codes in a system permits the association with the medical code, which is usually more specific, while simultaneously maintaining the existing codes, which is often a classification-type code, used for reporting and analysis purposes. The HL7 standard provides a robust method for capturing, identifying, and transmitting standardized clinical values as well as for transmitting the local non-standard code when needed.

which the code was drawn. In the first OBX segment in Figure 13.4, the stage has a value of "T1^T1 STAGE^AJCC." In this case, "T1" is the code, "T1 STAGE" is a brief description of the code, and "AJCC" indicates the coding scheme from which the code was taken. In some situations, a coded field can contain two triplets. The first triplet represents the coded value of the field, and the second triplet represents a translation of the first code into another coding scheme, as shown for the value of laterality in the last OBX segment in the example. The coded value "1^Left^CR410^G-A101^Left^SNM" contains a code of "1" that means "left" as taken from the value set listed in cancer registry table 410 (CR410). This code can be translated as "G-A101," which means "left" in the Systematized Nomenclature of Medicine (SNOMED) coding system (Côté, 1977; Côté et al., 1993).

Vocabulary in HL7 Messages

Figure 13.5 shows the essential parts of an OBX segment, an important construct in HL7 messages. At its heart, the OBX segment is a name-value

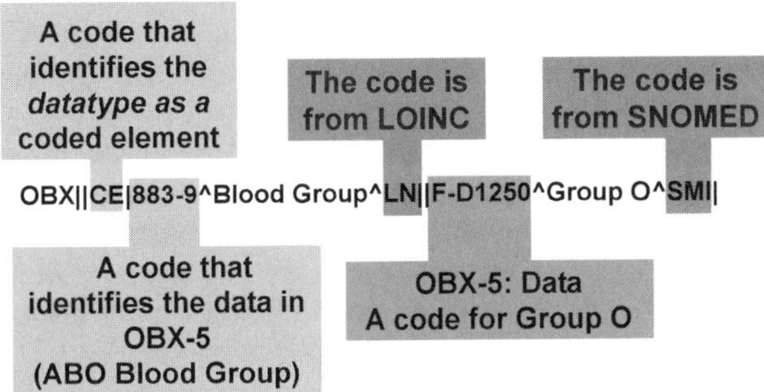

FIGURE 13.5. An OBX segment. An OBX segment is essentially a name-value pair. In this example, the third field in the segment is the *name* part of the name-value pair. In this case, the name has been set to the LOINC code "883-9" indicating that a blood group test was done. Included in the field is a text description of the code, and a label to show that the code came from the LOINC coding scheme. The fifth field in the message carries the *value* part of the name value pair. In this case, the value is the SNOMED code F-D1250, which indicates that the patient's blood type was found to be Type O.

pair. Field 2 of the OBX segment indicates the kind of value (format type) that the OBX segment contains. In this example, the format type is set to "CE," which means that this OBX segment contains a coded value. Field 3 of the OBX segment, called the observation, names the type of observation being reported. In the example, the observation identifier (OBX 3) is set to the Logical Observation Identifier Names and Codes (LOINC) code "883-9" (Forrey et al., 1996; Huff et al., 1998). This means that the OBX segment is reporting the patient's ABO blood group. Field 5 of the OBX segment, called the observation value, contains the value of the observation being reported. In this case, the observation value has been set to "F-D1250," which in the SNOMED coding scheme means "Blood Group O." Taken as a whole, this OBX segment states that the patient's blood type was evaluated and found to be Type O.

The name-value pair construct that the OBX segment offers is a versatile mechanism for data representation. It means that new kinds of data can be sent in an HL7 message by adding terms to the vocabulary, rather than by adding new fields to a message. If a new data element (for example, a new tumor antigen) must be sent in a message, a new field need not be added to a fixed record structure. Instead, a new LOINC code can be added, and the new data element can be transmitted by sending an additional OBX segment that contains the new data element.

The versatility of the OBX segment can also have negative effects. It can lead to multiple possible representations for data. For example, if we return to the cancer information shown in Figure 13.4, we see that there are choices about how the data might have been reported. Ignoring the codes for the moment, the initial representation of the data can be written as:

Primary Site: *Upper-outer quad of Breast*

Laterality: *Left*

This initial representation represents the location of the lesion as a primary site, which is then further modified by the laterality. Alternatively, the same information could have been represented as a single statement:

Primary Site: *Upper-outer quad of Left Breast*

In this case, the value of the primary site includes the laterality as part of the expression. What was represented as two statements in the first instance has been represented as a single statement in the second statement. The two different styles of representation contain the same information, but if the different styles are mixed, data from different sources may not be comparable. The structure of a message depends to some extent on the possible values that exist in the coding system, and the contents of a coding system depend to some extent on the message structure in which the codes are used. The structure of the message and the code set must be considered part of a consistent whole.

Use of Standard Terminologies in Messages

As shown in the preceding example, a division of labor can be seen between LOINC codes and SNOMED codes. LOINC codes were created for the specific purpose of identifying the kind of test, evaluation, or observation made. The kind of value associated with a LOINC code could be a number, a date and time, or a coded (narrative/textual) value. When the value of a LOINC code is of a textual nature, a SNOMED code can be used as a representation of the value. Thus, LOINC codes represent the names of attributes or observations, like hair color or blood type, while SNOMED codes represent the values of the observations, like brown or blonde for hair colors or Type O, Type A, or Type AB for blood types.

Correlation of SNOMED and ICD-O

The International Classification of Diseases for Oncology (ICD-O), is the classification coding system used in cancer registration to code several important and different concepts relevant to a tumor (World Health Organization, 2000; World Health Organization, 1990). The tumor concepts, captured in the ICD-O coding scheme, are the morphological description and the primary site of the tumor. ICD-O is used extensively, both within the United States and internationally (World Health Organization, 1990). The third version of ICD-O, just released in the United States, includes many new morphologic and behavior terms or modifications (World Health Organization, 2000).

TABLE 13.1. A comparison of the granularity of SNOMED and ICD-O codes*

SNOMED	Clinical Concept	ICD-O2/3
T-63000	Gallbladder, NOS	C23.9
T-63000	Cholecystic	C23.9
T-63000	Cholecysto-	C23.9
T-63010	Fundus of gallbladder	C23.9
T-63020	Body of gallbladder	C23.9
T-63030	Neck of gallbladder	C23.9
T-63040	Valve of Heister	C23.9
T-63100	Mucosa of gallbladder	C23.9
T-63110	Mucous gland of gallbladder	C23.9
T-63200	Muscularis of gallbladder	C23.9
T-63300	Serosa of gallbladder	C23.9
T-63310	Subserosa of gallbladder	C23.9
T-63320	Luschka's ducts	C23.9

*In the topography axis, ICD-O has a single code for gallbladder, while SNOMED has many codes corresponding to macroscopic and microscopic subdivision of the gallbladder.

SNOMED and ICD-O coding schemes have a well-documented history (Côté, 1977; World Health Organization, 1990). Although the morphology codes as developed in the ICD-O are the same as the morphological axis in SNOMED, the topography axis in SNOMED is more specific than the classification of site described for ICD-O. Table 13.1 compares the detailed SNOMED breakdown of the gallbladder with the single classification of the ICD-O series. ICD-O codes and SNOMED codes can play complementary roles in a message: ICD-O allows all tumors of an organ to be grouped within a single code, while SNOMED can be used to capture the exact location of the tumor for use in clinical treatment planning.

The Value of HL7 in Cancer Surveillance and Reporting

Cancer surveillance in the United States has a long history, and it is carried out through many different U.S. organizations. Information about cancer cases resides in different types of cancer registries, including hospital-based and population-based registries (Austin, 1983; Menck & Smart, 1994; Swan et al., 1998). The desire to understand the nature and distribution of cancer throughout the United States has led to standards for data exchange between different cancer registries.

The North American Association of Central Cancer Registries (NAACCR), established in 1987, is an association of organizations involved in standards development and the methodological analysis of the surveillance data so crucial to cancer control and epidemiologic research, public health programs, and quality patient care. The sponsoring organizations include the Centers for Disease Control and Prevention, Association of American Cancer Institutes, American Cancer Society, American College of Surgeons, American Joint Committee on Cancer, Laboratory Centre for Disease

Control, Health Canada, National Cancer Institute, National Cancer Registrars Association, and Statistics Canada. By participating in various NAACCR committees, these groups support the definition and refinement of standards and procedures used for collecting and exchanging cancer data (North American Association of Central Cancer Registries, 2000). The NAACCR standard is the primary one used for data exchange between cancer registries.

One issue with the NAACCR standard is its use of a flat file record structure to transmit data. This means that as new types of diagnostic studies and treatments become available, the format of the file must change or data items must be added to the end of the file. In either case, programs that parse and process the data must be changed to accommodate the new data format.

Studies have been launched to assess the potential value of using HL7 to transmit data between cancer registries. Data described in the NAACCR data standard volume were submitted to the LOINC committee, and LOINC codes were assigned to the NAACCR data items. The LOINC codes were designed to map one-to-one with the NAACCR data elements and to unambiguously identify the data item within HL7 messages. When LOINC codes are used as the observation identifier in the name-value pair construct of the HL7 OBX segment, new data elements can be added to a message simply by making new codes. The overall structure of the HL7 message does not change, making it easier to maintain the software that must receive and store the data in an analytical database. It has not yet been determined if using HL7 as a messaging standard between cancer registries is more flexible and cost effective than using the current NAACCR flat file format.

Traditional methods of cancer surveillance are labor-intensive. As shown in Figure 13.6, data are collected via manual chart review of the patient's paper medical record and entered into a computerized cancer registry.

Increasingly, many kinds of patient data are being captured electronically. These include cancer-related information like anatomic pathology reports, drug levels of chemotherapeutic agents, blood counts, and tests for tumor markers and antigens. The electronic capture of these kinds of data heralds a new era for cancer surveillance techniques and cancer data collection. As shown in Figure 13.7, ancillary departments like the pharmacy, clinical laboratory, radiology, and pathology enter data directly into departmental systems. The data is then shared via HL7 messages with other computers.

This presents the opportunity for programs to monitor the stream of data that indicates diagnosis of a new cancer case. New cases could be found within results of x-rays, anatomic pathology studies, or tumor antigens and enzyme levels. Once a new cancer case has been detected, the same data streams can be monitored for treatment and outcomes information. This new mode of cancer detection and reporting is possible because of the increased use of data exchange standards within the clinical environment.

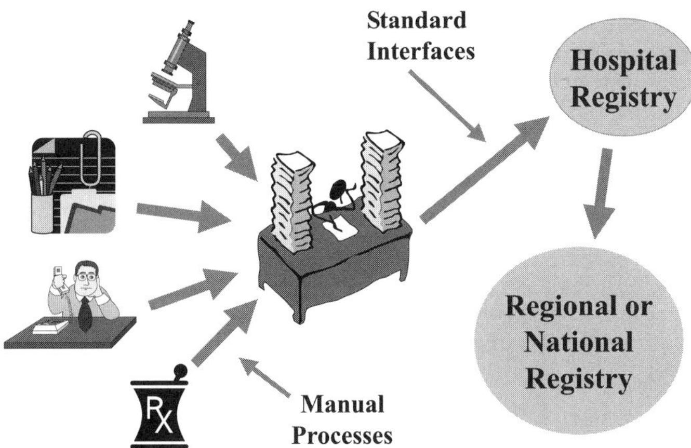

FIGURE 13.6. Typical cancer surveillance and data entry processes. Information is gathered by manual review of paper records. The information is then entered into a computerized hospital registry, and later it can be sent to a regional or national registry.

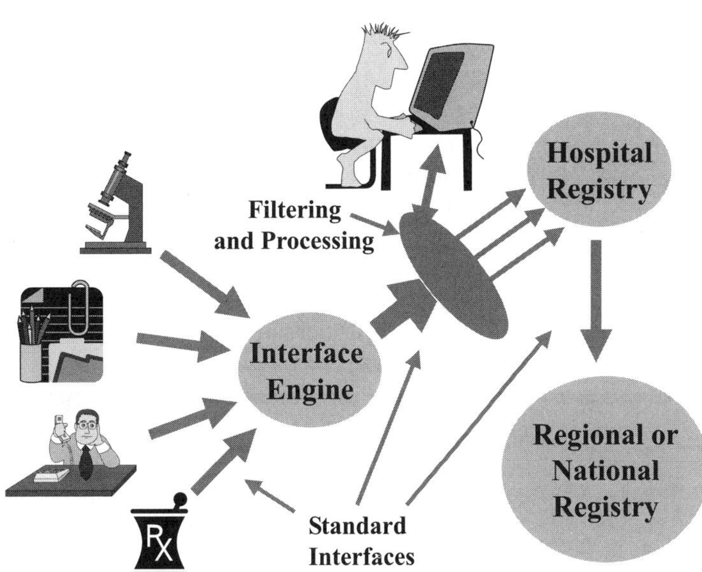

FIGURE 13.7. A potential strategy for cancer surveillance and data collection. In this future strategy, data will be entered electronically in ancillary departments, and programs used to filter and process the data rather than doing manual chart review. Specific filters can be used to monitor the data stream for diagnostic studies that lead to detection of new cancer cases. Once a case is identified, relevant treatment and outcomes data can be automatically added to the cancer registry.

The more consistently clinical information is identified, coded, and transmitted using standard messages and vocabularies, the more reliably it can supply additional information for uses like epidemiological or clinical outcome research. This reduces the effort of manual chart review, data entry, and the associated problems of inconsistent and idiosyncratic coding (Berman & Moore, 1996).

Because of the lack of conformity in the content of information needed, pathology reports have not been an ideal source for cancer information. Synoptic reporting protocols, developed by the Cancer Committee of the College of American Pathologists, are directed at increasing the accuracy and consistency of pathology reporting. There is a need to ensure correct capture of the critical information needed for high quality pathological diagnosis and for patient care and treatment. Incorporating these protocols in the surveillance aspects for cancer prevention and control activities will further streamline data capture and improve reporting timeliness (Compton, 1998).

Using controlled clinical terminologies like LOINC and SNOMED within standard HL7 messages will substantially improve timeliness and completeness of clinical data. These improvements will enhance the quality of cancer data available for effective surveillance. Promoting closer ties with clinically applicable vocabularies and standards groups will enable population-based decisions using clinically derived data.

The integration of hospital registry systems with electronic medical records systems has the benefit of capturing data from the medical chart and providing quality control opportunities for the medical chart. For example, verification of clinical staging information that a hospital registrar or registry system amalgamated from the medical record is needed as a prognostic indicator. Occasionally, a chart contains discrepancies regarding staging information captured by clinical information systems and a registry system (Commission on Cancer Information and Response System, 2000). Through integration and standardization of the registry systems, these quality control checks can benefit both provider and patient. Such discrepancies, if resolved at all, are manually adjusted into the cancer abstract.

Finally, certain activities in cancer registration help position cancer registry data to work in conjunction with standardized HL7 messages and clinical terminologies. A report created by Centers for Disease Control and Prevention (2000) outlines several steps through which cancer registries can apply industry standards. Several cancer registries in Pennsylvania and Washington have pilot projects using the HL7 standard to capture and transmit relevant information from laboratories and other facilities. In California, efforts are underway to develop a hospital registry system that will receive structured HL7 messages and report the information out to central population-based cancer registries.

The use and application of HL7 protocols will help registries open the interface standards so that data capture is streamlined, which can improve timeliness. The current limitations of flat-file reports of data to statewide population-based registries limit real-time reporting, reduce the amount of information, and do not support concise definition of the data contained in the transmission. HL7 standards using structured data types, standard identifiers, and standard vocabularies provide a superior structure for faster evolution to emerging technologies.

The application of HL7, LOINC, and SNOMED codes in cancer registries is not without controversy and challenges (Howe, 2000). Although resolving these and other challenges will certainly place demands on all participants in the cancer registry community, the benefits will strengthen the future of cancer surveillance and enhance the value of electronic medical records.

Looking Ahead

Although our discussion has centered on HL7 messaging standards and related standardized terminologies, the HL7 organization is involved in more than just message standards. There are also standards for visual integration of desktop applications, a standard for representing medical logic, and a standard for representing structured documents using eXtensible Markup Language (XML). Work is underway to create a standard for representing clinical guidelines. Each of these standards could play a role in improving the integration of cancer surveillance and reporting systems into the electronic medical record environment.

The visual integration standard, also known as CCOW (Clinical Context Object Workgroup), allows user context to be passed among multiple open applications on the desktop (Health Level Seven, 2001). For example, a physician might log in to a pharmacy application, select a patient, and review the list of current medications. Seeing that the patient is on Gentamicin, the physician would want to review laboratory data to ensure that the patient has appropriate renal function. When the physician opens the laboratory data review application, information is passed from the pharmacy application that tells the laboratory application who the physician is and which patient the physician is reviewing. The CCOW standard specifies how the user and patient context is shared between two or more open applications on the desktop.

The Arden Syntax Standard (Health Level Seven, 1999) is a language for describing medical logic modules. It allows medical rules to be stated in a formal syntax shareable across different facilities and enterprises. For example, Arden syntax can be used to state a rule that a patient on digoxin with a low serum potassium should receive a potassium supplement. Ongoing work within HL7 aims to define a standard for representing more complicated clinical rules, such as protocols and guidelines.

The Clinical Document Architecture Standard (Health Level Seven, 2000) specifies how different types of narrative reports can be shared between systems as structured XML documents. XML document type definitions

(DTDs) specify the structure for the clinical documents. By adhering to the standard, documents can be more readily processed in an automated fashion and incorporated into research databases or into the patient's electronic medical record.

References

American Society for Testing and Materials (ASTM). 1988. ASTM E1238-88: Standard Specification for Transferring Clinical Observations Between Independent Computer Systems. West Conshohocken, PA: ASTM.

Austin D. 1983. Cancer Registries: A Tool in Epidemiology. Review of Cancer Epidemiology 2:119–140.

Berman JJ, Moore GW. 1996. SNOMED-Encoded Surgical Pathology Databases: A Tool for Epidemiologic Investigation. Modern Pathology 9(9):944–50.

Bidgood WD, Jr, Horii SC. 1992. Introduction to the ACR-NEMA DICOM Standard. Radiographics 12(2):345–355.

Centers for Disease Control and Prevention. 1997. Electronic Reporting of Laboratory Data for Public Health: Meeting Report and Recommendations. Atlanta: Centers for Disease Control and Prevention.

Centers for Disease Control and Prevention. 2000. Working Toward Implementation of HL7 in NAACCR Information Technology Standards. Atlanta: Centers for Disease Control and Prevention.

College of Healthcare Information Management Executives (CHIME) and HCIA, Inc. 1998. The 1998 H.I.S. Desk Reference: A CIO Survey. Ann Arbor: CHIME and HICA, Inc.

Commission on Cancer. Information and Response System. 2000. Available at web.facs.org/coc/default.htm. Accessed November 2000.

Compton CC. 1998. Reporting on Cancer Specimens, Protocols and Case Summaries. Skokie, IL: College of American Pathologists.

Côté RA. 1977. Systematized Nomenclature of Medicine. Skokie, IL: College of American Pathologists.

Côté RA, et al. 1993. The Systematized Nomenclature of Human and Veterinary Medicine—SNOMED International. Northfield, IL: College of American Pathologists.

Effler P, et al. 1999. Statewide System of Electronic Notifiable Disease Reporting from Clinical Laboratories: Comparing Automated Reporting with Conventional Methods. JAMA 282(19):1845–1850.

Hammond WE. 1988. Transferring Clinical Lab Data Between Independent Computer Systems. ASTM Standardization News: (November):28–30.

Forrey AW, et al. 1996. Logical Observation Identifier Names and Codes (LOINC) Database: A Public Use Set of Codes and Names for Electronic Reporting of Clinical Laboratory Test Results. Clinical Chemistry 42(1):81–90.

Health Insurance Portability and Accountability Act (HIPAA). 1996.

Health Level Seven. 1987. Health Level Seven Standard Version 1.0. Ann Arbor: Health Level Seven.

Health Level Seven. 1999. Arden Syntax for Medical Logic Systems. Ann Arbor: Health Level Seven.

Health Level Seven. 2000. Version 3 Standard: Clinical Document Architecture Release 1.0. Ann Arbor: Health Level Seven.

Health Level Seven. 2001. CCOW Version 1.3. Ann Arbor: Health Level Seven.

Howe H. 2000. Adopting the HL7 Standard for Cancer Registry Work: Clarifying Unresolved Issues. One: Incidence. In Cancer Incidence in North America, 1993–1997. Springfield, IL: North American Association of Central Cancer Registries (NAACCR) www.naacr.org/data/cina9397/vone-7.pdf

Huff SM, et al. 1998. Development of the LOINC (Logical Observation Identifier Names and Codes) Vocabulary. Journal of American Medical Informatics Association 5(3):276–292.

Institute of Electrical and Electronics Engineers (IEEE). 1990. IEEE Standard Computer Dictionary: A Compilation of IEEE Standard Computer Glossaries. New York: IEEE.

Lindberg DA, Humphreys BL, McCray AT. 1993. The Unified Medical Language System. Methods of Information in Medicine 32(4):281–91.

Logical Observation Identifier Names and Codes (LOINC®) Committee. 1995. Logical Observation Identifier Names and Codes (LOINC®) Users' Guide vs. 1.0 – Release 1.0j. Indianapolis: Regenstrief Institute.

Menck H, Smart C. 1994. Central Cancer Registries Design, Management and Use. Newark, NJ: Harwood Academic.

McDonald CJ. 1984. The Search for National Standards for Medical Data Exchange (Editorial). MD Computing 1(1):3–4.

McDonald CJ, Hammond WE. 1989. Standard Formats for Electronic Transfer of Clinical Data (Editorial). Annals of Internal Medicine 110(5):333–335.

National Electrical Manufacturers Association (NEMA). 1997. NEMA PS 3.1–PS 3.12: Digital Imaging and Communications in Medicine (DICOM). 1997. Rosslyn, VA: NEMA.

National Library of Medicine (NLM). 1993. UMLS® Knowledge Sources. Bethesda, MD: NLM. p. 157.

North American Association of Central Cancer Registries. 2000. Springfield, IL: North American Association of Central Cancer Registries.

Simborg DW. 1984a. Local Area Networks: Why? What? What If? MD Computing 1(4):10–20.

Simborg DW. 1984b. Networking and Medical Information Systems. Journal of Medical Systems 8(1–2):43–47.

Swan J, et al. 1998. Cancer Surveillance in the US: Can We Have a National System? Cancer 83(7): 1282–1291.

World Health Organization (WHO). 1990. International Classification of Diseases for Oncology, 2nd ed. Geneva: WHO.

World Health Organization (WHO). 2000. International Classification of Diseases for Oncology, 3rd ed. US Interim Version 2000 Edition. Geneva: WHO.

14
The Health Level Seven Reference Information Model

Abdul-Malik Shakir

An information model documents information from a particular functional domain, for a specific purpose, using a formal specification language. It consists of a graphical expression accompanied by a data dictionary, both of which use predefined symbols, semantics, and rules of construction.

Information models have several uses. Primarily, they increase understanding of information in a domain by unambiguously communicating the modeler's understanding. Information models help reconcile multiple perspectives on information into a single specification. They can document the design of an information system's data component so the design can be evaluated and enhanced. Information models also help reveal assumptions, reduce ambiguity, reconcile and expand understanding, and consolidate ideas.

The Health Level Seven (HL7) Reference Information Model (RIM) is the model from which the information-related content of HL7 version 3.0 protocol specification standards is drawn. The HL7 RIM, which documents information from the healthcare domain, is the consensus view of information from the HL7 working group and international affiliates. It uses notation based on the Uniform Modeling Language (UML) and the information modeling conventions outlined in the HL7 message development framework. In this chapter, we provide an introduction to the HL7 RIM, including its history and purpose, a description of its structure and content, a summary of its maintenance process, its use by HL7 and others, and a glimpse of future directions.

History of the HL7 RIM

Development of the HL7 RIM began in April 1996. As Table 14.1 indicates, the model combined the content of specific information models developed by HL7 technical committees, standards development organizations, and HL7 member organizations.

The HL7 Technical Steering Committee received a preliminary version of the RIM at the HL7 working group meeting held in August 1996 in

TABLE 14.1. Information models used to develop the HL7 RIM

HL7 Technical Committees	• Admission/Discharge/Transfer • Finance • Medical Records • Orders/Results • Patient Care
Standards Development Organizations	• CEN TC251 • DICOM
HL7 Member Organizations	• Eli Lilly and Company • HBO and Company • Health Data Sciences • IBM Worldwide • Kaiser Permanente • Mayo Foundation • Hewlett Packard

Washington, D.C. The first release of the RIM, intended for use in developing version 3.0 messages, was distributed to the HL7 technical committees at the January 1997 working group meeting in Tampa, Florida. This release was known as the HL7 draft RIM version 0.80.

The next two working group meetings focused on gaining familiarity with the draft RIM and implementing a process for obtaining and reconciling the technical committee's proposed enhancements to the model. The RIM maintenance process became known as "RIM harmonization."

The HL7 RIM Harmonization Process

The HL7 RIM harmonization process is a major source of strength for the model. Through this process, HL7's vast community of subject matter experts validate the content of the RIM and shape it into a comprehensive, consistent, and credible representation of healthcare information needs. The harmonization process ensures that the model is a consensus view of the entire HL7 workgroup. Following is a step-by-step outline of the process.

- **Prepare a RIM change proposal.** HL7 technical committees, special interest groups, and international affiliates propose changes to the RIM to enhance its content and make it more suitable for producing protocol specification standards. Accredited standards developing organizations and HL7 individual or corporate members may also submit changes. The change proposal identifies the affected components of the RIM and the rationale for the change.
- **Review the change proposal with steward technical committees.** For each component of the RIM, the technical committee that has primary accountability for the component's subject matter is assigned to serve as steward. These stewards review the change proposals and acknowledge support or opposition. The submitter considers this input and may choose to revise or withdraw the proposed change.

- **Submit the change proposal for harmonization.** If the change proposal is not withdrawn, it is submitted to HL7 headquarters for consideration at the next harmonization meeting. Submitted change proposals are posted to the HL7 Web site, and HL7 members are notified of the posting via e-mail. In this way, members are able to comment on the proposal and prepare their arguments for or against it prior to the harmonization meeting. All proposed changes to the RIM are posted at least 30 days prior to the meeting.
- **Discuss the change proposal at the harmonization meeting.** The RIM harmonization meeting, scheduled approximately midway between working group meetings, is open to all HL7 members and members of accredited standards developing organizations. Submitters of change proposals, representatives of steward committees, and modeling/vocabulary facilitators must attend the harmonization meeting.

  Attendees discuss each proposed change to the RIM in detail. Submitters share the rationale for the changes they propose. The steward technical committees then share their views on the proposed change and indicate support or opposition, and the remaining participants also contribute comments for or against the proposal.

  Following this discussion, the submitter has several options. He or she may revise the change proposal in response to objections, table the changes, or withdraw the proposal.
- **Vote on the RIM change proposal.** Change proposals that are neither tabled nor withdrawn are subjected to a vote to determine their disposition. If the steward technical committee favors the change, a simple majority can approve the change. If the committee opposes the change, two-thirds of the voters must vote favorably before the change can be approved. Only technical committee steward representatives and a representative from the International Committee can vote.

  The vote and disposition of each change proposal is recorded. Possible dispositions are "approved," "approved with changes," "tabled," "withdrawn," and "rejected." All approved changes are applied to the RIM for use at the next working group meeting.

Major Themes of the HL7 RIM Harmonization Meetings

Between 1998 and 2000, there were nine harmonization meetings to consider proposed enhancements to the draft RIM. The meetings culminated in version 1.0 of the HL7 RIM, unveiled at the HL7 working group meeting held in January 2001 in Orlando, Florida. The harmonization meetings focused on five major themes:

- **Ensure coverage of HL7 version 2.x.** This set of change proposals introduced content to the draft model to ensure that it included all the information content of HL7 version 2.x. Several technical committees continue to maintain a mapping from the RIM to the 2.x standard.

- **Remove unsubstantiated content from the model.** This set of change proposals focused on removing content from the draft model that the steward technical committee did not originate and could find no rationale for retaining.
- **Unify service action model.** This set of change proposals was the result of collaboration between multiple technical committees to simplify the way clinical information is represented in the draft model. It introduced a concise, well-defined set structures and vocabularies that address the information needs of a wide variety of clinical scenarios.
- **Ensure quality.** This set of change proposals addressed inconsistencies in the draft model and conflicts between the model and the modeling style guide. It began the practice of recording and tracking open issues in the model. The steward technical committee must close all open issues before using the model component in a balloted protocol specification. Open issues are generally resolved within one or two working group meetings.
- **Address the left hand side of the model.** This set of change proposals introduced powerful structures and vocabularies for the non-clinical portions of the model (patient administration, finance, scheduling). Like other efforts, this proposal involved the combined effort of multiple technical committees.

The harmonization process and themes have produced an HL7 reference information model that is credible, clear, comprehensive, concise, and consistent. Its structure is both flexible and extensible, and its contents can be readily mapped to the HL7 2.x message standard and other widely used healthcare dataset specifications.

Structure and Content of the RIM

To fully understand the structure and content of the HL7 RIM, we must first understand the Unified Modeling Language (UML). The UML specifies a set of constructs and symbols for use in constructing an information model. Figure 14.1 illustrates the components of a UML-based information model.

A class, the major component of a UML-based information model, represents a classification of objects that have common characteristics. There are 112 classes in release 1.0 of the RIM. Subject areas partition the model into convenient class groupings. Many subject area collections in the RIM are used to administer and aid in understanding of the model. The primary partitioning of the model separates its semantic content from the structural content. The major partitions are semantic content, structured documents, and message control. The semantic content partition contains 64 classes, the structured documents partition contains 27 classes, and the message control partition contains 20 classes.

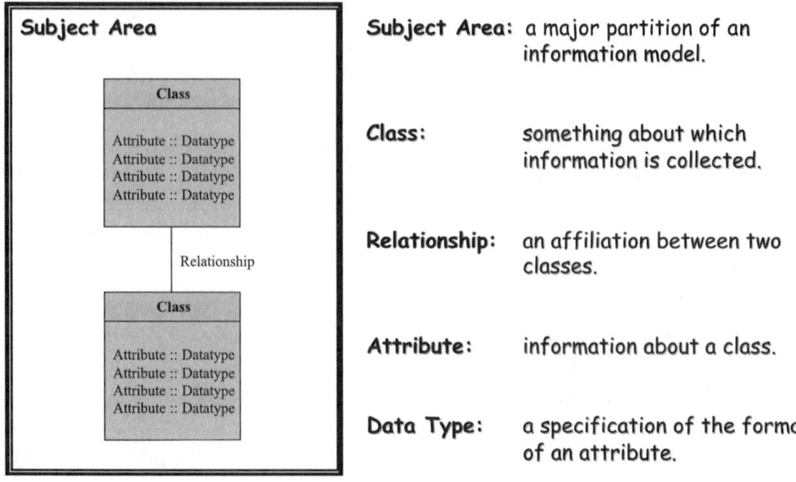

FIGURE **14.1.** Components of a UML-based information model.

RIM Classes and Relationships

There are four primary classes in the semantic content partition of the RIM.

- **An entity** is a physical thing, organization, or group. The concept of entity includes human beings and other living organisms, devices, pharmaceutical substances, and other materials, organizations, and places.
- **A role** is a timebound named function of an entity. The concept of role includes healthcare provider, military person, and notary public.
- **An act** is an intentional action. The concept of act includes patient encounters, referrals, procedures, observations, and financial acts.
- **A participation** is a link between an act and a role. The concept of participation includes actor, target, and primary participant.

There are also four basic relationship types used in the RIM: association, generalization, composition, and aggregation. An association relationship, which indicates dependence between classes, is the least complex type. Association relationships link the four primary classes. Entity and act are independent classes, role depends on entity, and participation depends on role and act. Figure 14.2 illustrates this with a straight line drawn between the classes.

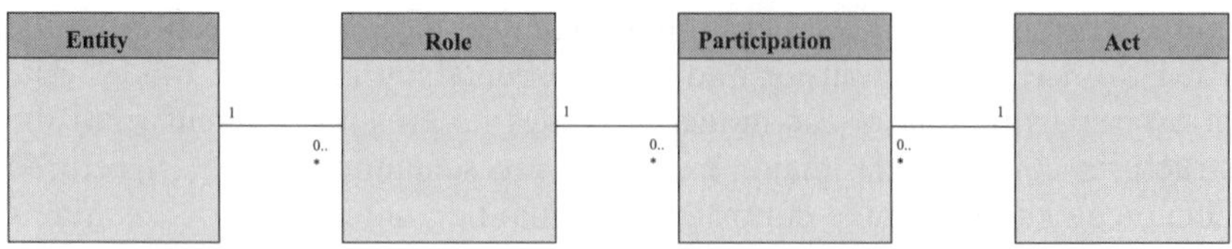

FIGURE **14.2.** Association relationships of the four primary classes.

The association line is annotated with multiplicities indicating the ratio of classes involved in the relationship. The annotation "1" signifies one and only one, "0..1" indicates zero or one, "0..*" signifies zero or many, and "1..*" indicates one or many. Association relationships among the four primary RIM classes have the following multiplicities:

- Each **entity** is associated with zero or many [0..*] **role.**
- Each **role** is associated with one and only one [1] **entity**.
- Each **role** is associated with zero or many [0..*] **participation**.
- Each **participation** is associated with one and only one [1] **role**.
- Each **act** is associated with zero or many [0..*] **participation**.
- Each **participation** is associated with one and only one [1] **act**.

Two additional core classes are **role relationship** and **act relationship**. A role relationship captures the linkage between one instance of role and another instance, and an act relationship captures the linkage between one instance of an act and another.

Figure 14.3 depicts the six core classes on which the rest of the RIM is built. Entities assume roles and participate in acts. Some acts are related to other acts, and some entity roles are related to other entity roles.

The remaining classes of the RIM are related either directly or indirectly to these core classes. Most classes are related to these core classes by way of a generalization relationship, which depicts a special kind of relationship between classes. On one end of the relationship is a general concept, and on the other end is a specialization of that concept. For example, the class entity has a generalization relationship with the classes living subject, material, organization, and place. The relationship indicates that a living subject, a material, an organization, and a place are all types of entities. Figure 14.4 depicts the generalization relationships by a line with an arrowhead on one end pointing toward the generic class.

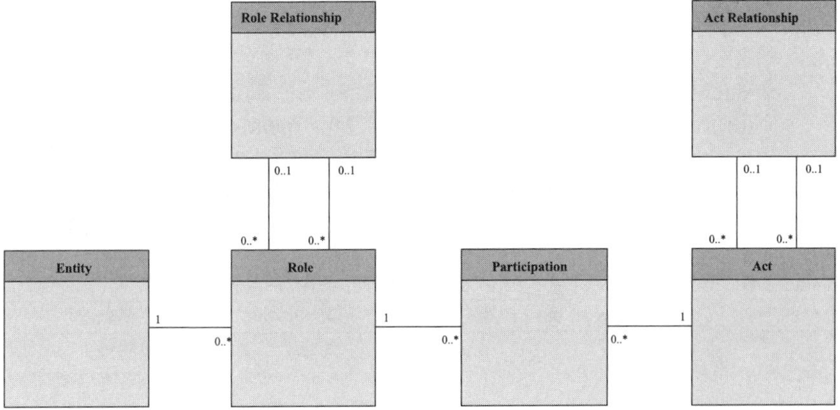

FIGURE 14.3. The six core classes of the RIM.

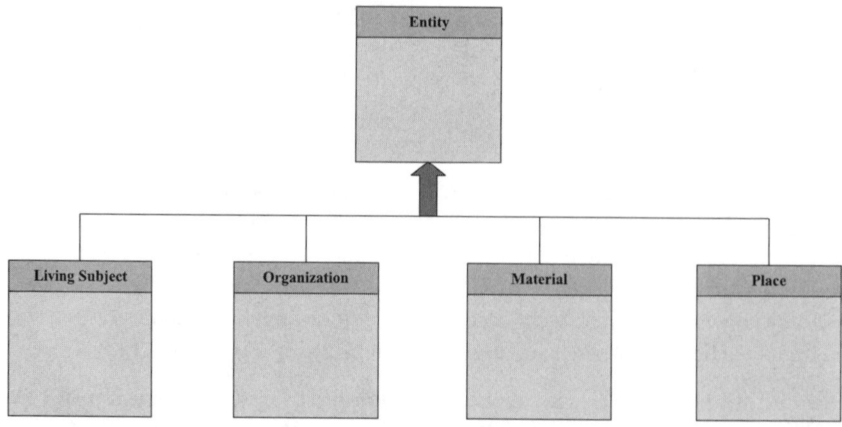

FIGURE 14.4. The generalization relationship in the RIM.

The RIM contains generalization relationships to the classes entity, role, role relationship, and act. Some of the special types of role are notary public, military person, and healthcare provider. The role type "healthcare provider" has a generalization relationship with the class "individual healthcare practitioner," a special type of healthcare provider. Generalizations have specializations, and the specializations may have specializations of their own. The collection of classes, connected in the tree-like structure of generalizations and specializations, are known collectively as a generalization hierarchy.

A generalization hierarchy has both depth and width. The depth is a measure of the maximum number of levels in the tree, and the width is a measure of the number of branches stemming from the root class. The act generalization hierarchy contains 27 classes and has a depth of 3 and a width of 12. By far the most expressive in the model, this hierarchy defines the information content of all clinical, administrative, and financial acts. Table 14.2 summarizes the dimensions of the four RIM generalization hierarchies.

The generalization hierarchies contain 51 of the 64 classes that comprise the semantic content portion of the RIM. This means that by focusing on the four root classes, we can conceptualize 80% of the model. All the specializations within the generalization hierarchy inherit the semantic properties (definition, attributes, and relationships) of the root classes.

TABLE 14.2. Dimensions of the four RIM generalization hierarchies

Root Class	Number of Classes	Depth	Width
Entity	13	3	6
Role	5	2	3
Role relationship	6	1	5
Act	27	3	12

RIM Attributes and Datatypes

The classes and relationships of the RIM provide a structural framework and semantic context for its information content, comprised of attributes and datatypes. An attribute is a property of a class. It is an abstraction of the relevant information about a class—information that can be communicated, stored, modified, and queried. Attributes make up the information in HL7.

Datatypes are the basic building blocks of attributes. They define the structural format of the data carried in the attribute and influence the set of allowable values an attribute may assume. Datatypes have very little intrinsic semantic content. The semantic context for a datatype is carried by its corresponding attribute. Every attribute in the RIM is associated with one and only one datatype, and each datatype is associated with zero or many attributes.

There are 466 attributes in the RIM: 348 in the semantic content partition, 62 in the message control partition, and 56 in the structured document partition. The 348 attributes in the semantic content partition are associated with 21 unique datatypes. Figure 14.5 includes 16 essential attributes of the core classes.

Just as understanding the semantics of the six core classes helps us understand the structure and context of the entire model, understanding these 16 attributes helps us understand the information content of the model. The following are brief descriptions of the 16 essential attributes, grouped by the six core classes.

- **Entity**
  - **Type_CD : CC.** A code indicating the category of entity and the specific type within that category. Broad categories included in the domain

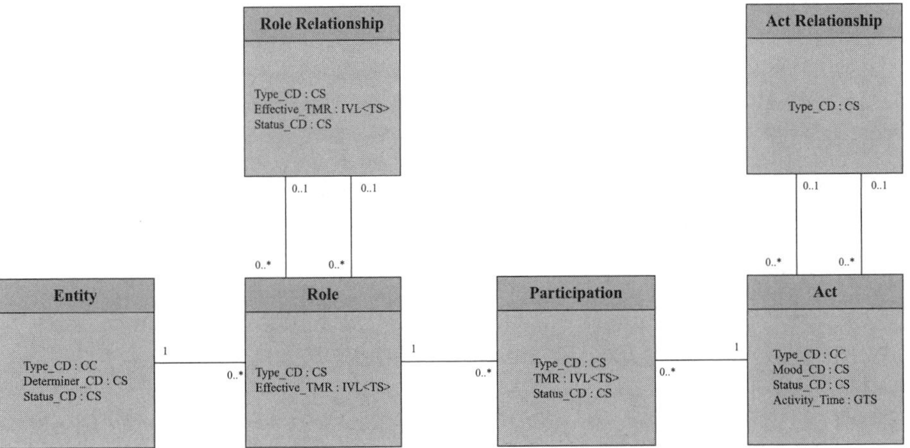

FIGURE 14.5. Sixteen essential attributes of the core classes.

  specification for entity type include material, living subject, animal, plant, human being, chemical substance, organization, and place.
  - This attribute provides great flexibility and extensibility for the concept of entity. Because the coding system for Type_CD is hierarchical, an entity can be declared at any level of specificity. This code can expand the concept of entity beyond the specializations included as classes in the RIM.
- **Determiner_CD : CS.** A code used to denote if the entity represents:
  - a class of thing, such as animal, human being, and state
  - a particular instance of a thing, such as Francis the talking mule, Fredrick Douglas, and California, or
  - a qualified grouping of things, such as a herd of cows, members in a health plan, or counties in a state.

This attribute helps keep the RIM concise by reusing the structure for entity instead of including additional classes for these variations in perspective.

- **Status_CD : CS.** A code indicating the state of the entity. Possible states include proposed, pending, existing, terminated, and imagined. This attribute allows the distinction between real and imagined, existing and non-existing entities.
- **Role**
  - **Type_CD : CC.** A code indicating the role an entity assumes over time. Possible roles include notary public, military person, healthcare provider, and individual healthcare provider. This attribute is another way to extend the concept of entity. It allows an entity, such as a person, to assume the role of patient, individual provider, donor, or next of kin.
  - **Effective_TMR : IVL < TS >.** The effective time range in which the entity assumed the role indicated by Type_CD. The time range, specified as a low and a high, constrains the period of time the entity role is in effect.
- **Role Relationship**
  - **Type_CD : CC.** A code indicating the type of relationship that exists between two entities. Possible relationship types include has, has part, has generalization, has dependent, and has owner. The vocabulary domain for this attribute does not specify the entity roles on either side of the relationship. The role relationship class is associated with a source and target entity role.
  - **Effective_TMR : IVL < TS >.** The time range that the relationship between the entities was in effect, noted as a low to high time specification.
  - **Status_CD : CS.** A code indicating the state of role relationship. Possible role relationship states include proposed, pending, existing, terminated, and imagined. This attribute allows the distinction between real and imagined, existing and non-existing role relationships.
- **Participation**
  - **Type_CD : CS.** A code indicating the type of participation the entity has in an act. Possible participation types include performer, reviewer,

subject, and tracker. This attribute captures participation in an act, and the vocabulary domain for this attribute must consider the distinction between this act participation type and an entity role type code.
  - **Status_CD : CS.** A code indicating the state of act participation. Possible act participations states include proposed, pending, existing, terminated, and imagined. This attribute allows distinction between real and imagined, existing and non-existing act participations.
- **Act**
  - **Type_CD : CC.** A code indicating the type of act. Possible types of act include observation, procedure, referral, billing, authorization, and consent. This attribute provides great flexibility and extensibility; because the coding system for Type_CD is hierarchical, an act can be declared at any level of specificity. This code expands the concept of act beyond the specializations included as classes in the RIM.
  - **Mood_CD : CS.** A code used to denote if the act is:
    - a definition, such as a master list of possible acts
    - an intent, such as a plan, goal, or objective
    - an order, such as a directed request for a clinical service
    - an event, such as the occurrence of an actual act
    - a criterion, such as a pre-condition or qualification.

This attribute is an essential property of the act class. It enables the RIM to concisely represent clinically relevant information.

  - **Activity_Time : GTS.** The time of an act. The general-timing-specification (GTS) datatype of activity time specifies the act as a single point in time, a series of points in time, a period of time, or an arbitrary collection of points in time and time periods. This attribute is not relevant for all moods of act. Depending on mood of act, this attribute may represent points in time or time periods that have not yet occurred.
  - **Status_CD : CS.** A code indicating the state of act. Possible act states include active, suspended, cancelled, aborted, and completed. This attribute specifies the allowable states of an act and defines allowable state transitions, such as active to suspended, suspended to cancel, suspended to active, and active to complete. The state transitions become the basis for trigger events, interactions, and messages.
- **Act Relationship**
  - **Type_CD : CS.** A code indicating the type of act relationship. Possible types of act relationships include the following: has component, has precondition, has outcome, is pertinent to, is revision of, replaces, and fulfills. This attribute allows multiple acts to relate to each other. Relating acts of different types, moods, times, and status can result in an infinite range of clinical concepts.

HL7 maintains the vocabulary domains for these essential RIM attributes. Some of the vocabulary domains (those for attributes with a datatype of CC) combine HL7 categories and external vocabulary domains. These coded attributes are known as "structure attributes," because they provide an alternative to using data modeling structures (i.e., classes and relationships) to convey the same concepts. This modeling style makes the RIM much more concise and provides tremendous flexibility and extensibility. New concepts can be easily introduced to the RIM through HL7 controlled vocabulary domains without affecting the structural validity of the model. The result is model stability.

Using the RIM

The HL7 Message Development Framework (MDF) documents the process for constructing, maintaining, and applying the RIM for use in developing HL7 message specifications. Using the RIM for message development involves three steps, depicted in Figure 14.6:

- defining the Message Information Model (MIM)
- defining the Refined Message Information Model (R-MIM)
- creating a Hierarchical Message Definition (HMD).

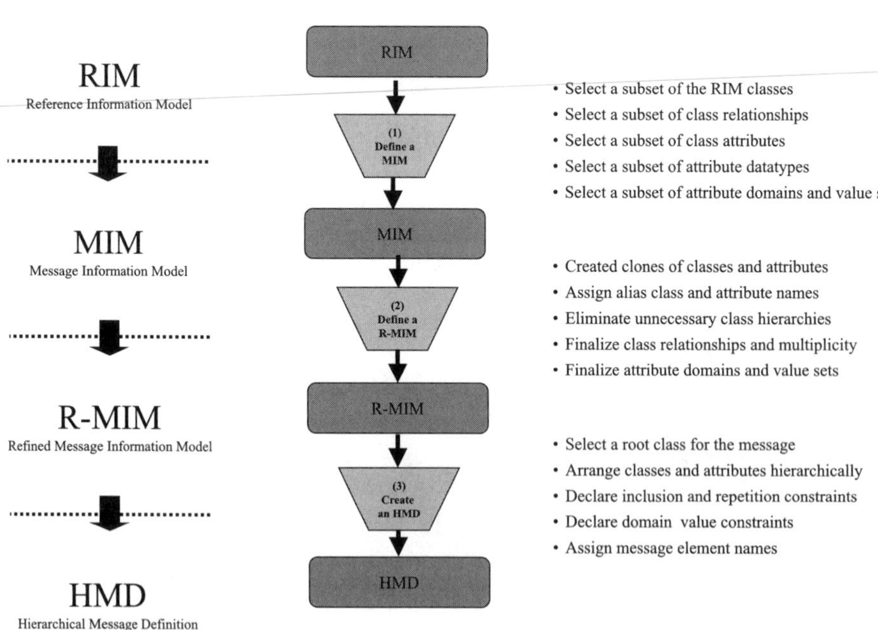

FIGURE 14.6. Steps in using the RIM for message development.

The HL7 Development Framework (HDF), which replaces the Message Development Framework, includes processes for developing non-message HL7 standard specifications like structured documents, components, and clinical decision support specifications using the RIM. As of this writing, the HDF is still in development.

The RIM is a tool to define version 3.0 message specifications and influence the content of the HL7 Clinical Document Architecture and the HL7 visual integration component specification. U.S. government organizations also use the RIM; examples include the Veterans Association (VA), Health Care Financing Administration (HCFA), the Centers for Disease Control and Prevention (CDC), and HL7 joint activities with other standards developing organizations like the European Committee for Standardization *Comité Européen De Normalisation* (CEN), the X12 Insurance Subcommittee Healthcare Taskgroup, and the American College of Radiology (ACR) and National Electrical Manufacturers Association (NEMA).

Looking Ahead

The HL7 RIM version 1.0 took five years to develop. Its modeling style is easy to understand and strikes a balance between extensibility and stability. The major strength of the model is the HL7 development methodology, which includes an open consensus-driven process for leveraging and harmonizing the clinical, administrative, and technical expertise and perspectives of HL7's large and diverse membership.

The HL7 RIM provided information-related content for HL7 version 3.0 protocol specification standards, but it can do much more. In the near future, vocabulary domains will emerge for coded RIM attributes, vendors will incorporate the RIM in the design of their software products, and other standards developing organizations will base the information component of their standards specifications on the HL7 RIM. As these developments unfold, the HL7 RIM will be further enhanced as part of a continuous quality improvement process.

References

Health Level Seven, Modeling and Methodology Technical Committee. 1999. HL7 Message Development Framework. Ann Arbor: Health Level Seven.

Health Level Seven, Modeling and Methodology Technical Committee. 2000. HL7 Reference Information Model. Version 1.00-20001220. Ann Arbor: Health Level Seven.

Health Level Seven, Modeling and Methodology Technical Committee. 2000. HL7 Vocabulary Domain Listings for RIM 1.0. Ann Arbor: Health Level Seven.

Health Level Seven. 2001. HL7 V3.0 Datatype Specification Version 0.90. Ann Arbor: Health Level Seven.

15
HIPAA Administrative Simplification Standards: Provisions of the Final Privacy Rule Related to Clinical Trials

William R. Braithwaite

Background

On December 28, 2000, the U.S. Department of Health and Human Services (HHS) published a final rule that set standards for health information privacy. This rule implements the privacy requirements of the Administrative Simplification subtitle of the Health Insurance Portability and Accountability Act of 1996 (HIPAA) and has three major purposes:

- to protect and enhance the rights of consumers by providing them access to their health information and controlling the inappropriate use of that information,
- to improve the quality of health care in the U.S. by restoring trust in the healthcare system among consumers, healthcare professionals, and the multitude of organizations and individuals committed to the delivery of care, and
- to improve the efficiency and effectiveness of healthcare delivery by creating a national framework for health privacy protection that builds on efforts by states, health systems, and individual organizations and individuals.

Other rules issued under the Administrative Simplification provisions of HIPAA set standards for administrative transactions, code sets, identifiers, and electronic information system security. This chapter discusses only the privacy provisions relevant to the conduct of clinical trials that are different from those that apply under all other situations.

Research

The rule defines *research* to mean a systematic investigation, including research development, testing, and evaluation, designed to develop or contribute to generalizable knowledge. This definition distinguishes research from similar activities (from the perspective of data collection and analysis) commonly used in healthcare operations, marketing, quality assessment, and oversight. The rule further distinguishes between research that only uses protected health information, such as records review, and research that includes treatment of research participants, such as clinical trials.

General Rules

The rule covers only the following entities: health plans, healthcare clearinghouses, and healthcare providers who transmit health information in electronic form in connection with a transaction for which a standard has been set under HIPAA. Such covered entities may not use or disclose protected health information for use in clinical trials research except pursuant to permission from the patient or as permitted by the sections of the final privacy rule that describe uses and disclosures allowed without patient permission. There are four types of patient permission relevant to clinical trials:

- consent to use or disclose information for treatment, payment, and healthcare operations
- patient authorization for use or disclosure of health information created for research that includes treatment
- authorization obtained for patient participation in the clinical trial
- if protected health information from old records is required for the research project, separate authorization may be required to obtain the necessary information from the previous provider(s).

A covered healthcare provider may condition participation in the research study and the provision of research-related treatment on the execution by the prospective research participant of an authorization permitting the researcher to use or disclose health information created for the research study.

Use of information for a clinical trial may proceed without this patient authorization if the researcher obtains documentation that an institutional review board (IRB) or similar board, called a privacy board, found that specified criteria were met and specified procedures were followed to grant a waiver. Criteria that must be followed for such decisions and documentation requirements are specified below. The Department of Health and Human Services (HHS) expects that researchers will rarely seek such waivers of authorization for clinical trials. There are other exceptions to the requirement for patient authorization (review of information preparatory to research, use of de-identified information, use of information on deceased) that may be more relevant to research other than clinical trials.

When using or disclosing protected health information or when requesting protected health information from another covered entity, a covered entity must make reasonable efforts to limit protected health information to the minimum necessary to accomplish the intended purpose of the use, disclosure, or request. This "minimum necessary" rule must be applied to the use of and requests for information for clinical trials, per se, but not to information used or disclosed for treatment purposes or otherwise with patient authorization. The minimum necessary rule can be satisfied by documenting a brief description of the protected health information for which the IRB or privacy board determined that use or access is necessary for the research.

Notice of Privacy Practices

An individual has a right to adequate notice of the uses and disclosures of protected health information that may be made by the covered entity, and of the individual's rights and the covered entity's legal duties with respect to protected health information. A covered entity may not use or disclose protected health information in a manner inconsistent with such notice, including research. Although the notice must state that use and disclosure of protected health information for research is permitted by the rule, in its notice a covered entity may elect to prohibit the use or disclosure of protected health information for research. If a covered entity's notice contains such a prohibition, such notice is binding and such information may not be used for research purposes without patient authorization, unless the covered entity first changes its notice.

Authorization for Clinical Trial

A valid patient authorization for use or disclosure of protected health information for a clinical trial must be written in plain language and must contain at least the following elements:

- a description of the information to be used or disclosed that identifies the information in a specific and meaningful fashion
- the name or other specific identification of the person(s), or class of persons, authorized to make the requested use or disclosure
- the name or other specific identification of the person(s), or class of persons, to whom the covered entity may make the requested use or disclosure
- an expiration date or an expiration event that relates to the individual or the purpose of the use or disclosure
- a statement of the individual's right to revoke the authorization in writing and the exceptions to the right to revoke, together with a description of how the individual may revoke the authorization
- a statement that information used or disclosed pursuant to the authorization may be subject to re-disclosure by the recipient and no longer be protected by this rule

- signature of the individual and date
- if the authorization is signed by a personal representative of the individual, a description of such representative's authority to act for the individual
- a statement that the covered entity will not condition treatment, payment, or enrollment in the health plan or eligibility for benefits on the obtaining of the authorization—except as permitted by the rule
- a description of each purpose of the requested use or disclosure
- a statement that the individual may:
  - inspect or copy the protected health information to be used or disclosed, and
  - refuse to sign the authorization
- if use or disclosure of the requested information will result in direct or indirect remuneration to the covered entity from a third party, a statement that such remuneration will result
- a description of the extent to which such protected health information will be used or disclosed to carry out treatment, payment, or healthcare operations
- a description of any protected health information that will not be used or disclosed for purposes permitted under the rule without patient permission, provided that the covered entity may not include a limitation affecting its right to make a use or disclosure that is required by law, and
- if the covered entity has obtained or intends to obtain the individual's consent for treatment, payment, or healthcare operations, or has provided or intends to provide the individual with a notice of privacy practices, the authorization must refer to that consent or notice, as applicable, and state that the statements made are binding.

Such an authorization may be in the same document as: a consent to participate in the research; a consent to use or disclose protected health information to carry out treatment, payment, or healthcare operations; and the notice of privacy practices. A covered entity must provide the individual with a copy of the signed authorization.

Without Authorization

A covered entity may use or disclose protected health information for research without patient permission, regardless of the source of funding of the research, provided that the covered entity obtains documentation stating that a waiver of the individual authorization required for use or disclosure of protected health information has been approved by either an Institutional Review Board (IRB) or a privacy board. A privacy board must: have members with varying backgrounds and appropriate professional competency as necessary to review the effect of the research protocol on the individual's privacy rights and related interests; include at least one member who is not affiliated with the covered entity, not affiliated with any entity conducting or sponsoring the research, and not related to any person who is affiliated with any of such entities; and must not have any member participating in a review of any project in which the member has a conflict of interest.

Appropriate documentation includes a statement that the IRB or privacy board has determined that the waiver of authorization satisfies the following criteria:

- The use or disclosure of protected health information involves no more than minimal risk to the individuals.
- The alteration or waiver will not adversely affect the privacy rights and the welfare of the individuals.
- The research could not practicably be conducted without the alteration or waiver.
- The research could not practicably be conducted without access to and use of the protected health information.
- The privacy risks to individuals whose protected health information is to be used or disclosed are reasonable in relation to the anticipated benefits, if any, to the individuals, and the importance of the knowledge that may reasonably be expected to result from the research.
- There is an adequate plan to protect the identifiers from improper use and disclosure.
- There is an adequate plan to destroy the identifiers at the earliest opportunity consistent with conduct of the research, unless there is a health or research justification for retaining the identifiers, or such retention is otherwise required by law.
- There are adequate written assurances that the protected health information will not be reused or disclosed to any other person or entity, except as required by law, for authorized oversight of the research project, or for other research for which the use or disclosure of protected health information would be permitted by this subpart.

Access of Individuals to Protected Health Information

With few exceptions, under this rule an individual has a right of access to inspect and obtain a copy of protected health information about the individual in a designated record set, for as long as the protected health information is maintained. An individual also has the right to have a covered entity amend such information. Clinical trial information would typically fall into a designated record set and be subject to such access rights. An individual's right to access protected health information created or obtained by a covered healthcare provider in the course of research that includes treatment may be temporarily suspended for as long as the research is in progress, provided that the individual has agreed to the denial of access when consenting to participate in the research that includes treatment, and the covered healthcare provider has informed the individual that the right of access will be reinstated upon completion of the research.

Conclusion

Most clinical trials research will be affected by the Final Privacy Rule in marginal ways; that is, no significant barriers to clinical trials are introduced. The new rules require careful crafting and execution of notices and authorizations as well as additional criteria and documentation for IRB decisions. Patient access and amendment rights to clinical records are extended into research records.

Timely Update

In the time since this chapter was written, HHS has published guidance on the final rule and has announced its intent to publish a Notice of Proposed Rule Making (NPRM) proposing changes to this final rule. The guidance, published on July 6, 2001, has a section on research that summarizes the rule and answers some questions that have arisen from the research community and the public. The guidance does not change the content of the regulations or their effect on clinical trials.

Publication of the NPRM is not expected before the end of 2001, and I expect changes to be proposed in areas such as consent that will affect the process of conducting clinical trials in relatively minimal ways. To keep up-to-date on these regulations, I suggest monitoring the HHS Administrative Simplification or Officer for Civil Rights web sites and/or subscribing to the Administrative Simplification listserv described at http://aspe.hhs.gov/admnsimp/.

16
Toward a Shared Representation of Clinical Trial Protocols: Application of the GLIF Guideline Modeling Framework

ROBERT A. GREENES, SAMSON TU, AZIZ A. BOXWALA, MOR PELEG, and EDWARD H. SHORTLIFFE

The knowledge contents of clinical practice guidelines and clinical trial protocols have much in common. A guideline specifies a recommended set of decisions and actions and the optimal pathways or sequences for carrying them out. Although often written in narrative form, guidelines should imply an underlying flowchart. Ideally such a flowchart is made explicit to resolve ambiguities and ensure that all potential pathways are fully specified.

A clinical trial protocol also specifies a set of decisions and actions and pathways for carrying them out, but decisions and actions in clinical trials are prescribed, not recommended. Alternative pathways exist for different subjects, typically dependent on a randomized assignment to one arm of the clinical trial. Once patients are randomized to a study arm, the format and rules for managing them are similar to those of a clinical guideline. Both guidelines and clinical trial protocols have eligibility criteria specifying the groups of patients for whom the guideline or protocol is applicable. Precise specifications define toxicity criteria and adverse event management.

Other details typically included in a clinical guideline are the nature of the evidence on which it is based, citation of references, and elaboration on particular issues. In clinical trial protocols, other components specified include the nature and purpose of the trial, study design, statistical methods, and participants.

In this chapter, we focus not on those other aspects, but on the eligibility criteria and the decision and action flow that describe the care process. We focus on the requirements for modeling clinical processes, hoping to facilitate implementation of clinical trial protocols in actual healthcare environments. The intent is to support use by healthcare practitioners as part of operational information systems, and the goal is to optimize the clinical trial encounter, retrieval and presentation of relevant data, collection and validation of new data, automation of the prescribed actions, and completion of case report forms. Such information systems can minimize errors, avoid repetitive data entry required by separate record keeping for the trial and for patient care, and ensure consistency in trial compliance and case reporting.

We are considering guidelines and protocols together because considerable work is underway to structure the description of guidelines so computers can execute them, and to standardize the structure to enable guideline sharing. These goals are of interest to clinical trial protocol developers as well. Ideally, structure requires unambiguous authoring of the decisions and actions, using precise medical terminology and logic; the ability to validate the specification in terms of the syntax, semantics, and logical consistency; and the ability to map decision variables to data elements in an electronic medical record (EMR). Healthcare information systems require similar mapping from actions to processes, particularly for order entry and the delivery of alerts and reminders. Standardizing the structure specification will allow disparate systems implementers and vendors to incorporate applications that provide access to guidelines at the point of care.

The need for structure is the same for clinical trials as it is for guidelines: to enable unambiguous interpretation and execution at the point of care, and to enable the protocol's data references to be interfaced with host system EMRs and its actions to be interfaced with host order entry systems. After standardization, clinical trials can be conducted at multiple sites, implemented in many distinct systems and platforms, and provide this capability for protocols from different sponsors and trials groups. Structure and standardization can provide a more streamlined and consistent way of collecting data, monitoring it for quality, and reporting it. The obstacles protocol developers face in achieving these goals are similar to those facing guideline developers.

We begin this chapter with a review of the nature and history of clinical practice guidelines, issues in their use, the rationale for computer-based guidelines, and problems and challenges in developing computer-based approaches. After comparing those topics with the issues involved in clinical trial protocol design, we discuss recent experience with computer-based guideline modeling aimed at developing a common representation for use in various implementations. Our discussion focuses on the use of the GuideLine Interchange Format (GLIF), as well as challenges inherent in this approach. Finally, we describe the special issues of clinical trials and how computer-based protocols can benefit from leveraging the approach followed for computer-based guidelines.

Goals of Clinical Practice Guidelines

Clinical practice guidelines aim to reduce practice variation, avoid errors, and encourage best practices (Field & Lohr, 1990). Guidelines were developed for clinical use as early as the 1970s, when they were called clinical algorithms and were largely disseminated in paper form. Interest in guidelines surged in the 1990s as managed care and integrated delivery networks grew and placed greater emphasis on cost effectiveness and reduced variability of clinical practices. A major goal is now to reduce practice variation by improving access to information about best practices, including guidelines and evidence to support them. The recent Institute of Medicine report, *To Err is Human*, has stimulated attention to guidelines, both to prevent errors and to enhance care quality (Kohn, Corrigan & Donaldson, 2000).

Traditional Guidelines

Despite long-term interest in them, guidelines have been plagued with problems in their authoring, delivery, and use. Typically, professional specialty organizations, government agencies, or large healthcare delivery organizations sponsor guideline development. Because these entities wish to produce high quality, authoritative guidelines, guideline development focuses heavily on the evidence base for recommendations and discussion of circumstances and issues relating to their applicability. The formal structure of the guideline usually receives much less attention. Ambiguities often exist in published guidelines, most of which are authored in narrative form, occasionally augmented by a flowchart. Systematic identification of the actions to be carried out in all possible circumstances is often not done, nor is there even precise specification of the circumstances under which the actions are being recommended. Guidelines that are either too general or too specific to a particular situation may not apply to actual patients or may provide ambiguous recommendations for a condition.

Guidelines are disseminated usually in read-only form, whether via textbooks, journal articles, CD-ROMs, or the Web. The National Guideline Clearinghouse (http://www.guidelines.gov), sponsored by the Agency for Healthcare Research and Quality in collaboration with the American Medical Association and the American Association of Health Plans, provides a compendium of guidelines on the Web from many sources (http://www.guideline.com) with search capabilities and links to the original documents. Guideline sponsors and authors hope physicians will read and memorize published guidelines and use them to improve their practice, but guidelines have not yet had this kind of impact.

Computer-Based Guidelines

A number of objectives have been cited for computer-based implementation of clinical guidelines (Advani, Lo & Shahar, 1998; Dazzi, Fassino, Saracco et al., 1997; Fox, Johns & Rahmanzadeh, 1998; Lobach & Hammond, 1997; Nilasena & Lincoln, 1995; Ohno-Machado, Gennari, Murphy et al., 1998). These include the ability to structure them more precisely (Fox et al., 1998; Ohno-Machado et al., 1998); to share them among developers and users

(Ohno-Machado et al., 1998); to validate them (Fox et al., 1998; Shiffman, 1997); to document them and link them to appropriate literature or databases (Agency for Healthcare Research and Quality); to search for them based on various criteria; to navigate or browse them (Abendroth & Greenes, 1989); and to integrate them into applications. Among possible applications, guidelines can be used in educational settings as drivers for clinical simulations or patient management problems, or may be retrieved and reviewed or navigated dynamically as references for clinical questions.

With respect to integration into clinical settings, computer-based guidelines can be used to support workflow management by organizing the presentation of forms for data collection and action selection (Zielstorff, Teich, Paterno et al., 1989) and data communication to participants ("actors") when specific tasks are required (Dazzi et al., 1997). Guidelines can also aid in decision-making (Lobach & Hammond, 1997; Shiffman, 1997); facilitate clinical trials management (Fox, Johns, Lyons et al., 1997); determine appropriateness of referrals, tests, or treatments; and implement critical paths and utilization review procedures. Guideline rules triggered by event monitors can generate alerts and reminders (Hripcsak, Ludemann, Pryor et al., 1994), and guidelines may serve as benchmarks for quality assurance (Bell, Layton & Gabbay, 1991).

To address these possibilities, and especially to deliver patient-specific guideline recommendations at the point of care, we must integrate guidelines into the framework of the information environment.

Desiderata for Computer-Based Guidelines

Here, we cite five primary desiderata for computer-based guidelines. As we discuss later in this chapter, these requirements also apply to computer-based clinical trial protocols. The importance of the desiderata varies depending on the intended application setting and use of the guideline.

- **Definition and structure.** All decision criteria and actions must be expressed with an unambiguous terminology, and all logical expressions must be well structured and syntactically and logically correct. This requires specification of all data elements and actions using an agreed-upon vocabulary. Ideally, it should be possible to specify units, ranges, and other constraints and to validate that logical expressions are consistent and complete.
- **Eligibility.** Eligibility criteria for guidelines have generally not been subjected to the necessary rigor to be interpreted by computer. To do this requires the use of standardized terminology for clinical data elements and unambiguous logical statements. Without this, it is difficult to automatically trigger guidelines. Guidelines for a particular disease may differ with respect to the aspect of the disease (screening, diagnosis, management), state of the patient (initial evaluation, initial treatment, maintenance

followup, presence of comorbidities, etc.), the intended user (patient, nurse, primary physician, specialist), and setting (home, office, inpatient). The retrieval of guidelines relevant to a specific patient and situation should be able to use these attributes to narrow the range of possible guidelines (Bernstam, Ash, Peleg et al., 2000).

- **Adaptation to local characteristics.** Implementation at the point of care requires the recognition that local sites may have unique characteristics. Local workflow, setting, and customs may dictate that procedures be carried out in specific ways or that certain personnel or systems be used at various points. Guideline medical recommendations themselves may need to adapt to local requirements, particularly if certain resources, such as an MRI scanner, are not available or there is a local preference for one medication within a class of drugs.
- **Mapping to host platform.** Various software platforms have unique requirements for access to databases like the EMR and initiation of actions like order entry or alerts notification. Because of the lack of structure in the authoring process, the lack of common format for dissemination, and the difficulty in interfacing to local host environments, few guidelines have been implemented in practice.
- **User interface.** Various delivery settings have specific requirements for interface to the user (e.g., via the Web, on a handheld device, or in a wide variety of software/hardware environments).

Lifecycle of Computer-Based Guideline Development

Because it requires so much effort to develop high quality, well-documented guidelines and fulfill the implementation desiderata, we must optimize this process as much as possible. The guideline lifecycle begins with a conceptual model of the purpose of a guideline and how it will be used in patient care (e.g., integrated into workflow, as a consultation tool, or as an event-triggered reminder). This will dictate the kinds of attributes and characteristics of the guideline that authors or knowledge engineers must encode. Eligibility criteria must also be defined.

Once developed, a guideline must be validated for syntactic and logical correctness before it can be executed. This can be considered an extension of the authoring process itself. The guideline must be stored in a well-defined representation format and disseminated in a form that systems or environments can parse and interpret. This process could include further adaptation of the guideline by authoring tools based on local requirements.

Guideline data elements also must map to the host system's EMR, and actions must link with the order/processing functions if they are to be integrated into host systems. If a guideline is to be used interactively in the native work environment, user interface characteristics must be determined. After use, modifications of the modeling process may be appropriate and updates to the guidelines themselves may occur, requiring further authoring and editing, and triggering iteration of the downstream processes of the lifecycle.

Common Formats for Sharing Guidelines

Common formats for representation and dissemination will foster use of guidelines in many possible host environments. If the authoring tools that support different models produce varying formal representations, they will be useful only in environments that understand those representations. Agreement on a common format facilitates delivery from varying modeling environments to multiple host environments.

Without a common format, individual modeling approaches must be translated to individual implementation environments, a many-to-many process. With a common format (to the extent that it enables representation of the features in various models), a guideline can be translated to that common format, and developers of implementation environments can then translate it into the formats they require. The process thus becomes a many-to-one and one-to-many task, which is considerably simpler and can be supported by common tools. Another advantage of a common representation and dissemination format is that standard tools can be developed for use in host environments to facilitate parsing, mapping to local databases, and execution.

Because of the range of guideline development approaches and potential applications being explored, convergence on a single model has not yet occurred. As experience with application implementation in host environments increases, pinpointing the most useful applications and interface approaches, we should be able to identify which modeling features are most critical and implement them in the common model. Thus the development of a common shared model should be seen as an evolutionary process.

Distinctions Between Clinical Trial Protocols and Clinical Practice Guidelines

Unlike clinical practice guidelines, clinical trial protocols are heavily regulated scientific experiments that test the safety and efficacy of new interventions. Clinical trials should ensure that patients receive a consistent method of workup or treatment so that the proposed approach can be evaluated against alternatives. As scientific experiments, clinical trials have a lifecycle different from that of clinical practice guidelines. From its inception as an idea or hypothesis to be tested, a clinical trial goes through the phases of experimental design, approval, recruitment and execution, and data collection and analysis. The results may be subject to meta-analysis for incorporation into evidence-based clinical guidelines.

Nonetheless, with regard to specification of protocols, issues arise that are somewhat similar to those for guidelines. While the decisions and actions must be precisely specified, most protocol authoring has not been consistent. Terminology for clinical data elements has not been standardized, logical statements often are not fully analyzed for ambiguities, and interfacing to clinical systems has not been considered in the design.

Re-engineering the design and conduct of clinical trials to make the processes more distributed has led to refinements in the representation of the clinical guidelines in protocols. It has also refined the ways they should drive data collection and data validation processes. Explicitly specifying tasks in the different phases of a trial's lifecycle is a prerequisite for understanding the representation requirements for modeling trial protocols. Designing, deploying, and analyzing clinical trial protocols involve tasks beyond patient-specific actions and decision support. The design phase may focus on the soundness of statistical considerations and the adequacy of eligibility criteria and adverse events monitoring. The deployment phase may focus on inter- and intra-organizational communication and coordination requirements for conducting a trial. The data collection process must be highly structured with requirements regulated.

For analysis, the requirements for reporting trial results must be defined, as well as those for interim analysis before the end of study and for meta-analyses. These tasks impose modeling requirements not needed for patient-specific decision support. For example, analyzing statistical soundness of a trial design or results requires different knowledge than recommending dose changes when a patient is experiencing drug-related toxicity.

Since ONCOCIN (Shortliffe, Scott, Bischoff et al., 1981) pioneered patient-specific decision support for conducting cancer clinical trials, researchers and institutions have looked at computer-based support at different stages of trial design and management. Design-a-Trial (Wyatt, Altman, Heathfield et al., 1994) helps clinicians create scientifically and ethically sound clinical trials. Rubin (Rubin, Gennari, Srinivas et al., 1999) looked at the problem of tool support for authoring eligibility criteria. T-Helper (Tu, Kemper, Lane et al., 1993) screened large databases for patients potentially eligible for trials. Ocelot (Sim, 1999) proposed trial banks that collect results of trials and subject them to systematic meta-analyses.

With all the tasks involved in designing, conducting, and analyzing clinical trials, the research agenda cannot succeed without the participation of a large number of stakeholders. A single project can work only on one aspect of a much larger problem. A collaborative effort is needed to harmonize models used for tasks in different phases of the clinical trial lifecycle to ensure that information can pass from one phase to another.

Despite the added requirements noted above, protocols share the need to specify eligibility criteria for individual trials and carry out logic and pathways for all steps in the application of the protocol to specific patients. We focus on these aspects in the remainder of this chapter.

Toward a Shared Representation for Clinical Guidelines: GLIF

Adoption of a common format for representing guidelines is essential for sharing them. Using the same format to specify different types of guidelines can ease automation and implementation, because only a single format needs to be supported by the implementing institutions. Working on a single format can focus efforts to achieve a good representation format, useful and usable authoring tools, tools for facilitating eligibility determination and retrieval, and implementation as executable applications.

A common set of tools can aid the process of creating, publishing, and sharing guidelines. Different institutions could create guidelines using authoring tools to support standard vocabulary, editing, and visualization. A central server on the Internet could store the encoded guidelines, and medical institutions could browse and download them, and using other tools, adapt them to their local setting, map them to the host EMR, and execute them in their own healthcare systems.

History

The Guideline Interchange Format (GLIF) is an evolving model for representing and sharing guidelines (Ohno-Machado et al., 1998). GLIF was initially developed and is being further refined through InterMed, a collaboration among Stanford, Harvard, and Columbia universities using a consensus-based multi-institutional process. The GLIF specification consists of an object-oriented model and corresponding text syntax. It contains a set of classes that represent guideline content, each with specific data types and attributes.

GLIF version 2 (GLIF2), published in 1998 (Ohno-Machado et al., 1998), enabled guideline modeling as a flowchart of structured steps representing clinical actions and decisions. However, because the attributes of structured constructs were defined as text strings that could not be parsed, such guidelines could not be used for computer-based execution requiring automatic inference. Even in that form, GLIF spawned several tools for authoring, navigation and browsing, management and retrieval by a shared server, and execution, as well as early applications and prototypes (Zielstorff et al., 1998; Lussier, Kukafka, Patel & Cimino, 2000; Fox & Bury, 2000; Dubey & Chueh, 2000; Silverman, Sokolsky, Tannen, et al., 1999; Boxwala, Greenes & Deibel, 1999; Grosso, Eriksson, Fergerson et al., 1999; Greenes, Boxwala, Sloan et al., 1999).

Current Status

GLIF3 (Peleg, Boxwala, Ogunyemi et al., 2000), a developing version of GLIF, is designed to support computer-based execution. GLIF3 builds on the GLIF2 framework but augments it by introducing several new constructs and requiring a more formal definition of decision criteria, action specifications, and patient data. GLIF incorporates means for harmonization with complementary specifications like the Arden Syntax logic grammar (Hripcsak et al., 1994) and HL7's Unified Service Action Model (Schadow, Russler, Mead & McDonald, 2000), which can ease integration of GLIF-based systems into the clinical environment.

While Arden Syntax represents single-decision rules in self-contained units called Medical Logic Modules (MLMs), GLIF specifies entire guidelines generally intended to unfold over time. GLIF uses a modification of the Arden Syntax logic grammar to specify logical and temporal decision criteria, but includes constructs that support other elements, like sequencing of actions and decisions and extension over multiple encounters, required by complex clinical guidelines. GLIF also includes an MLM-macro class that enables encoding of specific guideline recommendations into MLMs for institutions that wish to use them (Boxwala, Mehta, Ash et al., 2000). Another important feature of GLIF3 is a medical domain object model that will allow guideline steps to refer to patient data items defined by a controlled terminology that includes standard medical vocabularies (e.g., the UMLS [Lindberg, Humphreys & McCray, 1993]) and standard data models for the medical concepts (e.g., HL7's Unified Service Action Model [Schadow et al., 2000]).

The inclusion of Arden Syntax logic grammar, the medical domain object model, and an action specification hierarchy, give GLIF3 a *computable* level of specification that formally defines the logical criteria, definitions of patient data items, clinical actions, and the flow of the guideline. This formal definition of guideline components allows the encoded guideline to be validated for logical consistency and completeness. The computable specification level is an intermediate between two other levels: a human-readable flowchart level, retained from GLIF2, and an implementation level.

Viewing a guideline as a human-readable and traversable flowchart facilitates the understanding of authors and clinical users. The implementation level currently being developed for GLIF3 includes non-sharable institution-specific details that help incorporate guidelines into operational information systems. The representation explicitly separates sharable components of a guideline from institution-specific or vendor platform-specific components.

GLIF3 guideline representations are exchanged in Resource Description Framework (RDF) format, chosen to facilitate an open process and to replace GLIF2's proprietary ODIF format (Pattison-Gordon, 1996). Developed under the auspices of the WWW Consortium (W3C), RDF is an infrastructure that enables the encoding, exchange, and reuse of structured metadata (http://www.w3.org). RDF has an explicit model for expressing object semantics (objects and attributes) using XML (eXtensible Markup Language) syntax.

An RDF schema defines the metadata definitions of GLIF3's object model, and RDF markup specifies guideline instances that conform to the RDF schema. The RDF instance files and the RDF GLIF schema are easily interchanged among institutions that use GLIF as the language for representing encoded guidelines. Currently, there are two GLIF authoring tools: Protége (Grosso et al., 1999), and the GEODE Authoring Tool (Greenes et al., 1999). Both of them provide a graphical environment for creating and editing guidelines visualized as flowcharts.

The GLIF3 Model

The GLIF3 model is object-oriented. It consists of classes, their attributes, and the relationships among the classes that are necessary to model clinical guidelines. The model is described with Unified Modeling Language (UML) class diagrams (Object Management Group, 1999). The Object Constraint Language (OCL), a part of the UML standard, specifies additional constraints on represented concepts.

A top-level view of the GLIF model is shown in Figure 16.1.

The guideline class is used to model clinical guidelines and sub-guidelines. A guideline contains an algorithm, or a flowchart of temporally sequenced nodes called steps. Different classes of steps (all derived from the Guideline_Step abstract class) are used for modeling different constructs. GLIF's guideline class specifies maintenance information (such as author, status, modification date, and version), the intention of the guideline, eligibility criteria, didactics, and the set of exceptions that interrupt the normal flow of execution. The guideline defines patient data items accessed by its steps and defined in the medical domain object model.

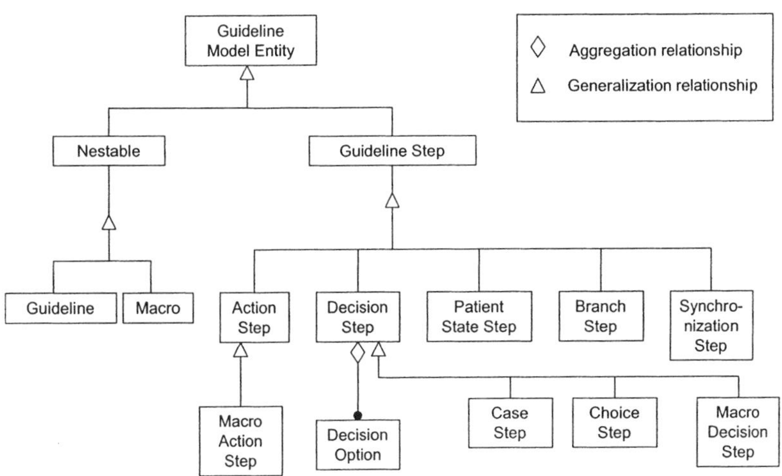

FIGURE 16.1. The GLIF model. A top-level view of the main GLIF classes.

Decision steps, an abstract class, conditionally direct flow from one guideline step to another. GLIF provides a flexible decision model through a hierarchy of decision step classes that distinguishes between case steps (which can be automated) and choice steps (which must be made by an external agent like a physician, other healthcare provider, or another program). For each subclass of the Decision_Step class, an associated subclass of Decision_Option is used to specify the decision options for a step of that class. The criteria in the decision options are written in an expression language derived from the logical expression grammar of Arden Syntax.

Currently, GLIF defines only case and choice classes. The decision hierarchy can extend to support different decision models and decisions that consider uncertainty or patient preferences.

The Action_Step class is used for modeling actions. Action steps contain two distinct types of tasks: medically oriented actions, like a recommendation for a particular course of treatment, and programming-oriented actions, like retrieving data from an electronic patient record. The tasks in an action can be iterated, and the iteration has a formal definition. Nesting decision and action steps allow recursive specification of actions and decision. In other words, through nested steps, we can specify details of high-level actions and decisions as sub-guidelines.

The Branch_Step and **Synchronization_Step** allow modeling of multiple simultaneous paths through the guideline. The paths may occur in parallel, or in any order.

Patient_State_Steps serve as entry points into the guideline and allow for labeling patient states (e.g., a state of taking one anti-hypertensive drug). Patient state steps contain formally specified logical criteria that define the patient state and can be used as eligibility criteria for entry into the guideline at that step.

The specification for supplemental material allows us to associate didactic material with the guideline itself or with sections of it. The supplemental material can be in different formats (like plain text and HTML) for different purposes (like rationale, further reading, and patient education).

As an example, Figure 16.2 shows a portion of a guideline for management of stable angina (ACC/AHA/ACP-ASIM, 1999), focusing on the "education and risk factor modification" sub-guideline.

The HL7 GLIF SIG

In March 2000, an invitational workshop called "Toward a Sharable Guideline Representation" was held in Boston. It was organized by the InterMed Collaboratory and sponsored by the U.S. Army, the Agency for Healthcare Research and Quality (AHRQ), the National Library of Medicine (NLM), the American College of Physicians-American Society of Internal Medicine, and the Centers for Disease Control and Prevention (CDC). The workshop included representatives from ten different coun-

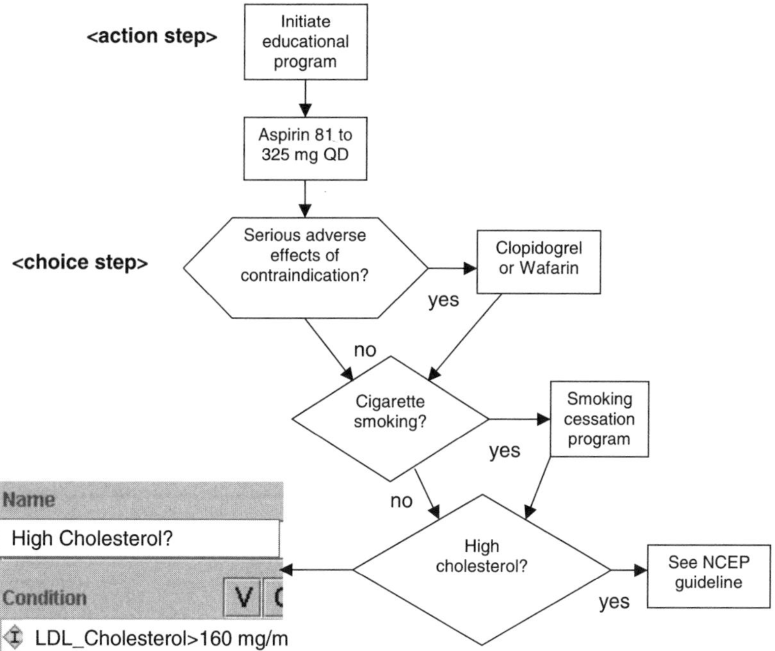

FIGURE 16.2. A portion of GLIF guideline authored with Protégé, for education and risk factor modification in stable angina.

tries—among them stakeholders from academia, government agencies, professional organizations, insurers, providers, and industry—who recognized the need for a standard shared computer-interpretable guideline representation format. The workshop resulted in five task forces to pursue a sharable guideline representation standard by exploring functional requirements of guidelines, modeling and representation, special needs of clinical trials, infrastructure and tools, and organizational framework for continuing these activities.

To elaborate on the model for guideline representation that could serve as a common basis for implementations and potentially serve as a standard, the InterMed team conferred with the HL7 organization about the benefits of furthering this activity under HL7 auspices. In September of 2000, the HL7 board of directors established a new technical committee on Clinical Decision Support (CDS), moved the existing Arden Syntax committee under the CDS committee as an Arden Syntax special interest group, and established a Clinical Guidelines special interest group, also under the CDS committee, to pursue standardization of GLIF. The HL7 Winter Working Group Meeting (http://www.HL7.org) in January 2001 was the first meeting of the CDS committee and the Arden Syntax and Clinical Guidelines special interest groups.

Several aspects of GLIF development make this relationship with HL7 desirable:

- GLIF specification of logic for both eligibility criteria and decision steps is intended to be compatible with Arden Syntax and extend it in various ways as the expression language for both MLMs and guidelines continues to be refined.
- GLIF's data model uses the USAM approach for modeling clinically relevant services and actions. It is developed under HL7 and models the clinical part of HL7's Reference Information Model (RIM).
- GLIF is an open consensus standard without proprietary interests or goals. This approach explicitly encourages involvement and participation by representatives from both the public and private sectors.
- Most commercial stakeholders and many academic and healthcare organization developers involved in implementing guidelines participate in HL7 and thus can participate in further refining a shared representation model.

The ideal is an open process in which specifications and other materials are made widely available to an open resource library. This already exists at a Web site maintained by the InterMed collaboratory (http://www.glif.org), but it will someday be available through HL7 and hopefully will include tools, example guidelines, and other documentation.

GLIF as a Model for Clinical Trial Protocols

GLIF is a guideline representation that can enact clinical guidelines in specific patient situations. As the Stanford EON project has shown (Tu & Musen, 1999), such a guideline representation can be used as a model for the enactment of clinical trials. Clinical guidelines and trial protocols share certain functions, such as sequencing actions over time, modeling decision criteria for choosing alternatives, making abstractions from primitive data, and checking applicability of guidelines to patients.

With a few exceptions (like grading evidence needed to describe guidelines), most modeling constructs required to represent guidelines are also needed to represent protocols. Their usage differs not in kind, but in degree of importance. For example, unlike guidelines that assist clinicians in decision making, clinical trial protocols emphasize the workflow aspect of patient management. They specify the sequencing and repetition of interventions, enumerate the studies that must be done on a regular basis, and define algorithms for adjusting interventions based on reactions to previous interventions. Even though they are more prescriptive and specify actions at a more detailed level than do most clinical practice guidelines, the algorithmic aspect of clinical protocols can be represented with existing GLIF modeling constructs.

Nevertheless, modeling clinical trial protocols to provide clinicians with point-of-care decision support requires attention to several issues not present in clinical practice guidelines.

- **Cancer protocols often have intrinsic timelines different from a calendar timeline.** "Day 8" in a chemotherapy trial may not be the eighth calendar day after the start of chemotherapy if, for example, treatment is delayed because of toxicity. The ONCOCIN program worked in terms of "cycles" and "sub-cycles." "Day 1" and "Day 8" were modeled as two sub-cycles of a chemotherapy cycle.
- **A clinical trial may be double-blinded.** An advice system that provides decision support cannot know the arm to which a patient is randomized. Such protocols must be modeled without regard for randomization. A protocol document may describe two arms of treatment, but a model should have only one branch, because the execution system will not know the arm to which a patient is assigned.
- **Cancer clinical trials have well-defined grading systems for toxicities.** These require mechanisms, such as Shahar's Resume system (Shahar, 1997), for making abstractions from observations into toxicity episodes.
- **Clinical trials adjust management of patients based on their reactions to previously administered treatment.** The modeling environment needs a rich language for making temporal queries. These queries depend on temporal context, require ordinal selection, and need to make temporal comparisons. Examples of temporal query systems designed to model temporal patterns of adverse events include Kahn's TNET system (Kahn, Tu & Fagan, 1991) (designed as part of ONCOCIN) and the Tzolkin system (Nguyen, Shahar, Tu et al., 1999), used in the EON project.
- **The most complicated part of a chemotherapy protocol may be the part that describes how to adjust treatment based on toxicities.** Because these treatment modifications are often organized by classes of toxicities, a protocol may reduce the chemotherapy dose if a patient's measured platelet count is below a certain range. One common problem in modeling the attenuation algorithm is that protocol authors often do not specify how to modify the dose-adjustment algorithm for multiple drug toxicities. A trial protocol may give conflicting algorithms for managing toxicities. For toxicity 1, it may suspend the drug until the patient recovers and then give 75% of the previous dose, and for toxicity 2, it may reduce the drug dose by 75% and escalate back to a full dose if the patient recovers. The protocol may not specify the appropriate management strategy if both toxicities occur.
- **The eligibility criteria of a clinical trial are entry criteria that, once a patient is enrolled, can be ignored.** Conceptually, eligibility criteria for clinical trials are somewhat different from eligibility criteria for guidelines. The latter are really applicability criteria that a patient must satisfy if the guideline is to be relevant.

- **A phase-1 clinical trial seeks to find the maximum tolerated dose of a drug regimen.** The dose given to a patient may depend on reactions other patients have to the drugs. A chemotherapy-dosing program must query data involving other patients when it computes the dose for a particular patient.

Looking Ahead

Despite the differences we have noted, the similarities between implementation issues for clinical practice guidelines and clinical trial protocols are compelling. The shared elements suggest that the clinical trial modeling community should build on the guideline modeling framework to incorporate modeling characteristics that clinical trials need. Because it has a robust design and its development is an open process, GLIF is a good candidate for this. By adopting this approach, clinical trial implementers can take advantage of the GLIF tools for authoring, validation, dissemination, term management, and mapping to local environments.

Acknowledgments. This work was supported in part by Grant LM06594 from the National Library of Medicine, with cooperative support from the Department of the Army and the Agency for Healthcare Research and Quality. Prior support was also provided by the Defense Research Projects Agency. The authors wish to acknowledge other members of the InterMed Collaboratory for their participation in the work described in this chapter, notably Lucila Ohno-Machado, MD, PhD, Qing Zeng, PhD, Vimla Patel, PhD, Nachman Ash, MD, Omolola Ogunyemi, PhD, and Elmer Bernstam, MD.

References

Abendroth TW, Greenes RA. 1989. Computer Presentation of Clinical Algorithms. MD Computing 6:295–299.

ACC/AHA/ACP-ASIM. 1999. Guidelines for the Management of Patients with Chronic Stable Angina. Journal of the American College of Cardiology 33:2092–2197.

Advani A, Lo K, Shahar Y. 1998. Intention-Based Critiquing of Guideline-Oriented Medical Care. Proceedings of the American Medical Informatics Association Symposium 483–487.

Bell D, Layton AJ, Gabbay J. 1991. Use of a Guideline Based Questionnaire to Audit Hospital Care of Acute Asthma. British Medical Journal 302:1440–1443.

Bernstam E, Ash N, Peleg M, Boxwala A, Mork P, Greenes RA, Shortliffe EH, Tu S. 2000. Guideline Classification to Assist Modeling, Authoring, Implementation and Retrieval. Proceedings of the American Medical Informatics Association Symposium 7(Suppl):66–70.

Boxwala AA, Greenes RA, Deibel SR. 1999. Architecture for a Multipurpose Guideline Execution Engine. Proceedings of the American Medical Informatics Association Symposium 6(Suppl):701–705.

Boxwala AA, Mehta P, Ash N, Lacson R, Greenes RA, Shortliffe EH, Peleg M, Bury J. 2000. Representing Guidelines Using Domain-Level Knowledge Components. Proceedings of the American Medical Informatics Association Symposium. Journal of the American Medical Informatics Association 7(Suppl):97.

Dazzi L, Fassino C, Saracco R, Quaglini S, Stefanelli M. 1997. A Patient Workflow Management System Built on Guidelines. Proceedings of the American Medical Informatics Association Annual Fall Symposium:146–150.

Dubey AK, Chueh HC. 2000. An XML-Based Format for Guideline Interchange and Execution. Proceedings of the American Medical Informatics Association Symposium 7(Suppl):205–209.

Field MJ, Lohr KN. 1990. Guidelines for Clinical Practice: Directions for a New Program. Washington DC: Institute of Medicine, National Academy Press.

Fox J, Bury JP. 2000. A Quality and Safety Framework for Point-of-Care Clinical Guidelines. Proceedings of the American Medical Informatics Association Symposium 7(Suppl):245–249.

Fox J, Johns N, Lyons C, Rahmanzadeh A, Thomson R, Wilson P. 1997. PROforma: A General Technology for Clinical Decision Support Systems. Computing Methods and Programs in Biomedicine 54:59–67.

Fox J, Johns N, Rahmanzadeh A. 1998. Disseminating Medical Knowledge: The PROforma approach. Artificial Intelligence in Medicine 14:157–181.

Greenes RA, Boxwala A, Sloan WN, Ohno-Machado L, Deibel SR. 1999. A Framework and Tools for Authoring, Editing, Documenting, Sharing, Searching, Navigating, and Executing Computer-Based Clinical Guidelines. Proceedings of the American Medical Informatics Association Symposium 6(Suppl):261–265.

Grosso WE, Eriksson H, Fergerson R, Gennari JH, Tu SW, Musen MA. 1999. Knowledge Modeling at the Millennium (the Design and Evolution of Protege-2000). In Gains BR, Kremer R, Musen M, eds. 1999. The 12th Banff Knowledge Acquisition for Knowledge-Based Systems Workshop. Banff, Canada 7(4):1–36.

Hripcsak G, Ludemann P, Pryor TA, Wigertz OB, Clayton PD. 1994. Rationale for the Arden Syntax. Computers and Biomedical Research 27(4):291–324.

Kahn MG, Tu S, Fagan LM. 1991. TQuery: A Context-Sensitive Temporal Query Language. Computers and Biomedical Research 24:401–419.

Kohn LT, Corrigan JM Donaldson S, eds. 2000. To Err Is Human: Building a Safer Health System. Committee on Quality of Health Care in America, Institute of Medicine. Washington DC: National Academy Press.

Lindberg DA, Humphreys BL, McCray AT. 1993. The Unified Medical Language System. Methods of Information in Medicine 32(4):281–291.

Lobach DF, Hammond WE. 1997. Computerized Decision Support Based on a Clinical Practice Guideline Improves Compliance with Care Standards. American Journal of Medicine 102:89–98.

Lussier YA, Kukafka R, Patel VL, Cimino JJ. 2000. Formal Combinations of Guidelines: A Requirement for Self-Administered Personalized Health Education. Proceedings of the Amercian Medical Informatics Association Symposium 7(Suppl):522–526.

Nguyen JH, Shahar Y, Tu SW, Das AK, Musen MA. 1999. Integration of Temporal Reasoning and Temporal-Data Maintenance into a Reusable Database Mediator to Answer Abstract, Time-Oriented Queries: The Tzolkin System. Journal of Intelligent Information Systems 13(1/2):121–145.

Nilasena DS, Lincoln MJ. 1995. A Computer-Generated Reminder System Improves Physician Compliance with Diabetes Preventive Care Guidelines. Proceedings of the Annual Symposium on Computer Applications in Medical Care:640–645.

Object Management Group. 1999. The Common Object Request Broker: Architecture and Specification. OMG Document Number 91.12.1. Needham, MA: OMG. See also www.omg.org

Ohno-Machado L, Gennari JH, Murphy SN, et al. 1998. The Guideline Interchange Format: A Model for Representing Guidelines. Journal of the American Medical Informatics Association 5:357–372.

Pattison-Gordon E. 1996. ODIF: Object Data Interchange Format. Boston, MA: Decision Systems Group, Brigham and Women's Hospital. DSG-96-04.

Peleg M, Boxwala AA, Ogunyemi O, Zeng Q, Tu S, Lacson R, Bernstam E, Ash N, Mork P, Ohno-Machado L, Shortliffe EH, Greenes RA. 2000. GLIF3: The Evolution of a Guideline Representation Format. Proceedings of the Amercian Medical Informatics Association Symposium 7(Suppl):645–649.

Rubin DL, Gennari JH, Srinivas S, Yuen A, Kaizer H, Musen MA, Silva JS. 1999. Tool Support for Authoring Eligibility Criteria for Cancer Trials. Proceedings of the American Medical Informatics Association Symposium 6(Suppl):369–373.

Schadow G, Russler DC, Mead CN, McDonald CJ. 2000. Integrating Medical Information and Knowledge in the HL7 RIM. Proceedings of the American Medical Informatics Association Symposium 7(Suppl):764–768.

Shahar Y. A Framework for Knowledge-Based Temporal Abstraction. 1997. Artificial Intelligence 90(1–2):79–133.

Shiffman RN. 1997. Representation of Clinical Practice Guidelines in Conventional and Augmented Decision Tables. Journal of the American Medical Informatics Association 4:382–393.

Shortliffe EH, Scott AC, Bischoff MB, Campbell AB, van Melle W, Jacobs CD. 1981. ONCOCIN: An Aid for the Outpatient Management of Cancer Patients. Vancouver, BC: Seventh International Joint Conference on Artificial Intelligence 876–881.

Silverman BG, Sokolsky O, Tannen V, Wong A, Lang L, Khoury A, Campbell K, Qiang C, Sahuguet. 1999. HOLON/CADSE: Integrating Open Software Standards and Formal Methods to Generate Guideline-Based Decision Support Agents. Proceedings of the American Medical Informatics Association Symposium 6(Suppl):955–959.

Sim I. 1999. Trial Banks: An Informatics Foundation for Evidence-Based Medicine. PhD Dissertation. Program in Medical Information Sciences, Stanford University, 1–246.

Tu SW, Kemper CA, Lane NM, Carlson RW, Musen MA. 1993. A Methodology for Determining Patients' Eligibility for Clinical Trials. Methods of Information in Medicine 32:317–325.

Tu SW, Musen MA. 1999. A Flexible Approach to Guideline Modeling. Proceedings of the American Medical Informatics Association Symposium 6(Suppl):420–424.

W3C. 2000. Resource Description Framework. http://www.w3.org/RDF/W3C

Wyatt J, Altman D, Heathfield H, Pantin C. 1994. Development of Design-a-Trial, a Knowledge-Based Critiquing System for Authors of Clinical Trial Protocols. Computer Methods and Programs in Biomedicine 43:283–291.

Zielstorff RD, Teich JM, Paterno MD, et al. 1998. P-CAPE: a High-Level Tool for Entering and Processing Clinical Practice Guidelines. Partners Computerized Algorithm and Editor. Proceedings of the American Medical Informatics Association Symposium:478–482.

17
Informatics for Cancer Prevention and Control

Robert A. Hiatt

Informatics promises to expand options for cancer prevention and control, and investigators and practitioners in these fields are beginning to embrace new technologies. At the same time, accessing information with new technologies is still complex and threatening to many Americans. For cancer patients and their families, the opportunities to learn about new treatments and where to find the highest quality care can outweigh any reluctance to become initiated. On the one hand, those who need prevention information the most—those at risk of getting cancer—may consider the new technology too daunting to be of practical value.

A Cancer Informatics Infrastructure (CII) in prevention and control can help transform the new technology, making it meaningful for everyone. In most cases, this promise is still unfulfilled. As suggested by other chapters in this volume, the value of technology can be realized in several ways, both in research and application. In this chapter, we explore aspects of National Cancer Institute (NCI) activities in cancer prevention and control research and discuss how developing an informatics infrastructure can better harness their potential.

Cancer Prevention and Control

Understanding how informatics can help in further advancing progress in cancer prevention and control requires a little background on how this field has evolved. Although organized public health efforts to prevent and control cancer date back a hundred years (New York City Cancer Committee, 1944), a more rigorous scientific approach began only 25 years ago (Breslow et al., 1977). In the mid-1980s, the development of a formal definition and framework placed the field on a sound scientific and research base (Greenwald & Cullen, 1985). Greenwald and Cullen (1985) defined cancer control as "the reduction of cancer incidence, morbidity, and mortality through an orderly sequence from research on interventions and their impact in defined populations to the broad, systematic application of the research results." They proposed a framework describing a linear series of phases: hypothesis generation, methods development, controlled intervention trials, studies in defined populations, and demonstration projects.

Greenwald and Cullen's framework focused investigators on building appropriate foundations before progressing to large scale intervention research and application. Modeled after the paradigm of drug development, this logical progression of discovery inspired a generation of cancer control scientists to tackle prevention and early detection as an hypothesis and evidence-based enterprise. They generated a large body of new cancer control knowledge, two salient examples of which were in tobacco control and dietary modification research (Hiatt, 1997; Glanz, 1997; Lictenstein, 1997; Lerman, 1997; Lewis, 1997; Kaluzny, 1997).

Since 1997, when the NCI formed a new division dedicated to cancer prevention and another focused on cancer control and population sciences, the perspective has expanded to include a wider range of scientific domains (Hiatt & Rimer, 1999). For example, cancer prevention now focuses heavily on chemoprevention, biomarkers, and early detection, while cancer control emphasizes epidemiology, behavioral science, health services, and surveillance research. Informatics applications have an important role to play across this spectrum.

The NCI now defines cancer control research as "the conduct of basic and applied research in the behavioral, social, and population sciences that, independently, or in combination with biomedical approaches, reduces cancer risk, incidence, morbidity, and mortality and improves quality of life" (Hiatt & Rimer, 1999; Abrams, 1997). As much as 50% to 75% of cancer mortality in the United States can be attributed to external, non-genetic factors, most of which are related to human behaviors like tobacco and alcohol use, improper diet, lack of physical activity, overexposure to sunlight, and sexual activity associated with the transmission of certain viruses. Cancer control strategies and their use of informatics must recognize the critical role of human behaviors and societal influences, many of which fall outside the reach of the healthcare system.

Conversely, cancer prevention research now emphasizes biomedical over behavioral and social aspects of cancer causation and prevention, with an increased focus on chemoprevention, nutritional science, cancer biomarkers, and early detection research based on discoveries in cancer biology, drug development, and other basic sciences (Bresnick, 1997).

Cancer control and prevention are closely linked, and most cancer centers and academic institutions do not distinguish between them. The scientific disciplines needed include epidemiology, nutritional sciences, molecular biology, clinical sciences, behavioral and social science, biostatistics, surveillance sciences, and health services research. This multidisciplinary mix, a hallmark of cancer prevention and control research, creates many opportunities for informatics innovation. We can envision the day when a national cancer informatics infrastructure will impact the daily lives of people at risk for cancer, those seeking diagnosis and treatment, and long-term survivors.

A Cancer Control Framework

Research findings in the cancer control arena translate into practice in the clinic and community, making new discoveries work for cancer patients, providers, and the public. Figure 17.1 is a framework, adapted from the Advisory Committee on Cancer Control of the National Cancer Institute of Canada (1994), illustrating how cancer control operates. In this framework, most cancer control research hypotheses emerge from fundamental research discoveries that, along with epidemiologic inquiry, answer the question "What do we know?" The framework encompasses discoveries from many health-related disciplines, including biomedical sciences, psychology, sociology, anthropology, and economics.

Intervention research builds on evidence from fundamental research and works to determine how to apply it throughout the health system and community. It answers the question "What works?" Although cancer control programs focus primarily on behavior, they can also combine with biomedical interventions or obtain support from public policy initiatives. Successful interventions are promoted at the community, state, and national levels, as well as by major health systems. The process is iterative, because any intervention generates new problems and questions and suggests hypotheses for further research, including basic bio-behavioral research. The most effective intervention programs also use innovations in communications and informatics to adequately disseminate results.

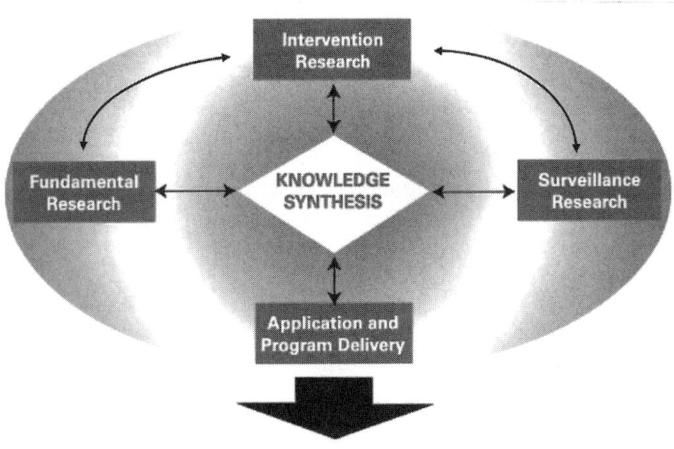

Figure 17.1. Cancer control research activities. Adapted from Advisory Committee on Cancer Control, National Cancer Institute of Canada 1994.

To generate hypotheses for cancer control research and assess outcomes of interventions, surveillance research is necessary. It answers the question "Where are we?" and helps determine where we need to go. Comprehensive and accessible cancer surveillance systems depend increasingly on informatics. Not only must we discover more efficient methods of registering cancer patients and collecting relevant data on them, we must also develop methods of linking data on risk factors and early detection behaviors to the outcomes. We must learn much more about the quality of cancer care, including information on outcomes like the quality of life and functional status of patients and survivors, patient satisfaction with care, and the economic burdens patients face after diagnosis and treatment.

Finally, in the cancer control research framework, information synthesis helps answer the question "What comes next?" and is at the interface of all other research activities. Future efforts must synthesize what we learn from each element of the cancer control process to inform the next stage and refine knowledge gained in earlier stages. This requires comparative analysis of accumulated research and increased efforts to standardize data elements into a dictionary that facilitates meta-analyses and other forms of data synthesis and review. Again, informatics will be at the heart of this endeavor.

Cancer prevention and control applications will advance with the adoption of common data elements (CDEs) and standardized data collection as formulated in the context of clinical trials and described elsewhere in this volume. Scientists, research communities, and others involved in cancer control activities must be integrated into the process. Once research leaves the laboratory and clinic and the knowledge stimulates research in human population sciences, the complexity of the task will increase as information systems interact with "uncontrolled" populations in various settings.

Like existing models—such as the Internet Engineering Task Force (IETF), the governing body for Internet standards—the principles suggested for developing and extending a successful CII into human population research and application will need to:

- provide mechanisms to facilitate stakeholder participation
- leverage sponsorship rather than subsidize the entire CII
- provide both a test bed and an infrastructure (Long Range Planning Committee, 2000).

Collaborating with partners like the Centers for Disease Control and Prevention and the American Cancer Society is perhaps more important in cancer prevention and control than in any other area of cancer research. These relationships are critical to disseminating and applying research results. Likewise, development and promulgation of a comprehensive CII must hold meaning for multiple stakeholders.

By providing examples of current and future initiatives that are or will be natural settings for new information technology, we can explore possible extensions of a CII into the three major domains of cancer control research. These domains follow the framework we use for cancer control: fundamental, intervention, and surveillance research. In the sections that follow, we explore them in detail.

Fundamental Cancer Control and Prevention Science

Informatics supports the foundation of cancer prevention and control sciences in several ways, all of which need substantial development to maximize the potential of a CII. Observational epidemiologic studies and prevention or early detection trials are the primary scientific approaches. Examples of current NCI-supported research illustrate the informatics requirements of fundamental research. Each of these examples is large and complex and requires an efficient informatics infrastructure.

The Cancer Genetics Network

The Cancer Genetics Network (CGN), a major NCI undertaking, is designed to support cancer genetics research that will impact medical practice (http://www-dccps.ims.nci.nih.gov/CGN/index.html). The CGN is one of several large infrastructures the NCI created to support fundamental research with applications in prevention, another being the Cancer Family Registries (http://www-dccps.ims.nci.nih.gov/EGRP/cfr.html).

The CGN illustrates the informatics needs of such large enterprises. Eight clinical sites, some single institutions, and other institutional consortia have come together in the CGN framework to share educational, clinical, and research resources. An informatics group provides a core resource to:

- design, implement, and maintain an information management system that supports large multicenter research protocols
- develop information systems that facilitate the exchange of human cancer genetics information and resources within the larger cancer genetics community.

An informatics core was deemed essential because the CGN needed to coordinate large amounts of data from multiple sites. The Informatics Center, located at the University of California at Irvine (UCI), designed a Central Information Management System (CIMS) to serve as a repository for data on participating individuals. Because protecting confidentiality was a vital concern, the Informatics Center developed a secure Web site with a firewall between the clients who use the Internet for access and the CIMS. The password-protected database uses data authentication and encryption and stores only non-confidential data.

Although the UCI Informatics Center contains information important to the CGN, the data could also be linked to other NCI-supported CII activities. Included are:

- core questionnaires
- a core data dictionary
- procedures for batch submission of data
- descriptions of reports and extract files
- information on the quality assurance system
- rosters
- meeting agendas and minutes.

The data dictionary items contain elements particular to four main areas: respondents, their family members, the study status, and descriptive information about the cancer. Each domain includes a participant and member identification number. The items within each domain and their definitions match the particular needs of the CGN, but current efforts are attempting to integrate them with the CII. In what may be an early model, CGN investigators are working with another major NCI initiative, the Early Detection Research Network, on research of joint interest. In the process, they are addressing uniform needs in informatics.

The Early Detection Research Network

The NCI designed the Early Detection Research Network (EDRN) for investigator-initiated, collaborative research on molecular, genetic, and other biomarkers for human cancer detection and risk assessment (http://edrn.nci.nih.gov/). Four components perform different but integrated functions:

- The Biomarkers Developmental Laboratories develop and characterize new biomarkers or refine existing ones.
- The Biomarker Validation Laboratories are an EDRN resource for clinical and laboratory biomarker validation, including technological development and refinement.
- The Clinical/Epidemiologic Centers conduct research on biomarker application.
- The Data Management and Coordinating Center provides logistical support for meetings and statistical and biocomputational research.

The EDRN, like the CGN, has specific informatics objectives that can link it to the CII. It has developed a secure Web site for data exchange and confidential communication and uses common data elements in conformity with existing NCI CDEs. The EDRN analyzes data that have been generated from geographically distinct systems and are difficult to locate, retrieve, and share. The data architecture in development will help integrate and analyze biologic data with epidemiologic profiles of human clinical responses. A first step in this endeavor is a pilot project of the EDRN Data Management and Coordinating Center (DMCC), which will build a prototype data set compiled from different EDRN centers using common data infrastructure and incorporating common data elements.

Cancer Prevention Trials

Prevention trials hold many of the same opportunities for informatics innovations as do clinical trials. The main differences are that the subjects are asymptomatic persons at risk, not cancer patients who need treatment options, and the trials are much larger. Still, once participants enroll in the trials, the information and data management elements are much the same.

For example, the Study of Tamoxifen and Raloxifene (STAR) trial is designed to determine whether the osteoporosis prevention and treatment drug raloxifene is as effective as tamoxifene in reducing breast cancer risk. More than 500 centers across the United States, Puerto Rico, and Canada are attempting to enroll about 22,000 participants in the NCI-supported trial. Women, who must be postmenopausal and at least 35 years old, are recruited to join STAR if they have a risk of developing breast cancer equivalent to the risk of an average 60-year old woman.

The STAR trial uses the World Wide Web through the NCI's clinical trials site (cancertrials.nci.nih.gov) and the site of the sponsoring cooperative group, the National Surgical Adjuvant Breast and Bowel Project (NSABP) (http://www.nsabp.pitt.edu). Both the general public and interested participants can learn about the nature of the trial, the locations of participating institutions, and how to enroll. Those with a more scientific interest can learn about the progress of recruitment, particularly recruitment by major race and ethnic group. Participating investigators have secure password-protected access to materials for patient enrollment and other relevant information.

The STAR trial is one of several large prevention trials managed by NCI-supported cooperative groups. Others include the Prostate Cancer Prevention Trial, which is testing the drug finesteride, a testosterone analogue, in the prevention of prostate cancer. This ongoing randomized trial, managed by the Southwest Oncology Group (SWOG) (http://swog.org/), has enrolled 18,882 men and will generate results in 2004. SWOG also manages the new Selenium and Vitamin E Cancer Prevention Trial (SELECT), which will evaluate the effect of selenium and vitamin E administered separately versus in combination on the clinical incidence of prostate cancer. SWOG maintains the information about the trial and how to enroll on a Web site. Investigators or members of the cooperative group have password-protected access to trial materials for entering participants and for other study-related information (http://www.swog.org/SELECT/).

Intervention Science

For scientists developing and assessing intervention programs to reduce the cancer burden, the CII can help determine "what works." Cancer preventive research and practice already benefits from such information technology as computer-based educational resources (Kreuter, Strecher & Glassman, 1999; Rimer & Glassman, 1999) and reminder systems (Mandelblatt & Yabroff, 1999) for both providers and patients. Increasingly, systems provide public access to information about cancer care, including descriptions of cancer research programs, the criteria for participation, and the enrollment process (http://cancertrials.nci.nih.gov/index.html; http://cancernet.nci.nih.gov/).

Newer technologies will soon enable the development of behavioral interventions not previously possible. We will see more Web-based health education programs, interactive cable TV and CDs, and portable digital assistants (PDAs). Some of these will cue and track health behaviors on a 24-hour basis regardless of patient location or activity, and they will connect networks of office practices to central data banks (Rakowski, personal communication, 2000). Because of the broad reach of communications technology like Web sites, kiosks, and other interactive media, even people far from cancer centers and other major medical care facilities will have easy access to information on prevention or treatment. Information technology also helps users overcome language barriers, meaning that chronically underserved populations will soon have access to culturally appropriate information on prevention and access to care. These remote sites can act as portals for patient recruitment, removing the distance barrier for willing participants in cancer research studies.

A CII can improve our ability to collect data from participants as events occur—not after the fact, when they are clouded by imperfect memory. This will allow us to give immediate feedback and construct and deliver precisely tailored interventions to individuals. We will know more about each person, reach and include more patients, and conduct more complex interventions closer to the time of the desired behavior. A CII will also help us track behaviors across settings and segment the population more precisely.

Because a CII can impact people where they live, it can effect changes in behavior and create new opportunities for cancer prevention. This requires a perspective that goes beyond cancer patients and their participation in trials to a concern for all persons at risk for cancer. While new information technology will allow us to construct such interventions, behavioral theory must evolve to accommodate the possibilities.

As an organizing principle, Rakowski proposed the development of new behavioral theory based on "focal points," defined as a function of the desired behavior, the population or individual targeted, and the setting (Rakowski, personal communication, 2000). The complex task of considering all three elements simultaneously will demand informatics innovations. Building on early developments in common data elements and standards of information transfer will become a substantial challenge when we move into this larger, less controlled, but critical setting.

With the formation of the Division of Cancer Control and Population Sciences (DCCPS), the NCI has increased its support for research in the behavioral sciences. New programs focus on intervention research in tobacco control, dietary modification, physical activity, sun exposure, avoidance of cancer-related sexually transmitted diseases, and early detection behaviors. Within behavioral research, the NCI recently highlighted new opportunities in cancer communications (http://dccps.nci.nih.gov/eocc/), a field at the heart of quality cancer care and all successful behavioral intervention efforts. One of its priorities is to "enhance and refocus NCI's communications activities to provide comprehensive, technology-supported capability for imparting information about cancer that is easily accessible, timely, and appropriate." The research focuses not only on increasing our understanding of how consumers use health information and how they assess health risks, but also on how to reduce the gap between what we know about communications and how that knowledge is applied.

More tools in development will extend the power of traditional media like radio and television and make sophisticated use of the Internet. Expert groups such as the DHHS Science Panel on Interactive Communication and Health have concluded that few health-related interventions have the power of interactive health communications to improve health outcomes, decrease healthcare costs, and enhance consumer satisfaction. Healthcare providers must have better information on the best treatment protocols, compassionate and cost-effective patient care, and care delivery within culturally and racially diverse populations.

The Agency for Healthcare Research and Quality is reviewing research evidence on cancer-related "decision aids," which are interventions that help people make choices by tailoring options to a person's health needs. Investigators are also developing new tools for communicating about cancer-related risks. An online Publications Locator allows users of the NCI Web site to view and order NCI publications on causes and types of cancers, genetics, environmental and behavioral risk factors, prevention, clinical trials, treatment options, and managing side effects and pain. The NCI is also exploring ways to improve access to cancer-related information through an online Cancer Information Service, currently accessed through the call-in number 1 800 4CANCER (http://cis.nci.nih.gov/).

Another initiative is Joining Organizations with Leading Technologies (JOLT), which is working to bridge the gap between emerging technologies and their application within cancer communications. The World Wide Web Consortium on Cancer supports the delivery of authoritative cancer information through Web sites operated by survivors and other private volunteer groups. NCI is working with an Internet access hardware and software provider to enable low income families to add cancer information to their Web portal. Novel devices customized for cancer patients are also being designed to support inexpensive Internet access.

Cancer Surveillance and Health Services Research

Critical to understanding "where we are" in reducing the cancer burden is the role of cancer surveillance. For many years, the gold standard for quality cancer statistics has been the NCI-supported Surveillance, Epidemiology, and End Results (SEER) Program (http://seer.cancer.gov/). SEER collects and publishes cancer incidence and survival data from 11 population-based cancer registries and three supplemental registries covering approximately 14% of the U.S. population. The National Center for Health Statistics provides the mortality data reported by SEER.

Since 1973, the SEER registries have routinely collected data on patient demographics, primary tumor site, morphology, stage at diagnosis, first course of treatment, and survival rates within each stage. This costly and laborious task is performed by trained cancer registrars, who systematically abstract data from hospital and outpatient pathology reports, discharge files, medical records, laboratory data, and other sources. Their ascertainment of new cancer cases are approximately 98% complete. Following new cancer patients to the first course of therapy and collecting evidence of survival on an individual basis added another layer of complexity.

SEER is now expanding coverage of population segments previously under-represented in the program. It is also working closely with the CDC's National Program of Cancer Registries (NPCR) to improve the coverage of the many states that are not part of SEER and to create a more coordinated national cancer surveillance system. The goal is for all states to establish comprehensive, quality registries that meet the needs of public health programs and cancer research.

The NPCR collects data electronically by age, sex, race/ethnicity, and geographic region (within a state, between states, and between regions) on cancer incidence, stage at diagnosis, first course of treatment, and deaths. CDC is developing a system that will:

- provide valuable feedback to help individual state registries improve the quality and usefulness of their data
- support important data linkages with other cancer databases
- facilitate studies in areas like rare cancers, childhood cancers, occupation-related cancers, and cancers among racial and ethnic minority populations.

Coordinated efforts by the NCI and the CDC are extended by nonprofit partners in cancer surveillance, such as the North American Association of Central Cancer Registries and the National Cancer Data Base managed by the American College of Surgeons. These organizations play a vital role in the complex task of maintaining a useful national cancer surveillance system.

An expanded CII can profoundly impact this cancer surveillance enterprise. An ideally functioning system will require common data elements that conform to a single standard and their consistent use by all national cancer surveillance partners. Such a system could rectify substantial efficiencies in data acquisition, storage, transfer, and protection of confidentiality. Diagnosing physicians in all states must report new cancer cases, but this requirement is currently honored with varying levels of compliance. In practice, the work of the cancer registrar is essential to achieve nearly complete ascertainment. Looking to the future and an intergrated CII for the entire country, new technologies should dramatically streamline the current process and improve data capture for all new cancer cases.

Standard data entry screens, either on desktop systems or personal digital assistants (PDAs), can enable registration and reporting in the physician's office. The physician might enter core data elements conforming to the NCI CDEs at the time of diagnosis. With appropriate confidentiality safeguards and informed consent, registrars could expand these core elements to complete the data collection needed for comprehensive surveillance. Physicians can use the core elements to automatically identify patients eligible for clinical trials. The core elements, supplemented by enhanced data collection appropriate for more in-depth studies, can also deepen our understanding of the quality of care and outcomes and assess quality of life for survivors. Linkages with other data, such as the Medicare database or other databases that include patients under 65 years old, would markedly improve key health service research studies. The SEER-Medicare Database (http://www-dccps.ims.nci.nih.gov/ARP/seermedicare.html) links data reported to registries that participate in SEER to Medicare records and allows researchers to address areas like the economics of cancer care, patterns of care from diagnosis through treatment, variation in care across diverse healthcare systems, and changes in cancei care over time.

The Breast Cancer Screening Consortium (BCSC), a multicenter cooperative investigation coordinated by the NCI, links mammography results to cancer diagnoses (or lack of them) in geographically defined areas with high-quality cancer registries (http://www-dccps.ims.nci.nih.gov/ARP/breastcancer.html). This project, which has continued for several years, will soon produce information on the practice and quality of mammography screening operations in real-world settings. To make comparisons across sites and pool data for studies, the BCSC has also developed common data elements across participating centers and standard procedures for data collection. Different data collection methodologies are being explored to optimize efficiency and reduce the requirements for radiologist participation, especially in high-volume settings.

The future of cancer surveillance also holds the potential for linking information on persons at risk of cancer with that of registry data on cancer incidence and outcomes. Ideally, we would like to track personal behaviors that put people at risk, such as tobacco use and lack of physical activity, and link them to cancer incidence and outcomes. Linking risk factors with cancer outcomes is more difficult than linking screening behavior because of the long lag between a behavior change like smoking and the onset of a tobacco-related cancer. There are also problems with population migration and tracking behavior change over time.

Still, information technology and our expanding national cancer surveillance system promises to someday allow such meaningful linkages, even at an individual level. This will greatly improve cancer surveillance, not only because it helps prove the link between behavior and outcome, but also because such information will be a rich source of hypotheses generation for etiologic research and improvements in interventions.

The Potential of the CII

Informatics has not yet had a substantial impact on cancer prevention and control, although multiple opportunities exist for its application. Applications in the realm of prevention and control will assume various forms, each introducing far more complexity than that of the tightly controlled clinical trials setting. Because this kind of research depends on very large data sets of complex and interrelated factors, this area is particularly well suited to informatics applications. As we have demonstrated through this overview of cancer prevention and control applications, an integrated cancer informatics infrastructure holds exciting potential to increase our knowledge and enable and improve cancer prevention and control science.

References

Abrams DB. 1997. A New Agenda for Cancer Control Research: Report of the Cancer Control Review Group. Bethesda, MD: National Cancer Institute.

Advisory Committee on Cancer Control. 1994. Bridging Research to Action: A Framework and Decision-Making Process for Cancer Control. Advisory Committee on Cancer Control, National Cancer Institute of Canada. Canadian Medical Association 151:1141–1146.

Breslow L, Agran L, Breslow DM, Morganstern M, Ellwein L. 1977. Cancer Control: Implications from its History. Journal of the National Cancer Institute 59:671–686.

Bresnick E. 1997. Report of the National Cancer Institute: Cancer Prevention Program Review Group. Bethesda, MD: National Cancer Institute.

Glanz K. 1997. Behavioral Research Contributions and Needs in Cancer Prevention and Control: Dietary Change. Preventive Medicine 26:S43–S55.

Greenwald P, Cullen JW. 1985. The New Emphasis in Cancer Control. Journal of the National Cancer Institute 74:543–551.

Hiatt RA. 1997. Behavioral Research Contributions and Needs in Cancer Prevention and Control: Adherence to Cancer Screening Advice. Preventive Medicine 26: S11–S18.

Hiatt RA, Rimer BK. 1999. A New Strategy for Cancer Control Research. Cancer Epidemiology, Biomarkers, and Prevention 8:957–964.

Kaluzny AD. 1997. Prevention and Control Research Within a Changing Health Care System. Preventive Medicine 26:S31–S35.

Kreuter MW, Strecher VJ, Glassman B. 1999. One Size Does Not Fit All: The Case for Tailoring Print Materials. Annals of Behavioral Medicine 21:276–283.

Lerman C. 1997. Translational Behavioral Research in Cancer Genetics. Preventive Medicine 26:S65–S69.

Lewis FM. 1997. Behavioral Research to Enhance Adjustment and Quality of Life Among Adults with Cancer. Preventive Medicine 26:S19–S29.

Lictenstein E. 1997. Behavioral Research Contributions and Needs in Cancer Prevention and Control: Tobacco Use, Prevention and Cessation. Preventive Medicine 26:S57–S63.

Long Range Planning Committee. 2000. Final Report of the Long Range Planning Committee: Translating Cancer Research into Cancer Care. Bethesda, MD: National Cancer Institute.

Mandelblatt JS, Yabroff KR. 1999. Effectiveness of Interventions Designed to Increase Mammography Use: A Meta-Analysis of Provider-Targeted Strategies. Cancer Epidemiology, Biomarkers, and Prevention 9:759–767.

New York City Cancer Committee. 1944. History of the American Society for the Control of Cancer, 1913–1943. New York: New York City Cancer Committee.

Rakowski W. 2000. Personal communication.

Rimer BK, Glassman B. 1999. Is There a Use for Tailored Print Communications in Cancer Risk Communications? Journal of the National Cancer Institute Monographs 25:140–148.

Shea S, DuMouchel W, Bahamonde L. 1996. A Meta-Analysis of 16 Randomized Controlled Trials to Evaluate Computer-Based Clinical Reminder Systems for Preventive Care in the Ambulatory Setting. Journal of American Medical Informatics Association 6:399–409.

Section 4
Theory into Practice

Joyce C. Niland
Section Editor

Introduction
Moving Toward the Vision: Putting Applications in Place

JOYCE C. NILAND

This text is unique in that it addresses multiple audiences involved in cancer research and cancer care, including investigators, pharmaceutical companies, patients, and their families. In Section 4: Theory into Practice, we describe how the concepts, technologies, models, and infrastructure described in Sections 1 to 3 apply to real world examples of cancer informatics.

The chapters in this section take us step-by-step through the issues one needs to consider in moving from a concept to the realization of informatics applications in support of cancer care and research. The questions addressed in this section are:

- Is it better to build or buy clinical research systems?
- What is the appropriate unifying model for clinical research systems?
- How are informatics tools being used to help patients, families, and physicians discover available clinical trial options?
- How can we manage accumulating clinical research data electronically?
- What informatics tools should be made available to physicians and patients?
- How best can we use informatics to provide support to patients and their families during the process of receiving cancer care?
- What are the goals and provisions for the emerging area of Consumer Health Informatics?
- How is the Internet being used to deliver clinical trial information, and to measure the final outcomes of translating clinical research into standard practice?

When conceptualizing the design and deployment of informatics applications, the mnemonic "HIT" helps us keep in mind the three essential components: the *human*, *information*, and *technological* aspects. These components are presented in decreasing order of complexity, with the technology generally being the most conquerable, the information structure and content being more formidable to manage, and the human and organizational issues presenting the greatest challenges of all.

This point is amplified by several authors within Section 4, beginning with Chapter 18. Here Mitchell Morris provides us with his experience and insights into the factors to be considered in making the often difficult decision of developing an application inhouse versus purchasing a "ready-made" system from a vendor. Each solution has its pros and cons. The advent of Web-based tools has greatly expanded the flexibility and lowered the cost of creating inhouse applications. On the other hand, leveraging the investments and experience of a company often may make the most sense. However, even "ready-made" systems require a great deal of time, effort, and institutional resources to install and customize the application. The chapter includes a useful inventory tool to assist readers in compiling and organizing the relevant decision factors for their particular situation and institution. Long-term maintenance and operation of such applications must be factored in to the institutional costs and the organization must be willing and able to take this on. Relying on a vendor for long-term support may prove more practical, provided the financial and industry position of the company is sound, so that it does not succumb to competitive pressures and is forced to withdraw long-term product support.

To create practical clinical research applications and, most importantly, to be able to link them across organizations, a common unifying model must be employed. In Chapter 19, John Gennari describes a primary component of such modeling, the clinical state diagram. He provides two practical examples, in breast cancer and in lung cancer, and shows how these would be applied to two key areas of cancer informatics: authoring protocol eligibility criteria and providing patient eligibility decision support. Such models could help speed the development and conduct of trials, leading to new medical discoveries being brought into actual practice much more rapidly. A theme noted here is reiterated throughout several chapters of this text as well, namely, the importance of standard vocabularies and common data elements. Such standardization will not only speed the development of applications, but allow them to be interoperable across disease entities and organizations in the future.

Chapter 20 describes innovative uses of informatics to serve the patient and their family during the intensive and often bewildering treatment processes they may undergo. A successfully deployed neonatal care system is described by Herbert Goldberg and Charles Safran, and the lessons learned are extrapolated to the area of cancer treatment. Internet technologies are exploited to break down physical and geographical barriers among patients, their families, and their care providers. The quality of the information available over the Internet is brought out as a key issue. User authentication and secure transmission become even more critical when individual patient data are exchanged over the Internet. While previous applications in this section focused on patient care or direct interventional research, making their value more obvious, the authors rightly state that the value of systems that perform population behavioral management become less obvious. They discuss the need for future innovative partnerships among payers, providers, government, and the public to develop and deploy comprehensive cancer informatics systems. If such partnerships become viable, perhaps the choice of "make versus buy" will become a moot point in the future.

Informatics tools to inform the public about the existence of ongoing cancer clinical trials is approached from both the government perspective and that of a national, comprehensive cancer institute in two complementary chapters. In Chapter 22, Alexa McCray describes the National Library of Medicine's development of *ClinicalTrials.gov*, a Web site designed to provide patients, families, and other members of the public with access to information about clinical research studies via the Web. Development of this site was mandated by the Food and Drug Administration Modernization Act of 1997, specifically charging the National Institutes of Health with creating such a resource for access to both federally and privately funded trials. This site could be linked to transactional Web sites, such as the one developed at City of Hope National Medical Center, dubbed "*Clinical Trials On-Line*" and discussed in Chapter 21 by Joyce Niland and Douglas Stahl. Because this Web site is driven by an interactive database, the public can obtain up-to-the-minute summaries of over 100 ongoing trials and search for trials by disease, physician, age category, treatment modality, or key word. Physician profiles and research program descriptions online further inform patients and help them make educated choices about their treatment course. Web sites such as these can facilitate patient enrollment, thereby speeding critical medical discoveries.

As research data accumulate during the course of a trial, the methods described in Chapter 23 will help manage the research data at the national level. In Chapter 23, Dianne Reeves and Douglas Hageman describe the NCI's steps in developing a clinical research system, including using Internet-based technologies, understanding the underlying problems and work processes, carefully evaluating the "build versus buy" decision (echoing advice from Mitchell Morris's chapter on this topic), incorporating standards and best practices such as the International Conference on Harmonisation (ICH), Good Clinical Practice (GCP) guidelines, utilizing the most robust terminology ontologies and vocabularies, and considering the principles of system architecture, security practices, training and user acceptance. In the process, NCI and other organizations must be mindful of the potential burden imposed by reporting and data requirements on the institutions performing the trials. The American Association of Cancer Institutes (AACI) has recently initiated a "bottom up" assessment to help establish the best way to proceed with unified informatics approaches across cancer institutions. The first meeting took place early in 2001, and assigned subcommittees are now performing the work of assessing and compiling the best recommendations for future informatics tools and standards to speed cancer discoveries.

In Chapter 24, Donald Simborg describes how the iKnowMed Network is attempting to meet the needs of patient care and clinical trials in a single informatics tool. The hope is to improve the currently inefficient patient processes of recruitment and case reporting, and piloting the use of point-of-care information for clinical research. These are laudible goals; yet the most difficult component will be gaining user acceptance, particularly by physicians in a busy oncology practice with not a minute to spare. (The "H" of the "HIT" mnemonic!) A novel feature is the patient-centric user interface of the iKnowMyChart application, which would allow patients to view their own medical information online. Physician acceptance of this open availability of information, as well as privacy and confidentiality concerns, will dictate the ultimate adoption of this form of electronic system. The application of rules and alerts to continually improve the safety and efficiency of practice is proposed, along with the recurring theme for standardized vocabularies and data interchange. The recently enacted Health Information Portability and Accountability Act (HIPAA) will be a driver of future privacy practices. iKnowMed also proposes making aggregate data available to pharmaceutical firms, which may help speed new drug discoveries, yet is not without potential privacy issues that must be addressed.

As more and more people access the Internet daily for medical information, consumer health informatics (CHI) and interactive health communications (IHC) become critical fields. In Chapter 25, Deborah Mayer and Susan Hubbard discuss the four major societal trends in cancer care that have affected our development and deployment of informatics, along with their impact on altering the information needs and options of cancer patients. CHI helps us analyze consumers' needs for information, and IHC allows these information needs to be met through electronic devices or communication technologies. Functions include providing learning tools, promoting health behavior, assisting informed decision making, facilitating peer exchange and emotional support, and managing the demand for health services. Once again issues such as the quality of information provided and security/confidentiality concerns are a theme of this chapter. The impact on physician-patient relationships and outcomes is explored.

This last concept of 'patient outcomes' is the theme of Chapter 26 by Joyce Niland, describing an Internet-based system that has been in use for over four years by the National Comprehensive Cancer Network (NCCN) in conducting patterns of care and outcomes research. The system was developed at City of Hope National Medical Center, using leading edge Web technologies to collect information on care patterns and outcomes for cancer patients treated in the nations' leading cancer centers. Digital certification, authentication, encryption, and de-identification are key features of the system, which has resulted in the successful collection and analysis of data on over 7,000 cancer patients to date. An integrated database model allows rapid scale-up to multiple cancer sites, and an extension of the system into the community oncology setting is underway, including the development of a graphical decision support interface and the testing of scannable forms as an alternative to Web methodology.

Taken together, the applications described in Section 4 represent our vision of utilizing cancer informatics in the facilitation of new drug discoveries, patient care, and assessment of long-term outcomes. Informatics is the key to integrating science and medical research to acquire and manage future knowledge regarding the causes, prevention, and ultimate cure of cancer.

18
Selection of Oncology Information Systems

Mitchell Morris

The notion that organizations should purchase rather than develop software whenever possible holds true for many healthcare applications. The unique aspects of cancer medicine, however, do not fit this simple approach. Oncology routinely involves clinical trials, multidisciplinary care, and a complex and variable set of disease processes unmatched by any other field of medicine. Often, the task of collecting clinical data—e.g., for clinical trials—spans from small private practice offices to large freestanding cancer centers and everything in between.

Because of oncology's complexity and the perception that general acute care is the most profitable market, many software vendors have not developed solutions for cancer medicine. Oncology information systems must often integrate with other enterprise systems from mainstream vendors, complicating the "build versus buy" decision (Lowe, 2001; McDonald, 1997). There is no black and white difference between purchasing and developing software, only variations that fall in between.

In this chapter, we explore how to select software that will support clinical oncology. We discuss how to analyze the options of building and buying and make a decision based on the value of the software. Throughout, we emphasize three project management principles:

- **Establish a partnership between clinicians and information systems staff.** Information systems projects should involve an appropriate mix of end user and information systems participation (Sjoberg & Timpka, 1998). If involvement occurs too late in the project life cycle, user results may not be satisfactory. Project structures should encourage early and ongoing partnerships among users, management, and information systems staff. Physician involvement is especially critical to the success of this process (Anderson, 1999).
- **Encourage effective project steering.** Without careful guidance, even well-managed projects may generate undesirable or unexpected results. The commitment and sponsorship of the executive leadership are crucial to success. Each project phase should lead to a logical decision point at

which information about the project is conveyed to a defined steering body. The resulting interaction ensures appropriate investment of time and effort in the project and prevents unpleasant surprises.

- **Enable ongoing understanding and assessment of risks and benefits.** Critical treatment decisions for cancer patients require a thoughtful balance of risk and benefit. Selecting an information system demands the same analytic approach. While technology decisions do not have such an immediate impact on patient health, they have long-term effects on the quality of care and the progress of cancer research. Those involved in technology projects must understand expected benefits, prioritize investments based on anticipated results, and monitor actual outcomes. Most large information technology projects never achieve the expected benefits; for others, we can only assume a benefit in the absence of objective measures.

Proposal Phase

Before investigating available commercial software systems, the organization should develop a solid understanding of its needs and determine if the proposed project is worthy of further investment. The proposal phase, a high-level review, should identify the problem the software will solve. Appropriate questions include:

- What are the expected benefits?
- What should the solution look like?
- What functions should it have?
- Who will use it?
- How much can we afford to spend?
- When do we need this solution?
- What types of risks might we incur?
- Who will sponsor this program?
- Who will do the work?
- Will our organization install and maintain the software?

We would not build a new clinic without answering questions like these, and no organization should shop for an information system before conducting a similar review. This exercise will narrow the field, easing the task of selecting an oncology information system.

Identify the Problem

Organizations should purchase or develop software because it will solve a particular problem, not simply because it is fresh or innovative. Identifying the problem to be solved should take the form of program objectives. For example, an organization may have multiple paper-based forms for clinical trials management, no data standards, and *ad hoc* usage of several statistical analysis programs. The objective may be to establish uniform data sets to enable faster completion of trials, enhance data quality, and speed data analysis. If the organization has no problems with clinical trials management, articulating clear objectives will be more difficult. Once defined, the remaining questions must be compared with the overriding objectives to ensure consistency.

Determine Necessary Software Functionality

A group of stakeholders should determine the desired high-level functions of the software, a task best accomplished in a brainstorming session using a white board. The description should communicate general concepts without intricate detail. For example, the stakeholders might conclude that the system should track laboratory and radiology results, allow physicians to enter chemotherapy orders, and permit pharmacists to document which medications were administered.

Define Expected User Base

The initial stakeholder group should determine who will use the new system. This is, to a great extent, related to software functionality. For example, some systems might only be used by data managers and research nurses and operate in the background for physicians. Determining system users will aid movement to the next phase, where representation from different stakeholders is important. This will also play a critical role in eventual user acceptance of the system (Gardner & Lundsgaarde, 1994).

Determine Expected Benefits

The team should perform a high-level determination of benefits. This exercise is best carried out with a facilitated group process (Chocholik, Bouchard, Tan, Ostro, 1999). Some examples include:

- **Cost avoidance.** This may include averting expenditures (e.g., purchasing paper goods and supporting a legacy system) or reducing the workforce with the help of automated processes.
- **Revenue enhancements.** This might mean improving collections or more accurately coding for services.
- **Competitive advantage.** Software implementations could improve a practice's market share, attract new patients, or put them in a better position to apply for grants and complete clinical trials faster.
- **Qualitative benefits.** Systems can also enhance the quality of patient care, reduce medical error and adverse drug reactions, and increase physician and staff satisfaction with the work environment. Although difficult to estimate in terms of cost, these factors offer tremendous value.

Define Project Risks

All projects carry significant risk. In most software projects, the greatest risks surround cultural issues, not technological challenges (although both are a factor). Using a matrix of common IT project risks (see Table 18.1), the group should determine whether they fall into the low, medium, or high category. If too many are in the high category, they should reconsider the project's feasibility. Subsequent project phases should revisit the risk matrix, as risks change over time.

Estimate Costs

Before deciding whether to build or buy the system, organizations must estimate the cost. This may be limited to the number of zeros in the dollar figure, or it can be more precise. The final figure should include not only software costs, but also hardware, personnel, and training. (It is important to note that, during the proposal phase, no one is held accountable for "guesstimates.")

Assess People and Skill Requirements

Does the organization have the people and skills to select, implement, and maintain the software? If the answer is no, then they must also consider the cost of outsourcing or hiring new people. People and skills are necessary components of project management and change management—probably even more important than the technology component.

At the end of the proposal phase, next steps should be clear. By weighing the high-level benefits, costs, and risks, the organization can either move to the next phase or do nothing. Thus far, they have probably expended relatively little effort, but they have established communication within a group of management, clinicians, and IT staff. After presenting the proposal to the decision-making team and gaining approval, they can move on to the analysis phase.

Analysis Phase

If a solution is needed, the funds are present, and the risk is manageable, the organization can begin a more detailed analysis of feasibility, functionality, and acquisition strategy. Regardless of the build versus buy decision, this next phase is essential. It also involves more work than the proposal phase, including in-depth research of high-level estimates, collaboration with vendors if off-the-shelf software products are available, and configuration and installation of ready-made software. The analysis phase is the basis of the Request for Proposal (RFP). If software must be developed, the organization must draw up a detailed road map that will form the basis of their contract with a software development group.

Table 18.1. Risk factor rating matrix. To complete the assessment of risk factors below, indicate the appropriate level of risk (i.e., high, medium, or low) for each of the risk factors based on the supplied definitions. Place an "H," "M," or "L" in the rightmost column to indicate the assessed level of risk for each factor

Risk Factor Rating Matrix				
Risk Factor	High Risk	Medium Risk	Low Risk	#
		Organization Risk Factors – Enterprise Wide		
Organizational Strategies	Project does not support any organizational strategies	Project indirectly or partially supports organizational strategies	Project directly supports one or more organizational straegies	
Organizational Project History/ Experience	Organization has poor history or little experience with automated systems	Organization has experience with systems or some successful projects	Organization has extensive history with successful projects	
Organization Mission and Goals	Project does not support or relate to any Organization missions or goals	Project will indirectly impact on Organization goal or mission	Project directly supports an Organization goal or mission	
Work Methods of Organization	Project will directly alter the work methods of one or more agencies	Project will alter parts of have slight effect on work methods	Project will have little or no effect on Organization work method	
Organization Clients	Project provides main support of delivery of services to primary Organization clients	Project will alter some service delivery to Organization clients	Project will have little or no effect on delivery of services	
		Organization Risk Factors – Management		
Executive Management Support	No support for project, or major unresolved issues	Roles and mission issues unresolved or in process of being defined or approved	Agreed to support project	
Performance Objectives	No established performance requirements or requirements ill-defined and not measurable	Some performance questions or question on measurement	Verifiable performance, reasonable requirements, and measures clearly defined	
Organizational Stability	Management rapidly changing or not clearly defined	Some management change expected	Little or no change in management experienced	
Commitment to Project	Organization has little or no support for project	Organization states support for project but demonstrates lack of support	Strongly committed to success of project	
Experience with Similar Projects	No experience with projects of this type of projects in general	Moderate experience or experience with different type projects	Very experienced with similar projects	

TABLE 18.1. (*Continued*)

Risk Factor Rating Matrix				
Risk Factor	High Risk	Medium Risk	Low Risk	#
Policies and Standards	No policies or standards in place or ill-defined and ineffective	Policies and standards in place but weak or not followed completely	Policies and standards in place and are strong, effective, and followed completely	
Organization Risk Factors – Oversight				
Project Plan	Project plan outdated and/or plan not followed by project team	Plan approved, complete, and used by most of project team	Comprehensive plan approved, monitored, updated, and used by all project team	
Customer Service Quality	No improvements in service	Minor improvements to customer service	Major improvement to customer service	
Monitoring Process	No process established or process is ignored	Process established, not well followed, or ineffective	Process well-established, procedures followed, and highly effective	
Project Size and Scope	Rapidly changing size or scope, requirements not defined and not signed off by customers	Requirements defined and customers signed-off but changes to baseline expected	Requirements well-established, baseline defined, customer acceptance high, and few or no changes	
Quality Assurance	No quality assurance process of procedures established	Procedures established, but not well-followed or effective	Quality assurance system established, well followed, highly effective	
Management Requirements	None in place, defined, or ineffective	Requirements defined, some inconsistencies remain, and requirements may not have been distributed to employees	Well-defined, consistent, established, well distributed, effective	
Budgetary and Cost Factors				
Funding Sources and Constraints	Budget allocation in doubt or subject to change without notice	Some questionable allocations or doubts about availability	Funds allocated with out constraints	
Cost/Schedule Review	No review process established or totally ineffective	Controls established but not all complete or in place	All controls in place and effective	
Cost Controls	Cost control system lacking or nonexistent	Cost control system in place but weak in some areas	Cost controls well established, in place, and effective	

Table 18.1. (*Continued*)

Risk Factor Rating Matrix				
Risk Factor	High Risk	Medium Risk	Low Risk	#
Economic Justification/ Cost	Not justified or cost effective	Justification questionable or cost-effectiveness not completely established	Completely justified and cost-effectiveness proven	
Budget Size	Insufficient budget available to complete project as defined	Questions remain concerning budget	Sufficient funds available to complete project as currently defined	
Incremental Payments Based on Deliverables	No set, agreed-upon incremental payments based on product deliverables	Some set of agreed-upon incremental payments based on product deliverables	Complete agreement on incremental payments based on product deliverables	
Customer Factors – Participation				
Customer Training Requirements	Requirements not defined or addressed	Customer training needs considered but training or training plan in development	Customer training needs considered, training or training plan in place and in process	
Customer Acceptance	Customers have not accepted any of the concepts or design details of the system	Customers have accepted most concepts and details of the system, and process in place for customer approvals	Customers have accepted all concepts and details of the system and process in place for customer approvals	
Customer Experience on IT Projects	Customers have no previous experience with IT project and are unsure how needs can be met	Customer justification provided, justificatiion complete with some questions about applicability	Customer justification complete accurate and sound	
Involvement of Custo-mers	Minimal or no customer involvement on development team or little customer input into process	Customers on project team play minor roles or have only moderate impact on system	Customers highly involved with project team, provide significant input and participation in system	
Customer Factors – Requirements				
Customer Justification	Customers have not provided any or satisfactory justification for system development	Customer justification provided, justification complete with some questions about applicability	Customer justification complete, accurate, and sound	

TABLE 18.1. (*Continued*)

Risk Factor Rating Matrix				
Risk Factor	High Risk	Medium Risk	Low Risk	#
Achievable Benefits	Benefits undefined, baseline not established, unattainable, or immeasurable	Some questions remain about benefits, or baseline changing and measurements doubtful	Benefits well-defined, baseline established, measurable, and verifiable	
Deliverable Requirements Defined	No requirements defined for deliverables or unreasonable requirements	Some deliverable requirements remain to be defined or vague and immeasurable	All deliverable requirements defined, reasonable, and measurable	
Customer Requirements Defined	Customer requirements not defined or are insufficient for a successful project	Customer requirements defined but changes anticipated	Customer requirements well-defined and no changes anticipated	
System Integration/ Interfaces	Extensive integration of systems, or exchange of information or interfaces are a major part of project	Some integration or interfaces required and/or of some importance to project	Little or no integration or interfaces required	
Fit with Existing Environment	Introduces new technology to the environment	Limited use of new technologies	Uses proven techn-ology that integrates well	
Quality Control	Time line likely to adversely affect quality and completeness	Has critical time line, but little to no impact on quality	Time lines are not critical	
Technology Factors – Operations				
Open Systems	Proprietary system with little or no communication with other technologies	System capable of communicating with other technologies on a limited basis	Completely open platform, capable of communicating with multiple other technologies	
Vendor History	Vendor has poor history or has little experience dealing with government business deliverable	Vendor has limited history dealing with government deliverables, or has some successful projects	Vendor has extensive and successful history dealing with government deliverables	
Vendor Support	Vendor provides little or no support for hardware/software, and only at high cost and with poor response times	Vendor provides adequate support for hardware/software at contracted price with reasonable response times	Vendor provides complete support for hardware/software at reasonable or contracted price and within contracted response times	

Table 18.1. (*Continued*)

Risk Factor Rating Matrix				
Risk Factor	High Risk	Medium Risk	Low Risk	#
Maturity of Solution	Leading edge (in operation less than one year) or aged technology (over five years old)	State-of-the-art (in operation from 1–3 years)	Mature technology well established and proven (in operation 3–5 years)	
Commercial Software Stability, Reliability, Maturity	New commercial software with unproven record	Relatively new commercial software with some proven record	Established commercial software with proven record	
Security	No security measure in place, backup of data and hardware lacking, disaster recovery not considered	Some security measures in place, backups of data and hardware being done, disaster recovery considered, but procedures lacking or not followed	All areas following security guidelines, data and hardware completely backed up, disaster recovery system in place, and procedures easily followed	
Multiple Vendors/ Major Contractors	No clear delineation between vendor responsibility, contractors in conflict with one another, no clear prime contractor	Prime contractor delineated, vendor responsibilities defined, but conflict between vendors/ contractors	Prime contractor in place and responsible for successfully implementing project, no conflict between vendors, and dispute resolution policy established	
		Project Management Factors – Manager		
Staff Productivity	Staff productivity is low, milestones are not met, excessive delays in meeting deliverable requirements	Most milestones met, some delays in deliverables, staff output is acceptable	All milestones, met, deliverables on time, and productivity high	
Manager Experience	Project manager without experience with this type of project or new to management	Project manager with moderate experience or with different types of projects	Project manager very experienced with similar types of projects	
Management Approach	Project management approach weak or ineffective	Project management approach good, but needs development	Project management approach strong and effective	
Manager Authority	Project manager is manager in name only	Project manager has support of most of staff with some reservations	Project manager has complete support of entire staff and executive management	

Table 18.1. (*Continued*)

Risk Factor Rating Matrix				
Risk Factor	High Risk	Medium Risk	Low Risk	#
Manager Commitment	Project manager shows no commitment to project	Project manager states support for project but priority given to project indicates otherwise	Project manager has strong commitment to success of project	
		Project Management Factors – Process		
Elapsed Time	Project has major schedule delays that threaten success of the project	Project is within schedule, minor delays on some parts or deliverables	Project is within reasonable schedule, following work plan with no delays	
Problem Determination and Evaluation Process	A process to determine and evaluate problems is nonexistent or inadequate	Evaluation process exists, but some questions remain about process, or minor inconsistencies in process	Problem determination process adequate, consistent, and solves problems	
Change Control Management	No change control process being used	Change control process in place but not being followed completely, or ineffective	Formal change control process in place, followed and effective	
Development Methodology	No formal project development methodology being used, either commercial or in-house	Project development methodology established, but not followed or ineffective	Project development methodology in place, established, effective, and followed by staff	
		Project Management Factors – Personnel		
Experience of Staff	Staff has little or no experience with projects of this type and lacks experience with hardware or software	Project staff has some experience with projects of this type but lacks experience with hardware or software	Project staff is highly experienced with projects of this type, and has experience with hardware and/or software	
Availability of and Experience with Productivity Tools	Productivity tools not being used or considered	Productivity tools available but not used to full potential, or in process of being implemented, and training needed	Productivity tools used and staff trained in use of tools	
Commitment of Staff	Project staff has little or no commitment to the success of project	Project staff states commitment to project, but commitment is not genuine	Project staff highly committed to success to project	

TABLE 18.1. (*Continued*)

Risk Factor Rating Matrix				
Risk Factor	High Risk	Medium Risk	Low Risk	#
Consultant/ Organization Personnel Mix	Complete reliance on contractor or consultant staff with no Organization staff being trained in new system	Small percentage of Organization staff or some Organization personnel being trained on new systems	A balanced mix of Organization and contractor staff with Organization personnel capable of taking over new system	
Available Personnel Resources	Project staff has high turnover rate, little or no experience, or not available for project	Project staff available but not all in place, training plan established	Project staff all available, in place, experienced, and stable	
Project Team Factors – Experience/Training				
Expertise with Hardware	New hardware, little experience, different technology	Technology similar to existing systems. And some in-house experience	Mature technology, current in-house experinece, high experience ratio	
Expertise with Software	New software, and no experience with software or similar products	Some experience with software or similar product	High experience ratio with software or similar systems	
Technical Training Staff	Training not readily available, or no training plan in place	Training for some disciplines not available, but training planned and available	Training plan in place and training ongoing	
Expertise with Methodology	Project staff has little or no experience with methodology or similar methodology	Project staff has some experience with methodology or similar methodology	Project staff has extensive experience with methodology or similar methodologies	
Technology Factors – Business				
Analysis of Alternatives	Analysis of alternatives not completed, not all alternatives considered, and/or assumptions faulty	Analysis of alternatives completed, some assumptions questionable, and alternatives not fully considered	Analysis of alternative complete, all alternatives and options considered, and assumptions verifiable	
Complexity of Requirements	Project is very complex with multiple requirements form many different customers; requirements are complex and hard to find	Project is fairly complex with some requirements more easily defined; several customer groups will be aiding in the design	Requirements are few and easily defined; few customers to provide input	

The team should perform the following steps, most in parallel, and clearly document the results. Because decisions made in the analysis phase will impact all the product users, full involvement of the stakeholders is critical.

Perform Workflow Analysis

While some managers may feel they fully understand their organization's workflow, a formal analysis often uncovers many additional details and issues. Line staff like nurses and clerks often create elaborate manual systems to work around inefficient technology. Their methods of handling unusual patient or billing situations, for instance, can vary significantly from the standard.

Workflow analysis is best done with charts that examine the path of information through the work process and clearly outline each decision point. This analysis should identify areas that can benefit from automation. The team should develop a common understanding of current deficiencies in both manual and automated systems.

Next is the more difficult task of outlining the desired workflow. If the exact capabilities of a software product are unknown, this will have to evolve later in the project. Understanding how the software can improve workflow is a good start.

Document Current Technical Environment

Before proceeding with the new system, the organization must understand its technical environment. This can be divided into three major areas:

- **Network.** The team should describe the network environment in terms of network protocols and speed, clearly identifying slow segments and noting network path redundancy for mission-critical systems.
- **Server.** The team should delineate the server operating systems and environment, including a description of facilities for expanding servers and mass storage, such as data centers.
- **Desktop.** The team should describe the desktop environment, including the prevalent operating system, the number of computers relative to the number of users, and computer accessibility. The "age of the fleet" is also important.

Define Desired Technical Environment

The definition of the desired technical environment can be divided into the three areas noted above. If the network infrastructure cannot move the types and amount of data (e.g., radiology images), then the team should describe an upgraded environment. If additional space in the data center or additional mass storage and servers are needed, the team should described these. Operating systems not consistent with market trends should be noted, as should the desktop environment, which often requires an upgrade. Changing the technical environment can drive costs far beyond mere purchase and implementation.

Define Organizational and Technical Impacts

In this section of the analysis, the team should describe the impact of automation on the organization. Reporting structures, the process of work, change management, and training management issues should be outlined here. Cultural issues and training, often underestimated in technology projects, are usually the most challenging components. The team should also describe the technical impact based on the desired technical environment.

Define Business Process Metrics

An important but often overlooked task in a software implementation is defining how to measure the anticipated benefits. The project team should develop detailed, objective business process metrics that can be used before and after the implementation and represent the value of the project. These metrics should relate to the expected benefits of the system, as outlined in the proposal phase. Suggested metrics include:

- the percentage of new patients entered in clinical trials
- the cost of downcoded charges due to poor documentation
- the number of clerical FTEs needed
- treatment in accordance with established practice guidelines
- the appropriate use of growth factors or anti-emetics
- decreased days in accounts receivable
- decrease in length of stay
- decrease in medical transcription costs.

Develop Detailed Functional Specifications

Based on the future workflow analysis and the high-level functional specifications from the proposal phase, the team should develop detailed functional specifications. As with the other steps, they must involve future users and the technical staff. Users know what they want the software to do, and technical staff know whether those desires are realistic.

Locate Vendor or Industry Solutions

Having decided what type of software is needed, the team can now assess the availability of off-the-shelf solutions. They can:

- contact similar organizations using the software and consider site visits.
- visit trade shows where software is displayed, such as the American Society of Clinical Oncology, the Oncology Nursing Society, the Health Information Management Systems Society, the National Managed Healthcare Congress, and regional trade shows.
- work with IT staff to review trade magazines and consider calling in vendor representatives for demonstrations.

At this stage, organizations must avoid committing to a particular vendor or spending too much time discussing requirements with them. Once they know the requirements, many vendors will claim they can deliver exactly that. Instead, organizations should let the vendor present the capabilities of its software. If there is not a good match, they should be cautious of vendors who promise to develop new functionality, because a vendor's sales and marketing force may not speak for the engineering department. Promises made to secure a sale may be very difficult to implement.

Develop the Recommended Acquisition Strategy (e.g., Build Versus Buy)

The last part of the analysis phase is an assessment of build versus buy strategies. If nothing in the marketplace can fulfill even a portion of the organization's functions, then the decision is simple. However, products more commonly fulfill some but not all of the desired functions, making the build versus buy decision complex. Table 18.2 summarizes the pros and cons of building and buying, and in the next section, we discuss this comparison phase.

Table 18.2. Build versus buy

Build	Buy
Pros Software optimized to the organization's specific processes	Pros • Lower cost • Lower risk of implementation • Shorter time period to implement • More likely to use standards
Cons • Commitment to long-term support and ongoing development • Usually higher costs • Longer time to implement • Must be familiar with data standards to integrate with other systems • Greater risk of project failure • Human resources issues	Cons • Will not be designed to fit the organization's best practices • Will be subject to design changes for the overall market

Comparison Phase: Build Versus Buy Strategies

We began this chapter by questioning whether organizations should ever develop software when they can purchase it from a vendor. The pros and cons outlined in Table 18.2 seem to strongly favor buying software. Once most organizations complete a detailed analysis phase, however, they find that off-the-shelf products rarely meet all the functionality requirements. As the following sections testify, there is much to consider (Clemons, 2000; Hayes, 1995).

Consider Process Issues

The biggest advantage to developing software inhouse is clear: the team can design it to fit an ideal process and workflow using the detailed functional specifications created in the analysis phase. However desirable this may sound, there are several caveats. Because cost or programming limitations may make the functional specifications technically impossible, the team may have to compromise on what it considers "best practice." Also, because the "ideal" process has not yet been tested, organizations may discover flaws post-development that went unrecognized on paper. Off-the-shelf software, conversely, has a built-in work process that has presumably worked well at other sites.

Although commercial software will never exactly match ideal processes, the software company's expertise in best practices merits strong consideration. The software has likely been developed in conjunction with another oncology organization, and it may have been implemented at several other sites. Organizations can derive immediate benefits from the time, money, and hard work the software company spent to develop these practices.

While wrestling with the decision, the team might construct a checklist of desired functional requirements and note which of these the potential vendor currently offers. Again, organizations must be wary of "under development" claims; although the vendor may indeed plan to develop the software, it has many other customers with different priorities. How the new customer's priorities rate in the final work plan may differ from the salesperson's initial claims.

One feature of commercial software to examine closely is the degree to which it can be configured. In general, organizations should avoid customizing software—in other words, changing the source code or the basic operating functions. Configuration is different from customizing because it uses established tools to adjust the software features to create particular work processes. Some commercial software is highly configurable, and some is more rigid.

All organizations must compromise to some degree on their ideal work processes and desired functionality. A crucial decision for the steering team is what level of compromise they can live with and which side—build or buy—best fits this level of compromise.

Compare Costs

In general, it costs far more to develop software inhouse than to purchase it. While vendors recoup their development costs among several customers, organizations that choose inhouse development bear the entire cost burden. An exception is the use of Internet-based technologies, which organizations can use to automate certain work processes for a relatively low cost. Because we are in a transition between technologic platforms, some vendor products may reflect the higher costs of development and implementation in the client server environment rather than the lower cost browser-based platform using standard industry tools.

When performing a comparison, the organization must include all the cost considerations of the analysis phase: development costs, software licensing, hardware, other third-party software, training, internal staff costs, and contractor costs. Often, the licensing costs of commercial software or the development costs of internal software are only a small part of the equation. Differences between those two may be minimized when the total project cost is estimated.

Provide for Ongoing Support

After implementing software, the organization will find its needs slowly changing. New data models, the impact of regulatory action, and new technology demand a commitment to ongoing software development, especially when organizations build software internally. Such organizations must maintain expensive software developers who both understand the software and can continue its creative development. Although this can significantly increase maintenance costs, this approach will ensure that all enhancements will be based on the organization's specific needs.

Issues across the healthcare industry drive most change. For example, the Health Insurance Portability and Accountability Act (HIPAA) demands significant architectural changes in most healthcare software systems. Common data elements and other standards outlined in this volume will also drive change in oncology software. Commercial software developers must keep pace with these changes if they wish to stay in business. While some of the development cost will be passed to the customers, those costs will be distributed across the vendor's customer base.

Another aspect of support is day-to-day product support and the ongoing cost of maintaining experts who can fix the system. Because individuals with development talent often do not enjoy this task, organizations should retain a separate staff of IT professionals who maintain the production system. A commercial vendor has a set of engineers working on development and a separate staff for day-to-day support. This factor increases the cost of inhouse development.

Consider Timing Issues

Developing inhouse software takes longer than purchasing commercial software; however, commercial software must be extensively configured to fit the organization. Finding out how long a vendor's software takes to install is crucial; in some cases, configuring and installing software takes almost as long as developing it. Inhouse software is actually being "configured" to the organization's processes from the first day of development.

Assess Human Resource Needs

Expert programming staff is expensive and difficult to retain. Individuals with polished development skills usually command six-figure salaries and expect benefits like stock options and 401(k) plans. Commercial vendors can afford such staff and retain them through a variety of incentives, but it is very difficult for healthcare organizations to do the same. Because building software is a multi-year commitment, organizations must carefully consider their ability to attract and (more importantly) retain programming staff. These human capital costs, which vendors can distribute across their customer base, are some of the highest for inhouse development projects.

An alternative to hiring programming staff is contracting with a software development firm for the expertise. While the hourly rate may be higher than that of inhouse employees, highly talented and experienced individuals may be able to complete the project faster, saving both time and money.

Satisfy Integration and Standards Requirements

Integrating data from different systems is important, particularly in oncology. When an oncology information system is installed, it is often desirable to integrate laboratory, pathology, radiology, demographic, and other information sources into an electronic record or clinical trials system (McDonald, 1997). Healthcare information systems are usually HL7 compliant, which simplifies data flow among them. Most commercial vendors have experience with integrating information from other departmental systems into the product and some major vendors may have scripts already written to accomplish this.

Those who choose to build inhouse will have to develop these data exchanges from scratch. Using an interface engine can simplify this process, and an organization's IT department may have already built outgoing information flow from all the major departmental systems to an interface engine. How far this infrastructure has been established is a significant factor in the final decision.

Data standards raise another issue, as information sharing among organizations and training issues for new doctors and clinicians will be increasingly important. Organizations with data models and clinician interfaces that match those of other organizations can more easily share data and engage clinicians in their work.

Determine Value

After studying these issues, the steering committee should decide between build and buy based on sound comparative data. Issues of process, cost, support, human resources, timing, and integration are different for each organization, so no precise formula exists. Value, however, should be the deciding factor. This chapter does not describe how to calculate internal rate of return and net present value, but these financial measures can be used in the decision process and to justify internal expense with senior management.

New Possibilities: Internet-Based Technologies and Application Service Providers

As noted in this chapter, Internet-based technologies help some organizations rapidly develop new applications. Using this technology, the user's computer houses a Web browser, not client software. The software resides on a server accessed by the browser, an approach that enables a development process different from traditional software. In the traditional development process (some components of which are outlined above) the software is not released until the entire project is completed. The Internet-based approach is an iterative development process that releases components of some applications incrementally. Because no client software resides on the user's computer, making incremental progress in a production system is reasonable. Organizations that use this approach selectively can begin to reap the benefits of automation almost immediately, even though completing the program may take several years.

Internet-based technologies often involve readily available software tools that are simpler to work with than the proprietary tools many vendors use. This means the Internet-based approach relieves some of the pressure to secure the necessary expertise.

In the past few years, new services known as application service providers (ASPs) have emerged. With the development of Internet technologies and reasonably reliable data transmission over long distances, ASPs are a viable alternative to maintaining inhouse hardware and software. The ASP model comes in a variety of formats, but essentially works as follows: a vendor (sometimes the software company, sometimes a third party) hosts the computers and software at an offsite facility, the client organization accesses the application via the Internet, and data is stored offsite.

This approach may spare an organization some problems with human resources, ongoing support, and possibly cost. Completely outsourcing the application to the ASP eliminates the need for a technical staff, but it remains unclear whether the ASP model will be cost effective. In theory, because of the hardware economies of scale and the ability to reuse the technology and software for different sites, ASPs should lower costs. In reality, savings on hardware may not materialize, and the implementing and configuring process makes it difficult to share applications among organizations. Most ASPs end up running multiple configurations of the same software package.

Another consideration is the cost of the Internet bandwidth required to transfer data. As we move into an era of large data sets and medical images, the cost of broadband may increase. The reliability and security of the Internet are also concerns. Still, the ASP model is worth investigating and will continue developing over the next few years. Using the preceding criteria to determine best value will aid decisions about the ASP model.

Vendor Selection Phase

After deciding to purchase commercial software, organizations must take the next step—vendor selection. They might take action as follows:

- **Visit sites where the software is working.** During site visits, talk to actual users, not just individuals the vendor selects. Find out if doctors and nurses are using the software in the organization, or if it is simply a pilot program. Speak to administrators at the site to understand their expected return on investment and whether the benefits have been achieved. Site visits can also reveal whether the vendor responds to ongoing customer needs and maintains the software appropriately.
- **Investigate the financial condition of the vendor.** Is the vendor a candidate for acquisition where the product may no longer be developed or even discontinued? Does the company have adequate capital to carry out additional development work? Is the leadership visionary and stable? Do they have a growing customer base?
- **Review information about the vendor.** Peruse the information in trade journals or access it through a group purchasing organization.
- **Issue a formal request for proposal (RFP).** In their response, the vendor should respond to all functional and technical requirements. Use the checklist approach so the vendor can indicate which functions are in the current release and which are planned for future releases. Be skeptical of "planned" functions and consider contractually obligating the vendor to develop them if they are crucial to successful implementation. Such an obligation may penalize the vendor if these features are not implemented in a timely fashion.

Looking Ahead

Organizations must select oncology information systems in a thoughtful, systematic manner that places primary importance on potential value. To help chart an appropriate course, cancer centers should work closely with consultants and vendors. A successful selection process should include all key stakeholders, including management, IT professionals, and clinicians. As common data elements and other standards are developed, we hope the software industry will consider oncology applications a solid market for further investment.

References

Anderson JD. 1999. Increasing the Acceptance of Clinical Information Systems. MD Computing 16:1–9.

Chocholik JK, Bouchard SE, Tan JK, Ostrow DN. 1999. The Determination of Relevant Goals and Criteria Used to Select an Automated Patient Care Information System. Journal of the American Medical Informatics Association 6:219–233.

Clemons EK. 2000 (December 1). The Build/Buy Battle. CIO Magazine.

Gardner RM, Lundsgaarde HP. 1994. Evaluation of User Acceptance of a Clinical Expert System. Journal of the American Medical Informatics Association 1:428–438.

Hayes F. 1995 (December 11). Corporate Development Puzzle: Buy vs. Build. Computerworld.

Lowe HJ. 2001. Oncology Informatics: Transforming the Cancer Center in the 21st Century. MD Computing, 16:1–6.

McDonald CJ. 1997. The Barriers to Electronic Medical Record Systems and How to Overcome Them. Journal of the American Medical Informatics Association 4:213–221.

Sjoberg C, Timpka T. 1998. Participatory Design of Information Systems in Health Care. Journal of the American Medical Informatics Association 5:177–183.

19
Clinical State Diagrams and Informatics Tools for Clinical Trial Protocols

John H. Gennari

Previous chapters in this book describe the general process of clinical trial research and some of the informatics infrastructure needed to improve it. In this chapter, we specify how informatics ideas and tools can improve protocol-based oncology research. In particular, we discuss the idea of a *clinical state* that defines the targeted patient population for clinical trial protocols, and show how this idea can be used in tools to help standardize and improve protocol-based research.

At present, few successful tools exist for protocol management or protocol-based research. One persistent challenge is that informatics systems must be integrated with other tools and medical information systems. Modern physicians already confront information overload, and adding yet another stand-alone tool simply further complicates their workflow. Unfortunately, building an integrated, unified view of a complex process like protocol-based research and care is extremely difficult.

In this chapter, we discuss how to establish definitions for clinical states and how these standard clinical states can unify the tools that assist protocol-based research. As examples, we use the tasks of authoring new clinical trial protocols and enrolling patients into them. Although these tasks have different users and need different decision-support tools, the tools that support these tasks should share a common model of the clinical trial and of clinical states.

Defining Clinical States

One goal of informatics research in oncology is to better organize the information within oncology clinical trial protocols. Although information in protocols has many dimensions, any protocol targets a particular patient population to best achieve the research objectives of that protocol. We claim that a relatively small set of patient characteristics can succinctly describe these target populations. Since these characteristics describe the state of disease in the patient, we label these target populations *clinical states* for oncology protocols (Silva & Wittes, 1999).

TABLE 19.1. Set of questions to determine the clinical state for a breast cancer patient

Is there a diagnosis of breast cancer?
Is the primary tumor resectable?
Is there evidence of metastatic disease?
Are there any positive lymph nodes?
How many positive lymph nodes are there?
What is the histologic grade of the primary tumor?
Has there been previous chemotherapy for this cancer?
Is the patient ER or PR responsive?

Although some characteristics of cancer are common to all its forms, we can more thoroughly characterize clinical states that are specific to a particular cancer site like the breast, lung, or prostate. For each of these sites, we define a set of attributes that can categorize the patient into a target population for clinical research. Table 19.1 lists a set of questions for breast cancer patients. Answers to these questions are the patient attributes that determine clinical state, and therefore suggest which protocols might be most appropriate.

To some degree, different clinical trial protocols direct their research at patients in a particular stage of the disease. Thus, the idea of cancer staging approximates the idea of a clinical state, and many of the questions used to determine cancer stage can also help determine clinical state. However, many clinical trials also need prior history information and details that staging information does not capture, such as the number of positive lymph nodes. By focusing our efforts on the targets of clinical research, we hope to produce clinical states that are more detailed and dynamic than cancer staging classes.

Although the questions in Table 19.1 are specific to breast cancer, most oncologists rely on a similar short list to broadly characterize the patients they treat. Some of the questions in Table 19.1 have dependencies among them; for example, if there is evidence of metastatic disease, then the tumor generally is not resectable. Because of these relationships, it is useful to arrange the questions into a clinical state diagram, both to indicate an ordering and to determine when clinical state is sufficiently defined.

Clinical State Diagrams: Breast Cancer and Lung Cancer

To illustrate our ideas, we provide two examples of clinical state diagrams. Figure 19.1 presents our diagram for breast cancer. This diagram includes the questions listed in Table 19.1 as decision points that lead to additional questions—or eventually, to the *leaves* of the tree (at the bottom of the diagram), which represent clinical states for breast cancer. The state diagram captures dependencies among the questions; e.g., one cannot ask

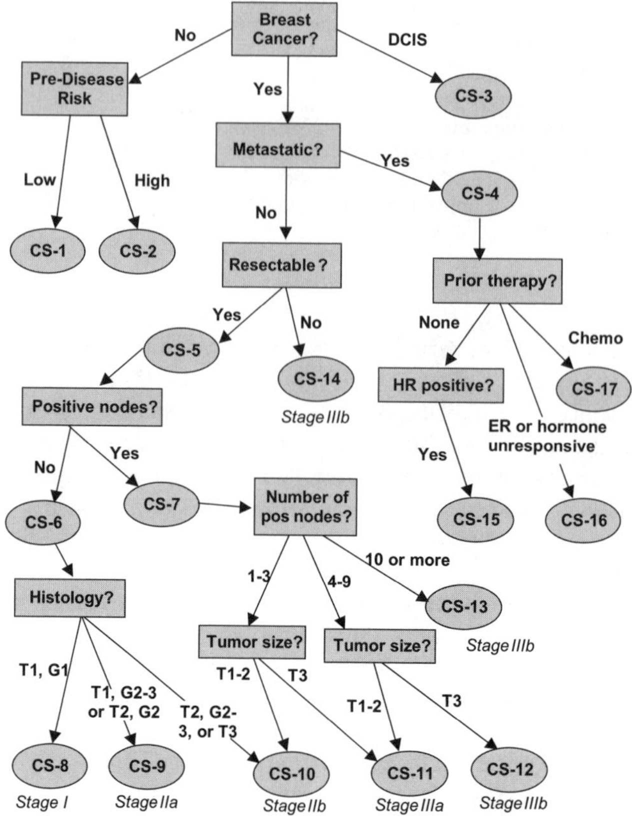

Figure 19.1. Clinical state diagram for breast cancer. The clinical states are the leaves of this tree (or any node indicated as "CS-x"), and the clinical questions are decision points that indicate what other questions should be asked and lead eventually to one of the clinical states.

how many positive lymph nodes exist before verifying that there are positive nodes.

As Figure 19.1 shows, not all clinical states are at the leaves of the tree; some are "internal nodes" of the diagram. These clinical states are broader classes of patients; for example, CS-7 represents a node-positive patient population without indicating the number of positive lymph nodes or the size of the primary tumor. We created these internal-node clinical states whenever they represented a general patient population that clinical trial protocols targeted for research.

As a second example, we include a clinical state diagram for lung cancer in Figure 19.2. As with breast cancer, we include questions important for staging the disease. More so than the one for breast cancer, this diagram is clearly a directed graph rather than strictly a "tree." The user can take multiple paths to reach states like CS7, CS9, and CS10.

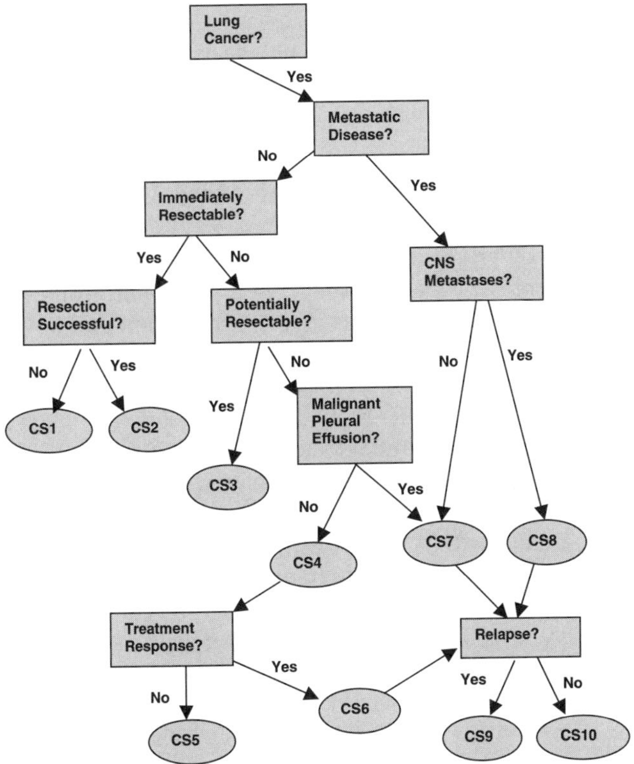

FIGURE 19.2. Clinical state diagram for lung cancer. As with Figure 19.1, all nodes labeled CSx are clinical states—categories of patients for clinical research in lung cancer.

Clinical States Versus Clinical Progression

The clinical state diagram should not be confused with a chart of disease progression or a guideline for diagnosis. Clinical state diagrams focus on the set of questions used to divide patients into groups suitable for clinical research. These broad groups do not fully characterize the state of disease progression in any single patient. To represent targets for clinical research, the clinical states must be broad; for Phase III clinical trial protocols, they must be broad enough to support enrollment numbers in the thousands of patients.

Although the clinical state diagram is not the same as a disease progression chart, the diagram should cover the common stages of disease because each stage may be a target for clinical research. In some cases, defining disease stage is itself a research task, but for most cancers, we already have a strong model of the disease and its progression through stages. The clinical state diagram cannot be a fixed, immutable structure. It must evolve as our understanding of the disease shifts and as the targets for clinical research change. For example, the discovery of a significant genetic marker may make it necessary to add questions and clinical states to a diagram for that disease.

Building Consensus for a Clinical State Diagram

The clinical state diagrams in Figures 19.1 and 19.2 are by no means final products. They represent a consensus from a particular group of clinicians and informaticians about what questions are important and how to classify patients into groups. Building a new clinical state diagram for another class of cancer would require collaboration with a group of clinical specialists in that domain. To build such a diagram, we would ask them for a set of critical questions that characterize patients, such as those listed in Table 19.1. We would review open clinical trial protocols for that cancer, examining how they describe their target patient populations. (These characterizations reside in the set of eligibility criteria for the protocol.) Using information from the protocols to establish the clinical states, we would arrange the questions into an initial clinical state diagram and present it to the clinicians for feedback, allowing as many revisions as needed to reach consensus.

Thus, the clinical state diagram depends both on clinician opinion and on the status of protocol-based research for that cancer. If the characterization of the disease is controversial, different specialists could create different clinical state diagrams. Similarly, if clinical research for that cancer shifts significantly with trials for new drugs or tests, then the clinical state diagram would reflect such changes. In this way, the diagram could evolve over time.

Clinicians may find the process of building a clinical state diagram illuminating, especially when defining clinical states and the set of critical questions. The tendency to characterize and classify patients into different categories may be a somewhat hidden practice with implicit understanding about how to do it. This implicit knowledge should be more explicit, so that clinicians can think constructively about the most critical questions and openly discuss how to categorize patients.

Benefits of a Clinical State Diagram

The principal benefit of building good clinical state diagrams is that they can help us apply clinical trial protocols and research in a more principled, consistent manner. As a standard, clinical state diagrams would also help developers build more unified informatics tools and applications that would help researchers and clinicians apply clinical trial protocols more effectively. In the subsections below, we describe how well-defined clinical states would benefit two specific applications, and we conclude with some broader implications of the clinical state diagram.

Clinical States and Authoring Protocol Eligibility Criteria

One goal of informatics for clinical trial protocols is to improve information flow across protocol-based research and health care. Building better protocols will help us produce conclusive research results faster, and thereby improve the standard of care more quickly. One way to improve the quality of clinical trial protocols is via the use of authoring tools that provide advice and standards for more consistent protocols.

One critical aspect of protocol authoring is defining the target population via the set of eligibility criteria. The descriptions of eligibility criteria relate closely to the definition of a clinical state, and any errors or problems in this phase can have major effects on clinical research. In current protocols, there is unnecessary variation in the wording and format of these criteria. By building a consensus clinical state diagram, and by associating those states with a set of canonical eligibility criteria, we can reduce the number of different criteria by about half without any loss of semantics (Rubin et al., 1999).

Thus, clinical researchers can use clinical state diagrams in conjunction with an authoring tool to help improve the quality of and standardize eligibility criteria for new clinical trial protocols. Of course, building a set of eligibility criteria is only one part of the protocol authoring process, but it is a crucial part where errors or problems can have major effects later in the clinical research process.

Because each clinical state in the diagram is associated with a set of standard eligibility criteria, once a researcher decides which clinical state is appropriate for a new protocol, an authoring tool can assume that this protocol will need all the associated eligibility criteria. These criteria are not sufficient for a protocol, but they form a useful "starter set." If all protocol authors agree to the use of a consensus clinical state diagram, then eligibility criteria in the protocols they write will be less varied in wording and format.

As we describe in Rubin et al. (1999), we have built an example protocol-authoring tool that provides this capability. Figure 19.3 displays a screen-shot from this tool. The panel on the left shows the clinical state diagram for breast cancer, and the one on the right displays a set of eligibility criteria. Clinical state diagrams for other disease sites are accessible from other tabs (the figure also shows the prostate cancer tab). In this case, the user is building a new breast cancer protocol and has selected clinical state CS-D. In the right panel, the tool lists the four eligibility criteria associated with this clinical state.

Selecting a clinical state is the first step in authoring a new protocol; the four criteria in Figure 19.3 are the starter set of eligibility criteria associated with state CS-D. Next, the researcher would select the tab marked "standard criteria" to add to the list of eligibility criteria. This tab allows users to select from other sets of standard eligibility criteria, organized by categories such as prior therapy, patient characteristics, and disease

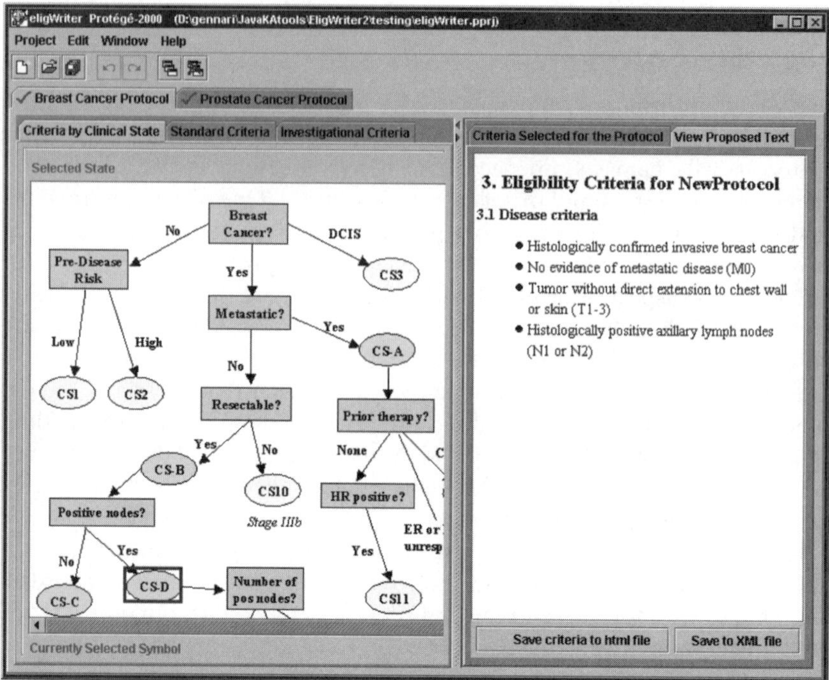

FIGURE 19.3. Screenshot of a prototype tool. The tool uses the clinical state diagram (on the left) to help generate a set of eligibility criteria for a new protocol (on the right).

characteristics. Any authoring tool must be flexible, since we cannot expect all researchers to use only the standard set of eligibility criteria. Therefore, the tool allows users to either modify one of the standard criteria or create new ones by selecting the tab labeled "investigational criteria." Although users have ultimate control over the wording of criteria, by providing standard criteria as defaults, this tool should improve the consistency of eligibility criteria across different protocols.

Although this type of application is not in use in real clinical settings, we have used it to test our ideas and our clinical state diagrams. We reviewed approximately 65 open prostate and lung cancer protocols and assigned primary clinical states to these protocols. We found that most clinical states had at least one protocol assigned to them and that protocols were not evenly distributed among the clinical states. In addition, about 20 to 25% of the eligibility criteria in these protocols were members of the "starter set" associated with the clinical states (Rubin et al., 1999).

Clinical States and Patient Eligibility

One noted problem with protocol-based clinical research is that patient enrollment rates often fall below what the protocol author expected or planned. Multiple factors contribute to low enrollment rates, but one reason is the difficulty of eligibility determination. A decision-support tool that helps match patients to trial protocols would increase enrollment, which in turn could speed the process of achieving research results and improving the standard of oncology care.

A decision-support tool for determining patient eligibility would also benefit from organizing patients and protocols into clinical states. If we can identify the critical questions for a given cancer, then we can assign patients to specific clinical states. Classifying patients into these states will simplify eligibility determination: patients will only be potentially eligible for clinical trial protocols that target their clinical state. In addition, once a patient matches the clinical state for a protocol, then he or she automatically satisfies all of the starter set of eligibility criteria.

Building a decision-support tool for determining patient eligibility in protocols is not a new idea (Tu et al., 1993), but previous tools have not achieved large-scale success, usually because they are not integrated with other information systems. If tools shared standards for information such as clinical state definitions and terminology standards, clinicians would consider them more useful and acceptable. For example, Chapter 24 by Donald Simborg describes a prototype system, iKnowChart, that includes an eligibility determination capability.

Although integration is still a work in progress, the iKnowMed Network tools can share information about terminology standards and definitions of clinical states and their associated eligibility criteria. If the iKnowMed Network shares the same definitions of clinical state with the eligibility criteria-authoring tool, the tools can work together. The iKnowMed Network includes a "high-level screening" capability that performs a partial match of patients to clinical trial protocols. This screening capability is exactly the process of matching clinical states between patients and protocols. If the tools share the same terminology and standards, the authoring tool can send the eligibility criteria for a new protocol directly into the iKnowMed Network, a crucial communication capability as ongoing protocols and eligibility criteria change. Electronic communication could ensure that protocol modifications and updates are more rapidly and accurately disseminated and applied than they are in today's paper-based environment.

Clinical States and Improving Research Coverage

Clinical research in oncology is not currently well organized or carried out in a principled manner. Advances are mostly incremental, driven by prior successes with related drugs or regimens, or by pharmaceutical companies that wish to develop particular agents. To look at clinical research more objectively and systematically, we can conduct a thorough review of the scope and direction of ongoing clinical trial protocols. For a broad review of research in a particular cancer, we can look at the organization of clinical states for that cancer.

Once we build a clinical state diagram, we can classify clinical trial protocols into the set of clinical states and pinpoint the most studied areas or target patient populations. This may uncover redundant (or nearly redundant) protocols in a heavily targeted area of study. Conversely, reviewing the entire clinical state diagram might highlight significant patient populations that are not the target of current protocols. Periodically reviewing this distribution of protocols across clinical states should help researchers and directors of oncology research programs think about which areas of disease progression are the focus of research efforts and which are less scrutinized.

Clinical States and Common Data Elements

As described in Section 3 of this volume, all clinical trials should share a medical terminology for describing common data elements, or CDEs. The idea of defining a set of clinical states is an extension of the CDE idea, since both concepts attempt to characterize commonalities among protocols. When developing the set of critical questions for determining clinical states, we also should note which CDEs can help answer those questions. Filling in the patient data for these CDEs may be most important: once we determine patient clinical state, then we can apply eligibility-determination tools to match the patient against appropriate clinical trials.

Common data elements were initially designed to describe data that must be captured and reported via case report forms as part of clinical trial results. However, CDEs also appear in eligibility criteria. In most cases, an eligibility criterion is simply a constraint stating that a CDE must have some particular value. A single eligibility criterion may require evaluation of several distinct CDEs. Therefore, in addition to associating every clinical state with a set of eligibility criteria, we can also associate each clinical state with a larger set of CDEs. This association helps us determine patient eligibility—we can focus on data elements that determine clinical state which will facilitate faster matches between patients and clinical trial protocols.

Looking Ahead

The challenge for oncology informatics is to build a unified view of information and knowledge for the entire protocol-based research and clinical care process. We must organize and streamline information flow and provide integrated decision-support tools that have clear and immediate benefit to users. In this chapter, we have explored one way to organize oncology knowledge about protocol-based research: defining a set of clinical states. We have demonstrated how to apply these definitions to two informatics applications: an authoring tool and a patient eligibility-determination tool.

However, this chapter provides only the foundation for clinical state diagrams and gives a few examples of how informatics tools could use clinical states. Much work remains; for example, ongoing efforts aim to demonstrate that these tools provide actual efficiency improvements in the workplace. Just as we must prove the efficacy of an experimental agent or a new treatment regimen, we must demonstrate that decision-support systems based on clinical state diagrams can increase efficiency and information flow in the clinical setting. Although we remain in the early stages of this process, we believe these ideas and applications can and will ultimately improve the process of clinical research in oncology.

References

Rubin DL, Gennari JH, Srinivas S, Yuen A, Kaizer H, Musen MA, et al. 1999. Tool Support for Authoring Eligibility Criteria for Cancer Trials. Proceedings of the American Medical Informatics Association Symposium 369–373.

Silva J, Wittes R. 1999. Role of Clinical Trials Informatics in the NCI's Cancer Informatics Infrastructure. Proceedings of the American Medical Informatics Association Symposium: 950–954.

Tu SW, Kemper CA, Lane NM, Carlson RW, Musen MA. 1993. A Methodology for Determining Patients' Eligibility for Clinical Trials. Methods of Information in Medicine 32(4):317–325.

20
Support for the Cancer Patient: An Internet Model

Howard S. Goldberg and Charles Safran

As consumerism permeates the practice of contemporary medicine, concepts regarding patient empowerment are rapidly evolving. Patients should actively participate in decisions that affect their lives and well being (Brennan & Ripich, 1994, Ferguson, 2000; Gustafson, McTavish, Boberg et al., 1999; Slack, 1977). No longer do physicians dictate a particular course of treatment based solely on training and experience. Instead, they are increasingly expected to educate patients and their families on illnesses, available therapies, potential outcomes, and complications, so that patient and physician can jointly make decisions based on the patient's preferences (Brennan, 1999; Brennan, 1996; Ferguson, 1995; Landro, 2000; Landro, 1999; Mandl, Kohane, Brandt, 1998; Safran, Jones, Rind et al., 1998; Slack, 1998; Slack, 1999).

This kind of patient activism can make significant differences in disease outcomes. The empowered patient is likely to comply with therapy, proactively report new or changing symptoms, and see him- or herself as a partner in the care process. Patient activism has the potential to improve lead times in discovering disease complications, reduce unnecessary service utilization like emergency room visits, and generally increase satisfaction (Brennan, Moore, Smyth, 1995; Brennan & Ripich, 1994; Goldsmith, Feldman, Cooney, Safran, 1998; Goldsmith & Safran, 1999; Gustafson, McTavish, Hawkins et al., 1998; Safran, Rind, Sands et al., 1996; Slack, 1998; Vandenberg et al., 1997).

However, patient empowerment also places additional resource demands on an already strained healthcare system. In the age of managed care and the seven-minute office visit, the healthcare system will struggle to adapt to new needs for increased patient education, feedback, and the kinds of interaction that foster empowering patients. At a time when patients are requesting increased participation in their own care, when healthcare enterprises have no additional resources to implement such a framework, and when third-party payers have no tangible incentives to financially support this kind of innovation, it is not surprising that the public views healthcare relationships as "broken."

Evolving Internet technologies can play a role in mending these fractured relationships among patients, providers, and payers. Systems designed to support the basic processes underpinning healthcare relationships can enable the evolution of the empowered patient (Ferguson, 1995; Goldsmith, Feldman, Cooney et al., 1998; Slack, 1999). All stakeholders in healthcare relationships are likely to embrace systems that can improve communication between patient and physician, improve access to clinical educational materials, and add efficiencies to the process of disease management (Slack, 1998).

In this chapter, we discuss the role of Internet-based information technologies in supporting the needs of patients and their families. Drawing from our experiences in the domains of neonatal intensive care and cancer care, we illustrate some common frustrations with healthcare delivery. Included is a basic framework for supporting patients and maximizing their participation in their own care, followed by a discussion of contemporary clinical information systems and their evolution into systems that incorporate patients in the process of care delivery. Finally, we present studies that demonstrate how clinical information systems that involve the patient can significantly impact clinical outcomes and patient satisfaction.

Encountering the Healthcare System

The Neonatal Intensive Care Unit (NICU)

The NICU is an overwhelming environment for parents, with the harried pace of the staff and the abundance of machinery used to keep sick infants alive. Parents' experiences with their children in the NICU are strikingly similar. They feel compelled to spend much of their day in the unit, at the hospital, or in frequent communication with the staff. They must become familiar with numerous physicians, nurses, and other professionals who may care for their children over an extended period. Parents must adapt their schedules to the staff's schedules in order to get updates or ask questions, and they must learn which staff members can provide what information. No matter how much time is spent at the hospital, questions always arise when no one is available: "They told me my baby was on the respirator, but breathing room air. What does that mean?"

Parents of premature infants essentially learn an entire curriculum (Gray, Safran, Weitzner et al., 2000). For example, they must learn about lung development, eye complications, and infection, as well as feeding, positioning, and car safety. Eventually, the child is ready to come home, and the parents suddenly realize that they themselves will be the caretakers, with responsibility for operating machinery, checking alarms, and keeping the routine that previously occupied an entire staff.

Cancer

Cancer patients also face significant challenges when entering the healthcare system (Slack, 1977). Patients with large or advancing tumors may have access to a variety of possible treatments, including surgery, radiation therapy, multiple chemotherapy regimens, and some combination of these options. Regimens may represent the current standard of care or they may be experimental protocols. There will likely be regional variation in available therapies, depending on the training and availability of various oncology specialists. To incorporate patients in decision-making, the caregiver presents them with a variety of statistics related to mortality, morbidity, and therapeutic complications. Patients have to make decisions within a very short timeframe to minimize the further spread of disease. Once patients begin treatment, they must begin to deal with the inevitable side effects of therapy, including pain, nausea, hair loss, and fatigue.

Chronic management of cancer involves a looser network of care and support. The care team follows their patients over intervals with periodic evaluations for disease progression, and over the long term, patients and their families take greater responsibility for symptom management and reporting. Patients become responsible for when and how the healthcare system is accessed, but they continue to rely on the specialist to determine when some new therapeutic intervention may help.

Managing bone marrow transplants also merits a special mention. Patients offered a bone marrow transplant face the same issues previously discussed in the acute management of cancer. Once they begin therapy, patients face the additional burden of isolation as their bone marrow reconstitutes itself over weeks to months. Families of bone marrow transplant patients face circumstances similar to those of parents with infants in the NICU. They tend to spend significant amounts of time at the hospital for both visitation and conferring with the staff. To some extent, the patient lives in an information vacuum. With limited access to the outside world, patients rely heavily on their care team for decision-making, and they have limited ability to gather additional information or network with peers.

Incorporating the Patient

The preceding examples underscore the fact that patient participation in medical care is information-intensive for patients and their families. Patients must become rapidly educated in medical domains that may be foreign to them. They must engage in an ongoing dialogue with specialists and the care team, and ideally, they have mechanisms for validating information presented to them. Over time, patients and their families assume greater responsibility in reporting and managing symptoms, as well as accessing the healthcare system.

Given the complexity of these interactions, there are numerous opportunities for breakdowns in the system. Because medicine is so complex, the care team must present information to patients at a level appropriate for them. Information transfer depends on synchronous communication between patient and care team, and since time is generally a scarce resource for medical specialists, they may relay information once with limited opportunity for review and assessment of comprehension. Scheduling time to speak with staff and specialists also places a great burden on patients and families, and regional variations in care may limit therapeutic options available to patients.

As diseases become chronic, the laxity of the care delivery framework becomes a major weakness in the system. Without a standard framework for symptom reporting and management, patients are left to their own devices. Absence of a framework can manifest itself in inappropriate use of resources: patients may not report symptom progression until they require acute hospitalization, or they may use emergency rooms as an alternate source of care. Ultimately, these breaks in the system manifest themselves in both additional costs and decreased patient satisfaction.

Incorporating patient participation in care delivery requires an underlying framework to help facilitate it. Without this framework, benchmarking and performance comparison are very difficult, as is designing clinical information systems that incorporate the patient. We believe that a valuable framework must include the following four elements:

- patient education
- information access
- facilitated communication
- community support.

Patient Education

Patients must begin with a basic understanding of their disease, its natural history, symptoms, and potential complications. This foundation will help them discuss what may be a wide range of treatment options, from standard therapies through experimental protocols. The care team should present and stage patient education in accordance with the patient's disease state; for example, the educational requirements of women with a newly discovered breast mass differ from those of women with recurrent breast cancer. Finally, the patient's provider should guide this educational process, so that the patient perceives it as an integral part of the overall treatment plan.

Information Access

Beyond this basic education, patients should have access to reference information on their disease. Each patient has a unique set of informational needs based on individual social, cultural, and familial backgrounds. An ideal library will offer materials geared to the layperson, plus access to clinical textbooks and medical literature for patients who have become knowledgeable about their diseases.

Because of the widespread availability of the Internet and the popularity of online health sites, many of today's patients bring their physicians stacks of printouts for further discussion. Physicians should guide information access based on the patient's particular context and needs. The need to participate in medical decision-making should guide information access, as even medical specialists have difficulty keeping up with the literature.

Facilitated Communication

Ongoing dialogue between patient and care team reinforces the education process. Patients and their families cannot be expected to rapidly integrate all the necessary information in an initial sitting or two. Invariably, the care team will have to repeat, re-explain, expand upon, or re-emphasize forgotten or misunderstood information.

Like the history-taking process itself, ongoing communication between the patient and the care team provides an opportunity to assess how much information the patient has absorbed. Patients encouraged to maintain an ongoing dialogue with the care team may also be timely, accurate self-reporters of new or perceived symptoms. Active patient participation in symptom management will help decrease discovery time of new complications, decrease unnecessary emergency room visits, and increase patient satisfaction with medical care (Mandl et al., 1998; Safran et al., 1998; Slack, 1998).

Community Support

Patients can augment their support systems by interacting with peers who are experiencing or have experienced similar illnesses and complications. Support groups complement and extend direct interactions between patients and care teams (Brennan et al., 1995; Brennan, 1999; Ferguson, 2000; Landro, 1999; McTavish, Gustafson, Owen et al., 1995; Pingree, Hawkins, Gustafson et al., 1996; Shaw, McTavish, Hawkins et al., 2000; Slack, 1999). From the perspective of the framework presented here, support groups can validate information received, provide additional relevant information sources, and supplement the patient-provider dialogue.

The collective experiences of a support group are likely to exceed those of any particular care provider; they are likely to be more vivid and practical for patients dealing with the day-to-day obstacles that an illness presents. A support group may also provide answers to questions more quickly than individual research, although patients should verify the accuracy of peer-supplied information with a physician.

Information Systems that Incorporate the Patient Clinical Record

Over the past 30 years, the creation of the electronic patient record (EPR) has been a major focus in the development of clinical information systems (Safran, Rind, Sands et al., 1996). The EPR broadly refers to the digital collection of clinical narrative and diagnostic reports specific to an individual patient. The purpose of the EPR is to improve clinical care, research, and aggregate data analysis by making clinical information available. A variety of clinical settings around the world have successfully implemented heterogeneous sets of EPRs with a variety of features.

A clinical information system (CIS) is a collection of applications and subsystems that support the process of care delivery. The CIS extends the EPR with additional functionality designed to streamline the flow of information related to clinical care. Clinically relevant applications include electronic mail, clinical results reporting, literature searching, and provider-based order entry. In combination with these applications, decision support subsystems generate alerts and reminders to providers based on clinical data and other events generated within the system. Of the many components that comprise a CIS, decision support systems can make some of the most significant differences in care delivery—for instance, in the detection of drug-induced renal injury or in the reduction of AIDS-related pneumonias (Safran et al., 1996; Safran et al., 1998).

While some single site locations have successfully implemented EPRs and CISs, the integrated delivery network (IDN) has not yet demonstrated the same success. The IDN, with its affiliated medical practices, community, and tertiary care facilities, circumscribes a logical geography in which care is rendered to a population. Streamlining the flow of information related to longitudinal care will ultimately require information integration throughout the IDN. Thus far, heterogeneous systems, organizations, cultures, and cost have remained major barriers to this degree of integration.

Internet technologies can help integrate the disparate entities that comprise an IDN. The World Wide Web supports integration of rich, multimedia data originating in disparate data sources through a set of standardized protocols and a common target presentation mechanism, the browser. Several groups have proposed and implemented solutions that use Internet technologies to assemble a "virtual" medical record and provide clinical information to healthcare providers. Following the merger of Beth Israel and New England Deaconess Hospitals in 1995, our group developed CareWeb, a set of components that virtually integrate clinical data from two disparate information systems (Halamka, 1999). The CareWeb architecture combines Internet transmission protocols and presentation standards with a common data model to support a single longitudinal view of clinical results. In combination with a strong authentication system and secure transmission protocols, the CareWeb system provides a working model for future distributed clinical information systems.

Notably, most technology innovation in clinical information systems has focused on supporting the needs of healthcare providers. While patients are the ultimate consumers of healthcare resources, and their satisfaction with these services determine the allocation of these resources, patients have been only minor players in the use of healthcare information technology. However, if improved information access and improved mechanisms for communication and collaboration can impact the use of healthcare services, then future healthcare information systems should focus on supporting the patient as well as the clinician. This technology can serve as a bridge to improved patient-doctor relationships, where "high tech" can enable "high touch."

To explore the hypothesis that enhancing patient participation can significantly improve measures of health outcomes, our group has created a system that supports the empowerment framework previously described. Our initial work has involved developing a system called Baby CareLink, designed to support the needs of families with premature infants. From this initial experience, we have generalized the technical framework to form the CareLink architecture. As proof of concept for reuse of the architecture, we have created prototype environments to support cancer patients in the domains of breast cancer and bone marrow transplant.

The CareLink architecture supports asynchronous communication, "prescribed" education, knowledge exploration, community collaboration, and data integration. The system also includes strong two-factor authentication methods that we developed for use in the CareWeb architecture. In its research implementation, Baby CareLink included real-time, ISDN-based videoconferencing. Patients and family can access the system over the Internet as a user-friendly Web site.

The CareLink architecture's support of patient empowerment is further explained in the following sections.

Secure, Workflow-Based, Asynchronous Communication

CareLink provides a secure Message Center to support dialogue between staff and families. The Message Center is secure because message routing occurs over trusted servers and store-and-forward does not occur over public servers, meaning that no readable artifact of confidential medical information exists. The Message Center is also "workflow-based," meaning that message relay follows the workflow of the supported clinical unit. In Baby CareLink, parents forward messages to the staff, and any staff member can reply to any of the individuals associated with an infant. Finally, communication occurs asynchronously, which means that messages can be written and answered at convenient, appropriate times. This asynchronous dialogue eliminates the burden of physically tracking down busy staff members. In combination with real-time videoconferencing, families can use these capabilities to stay in touch with their children and the staff without taking up residence in the hospital.

Prescribed Education

Typically, the hospital staff guides the process by which families learn about their childrens' conditions, complications, and care. A prescribed education module allows staff to assign educational material to families and receive structured feedback on their comprehension. Families receive the educational material in a timeline-appropriate fashion; e.g., families of 26-week old infants will be assigned material on topics like respirators, nutritional support, and infection, while families of older infants will be assigned materials on such subjects as positioning and car seat safety. This learning model allows families to receive just-in-time education appropriate to the status of their child, and it lets the staff gauge a family's comprehension and customize the pace and content. In the case of premature infants, continuous education prepares parents both cognitively and psychologically for the eventual homecoming of their infant.

Knowledge Exploration

A freestanding digital library complements the structured educational process. Reference materials describe medications, procedures, and conditions in lay language, and staff can customize the library to include additional materials or hyperlinks to recommended auxiliary materials. A staff-provided library facilitates guided exploration, so that families may access materials already judged clinically sound.

Community Collaboration

Patients and families who have undergone similar experiences can give valuable first-hand advice to others. Moderated chatrooms complement the knowledge and learning obtained from other CareLink modules and provide yet another form of support. Peers can quickly provide resource recommendations, validating and contrasting points of view, and crucial psychological support.

Data Integration

Beth Israel Deaconess Medical Center has integrated CareLink with clinical systems to share data with families. In Baby CareLink, this integration enables the creation of a multimedia record that includes a photo library of the infant and growth charts. By presenting a synopsis of relevant data from the patient record, this concept can also be extended to create a "personal" medical record.

In these ways, the CareLink architecture lays the groundwork for patients and families to actively participate in the care process. Information technology minimizes the additional workload on the clinical staff, lowering their resistance to adopting this new care model. Once adopted, these technologies can improve patient interaction and evaluation with little effect on staff workloads.

System Evaluation and Impact on Health Outcomes

While systems like CareLink have intuitive appeal to diverse groups of healthcare stakeholders, adoption of such systems will likely depend on their ability to demonstrate positive impact on outcomes (Brennan, Moore, Smyth, 1995; Brennan & Ripich, 1994; Brennan, 1995; Goldsmith, Feldman, Cooney, Safran, 1998; Goldsmith & Safran, 1999; Goldsmith, Chapman, Wandel et al., 1997; Goldsmith, Feldman, Cooney et al., 1998). The value of "traditional" clinical information system technology, such as decision support systems designed to reduce medical error, is obvious to decision makers. Less obvious is the value of systems that perform population behavioral management but do not perform a direct medical intervention.

One randomized controlled trial evaluated the effect of online pain management information on post-operative pain in ambulatory surgery patients (Goldsmith, Feldman, Cooney, Safran, 1998; Goldsmith & Safran, 1999; Goldsmith, Feldman, Cooney et al., 1998). In this trial, 195 surgical outpatients at Beth Israel Deaconess Medical Center were randomized to either a control group or intervention group. The control group had access to an ambulatory surgery nursing Web site; the intervention group had access to the same Web site with an additional section discussing pain management. Pre- and post-operative instructions were provided in accordance with usual care, and post-operative pain was measured using the 5-point Verbal Rating Scale portion of the McGill Pain Questionnaire.

The populations of the control and intervention groups were similar in age, sex, and American Society of Anesthesia (ASA) status. Ages ranged from 18 to 82, and the studied population was about 71% female. Forty-one percent of the studied population returned questionnaires. Patients in the intervention group reported significantly less post-operative pain upon arrival home, the first night following surgery, and the day after surgery ($p < 0.016$, $p < 0.013$, $p < 0.037$). The data suggest that the availability of just-in-time pain management information over the Internet enhanced the outcomes of care in this ambulatory surgery population. Although it would be interesting to compare outcomes between a paper-based group and a Web-based group, the study demonstrates that "...the Internet can successfully be used as a platform on which to deliver interventions to patients" that "... significantly enhance the outcomes of care for patients and their families."

Another randomized controlled trial evaluated the effect of the Baby CareLink system on length of stay in low birth weight infants and the satisfaction of the patients' families (Gray, Safran, Weitzner et al., 2000). Between November 1977 and April 1999, 30 control and 26 study patients were enrolled from a total of 176 eligible infants at Beth Israel Deaconess Medical Center. Families in the study group had access to Baby CareLink, while families in the control group received care as practiced in the unit. Within two weeks of enrollment, families in the study group had an ISDN line installed at their residence, and a configured Baby CareLink PC installed by a technician.

Average length of stay for the entire CareLink group was shorter (68.5+/–28.3 days vs. 70.6+/–35.6 days), and length of stay was lower for study patients born weighing less than 1000 grams (77 days vs. 93 days). Both of these differences trended toward but did not reach a statistical level of significance of $p < 0.05$. All study patients were discharged directly to home, while 17% of the control patients were transferred to a community hospital prior to discharge home ($p < 0.05$). Only 3% of study families reported one or more problems or issues with care, as opposed to 13% in the control group. Thirteen percent of study families reported problems with the unit's physical environment and visitation policy, as opposed to 50% of control families. Family visits, telephone calls to the unit, and holding of the infant did not differ between groups.

These results suggest that Internet support of the educational and emotional needs of families with low birth weight infants significantly improves satisfaction with care delivery and lowers costs associated with hospital transfers. The system may also facilitate earlier discharge to home. While it did not reach the level of statistical significance, the magnitude of difference in length of stay for the smallest of infants—those who generally require the longest periods of care—suggests that behavioral interventions can play a major role in preparation for discharge. Because system installation time could lag up to two weeks in study infants, rapid system availability could further impact length of stay. We should interpret the results cautiously: the sample size was small, the study was conducted at a tertiary referral center, and a dedicated team was available to support the system. Still, it is clear that actively engaging patients and families in the care process improves families' perception of that care and may positively impact transfers and length of stay.

Looking Ahead

Growth of the Internet has helped create new communications networks and a deluge of medical content, developments that are changing the way patients approach the healthcare system. When confronted with the onset of a new disease or frustrated by management of an ongoing disease, patients now have tools at their disposal to actively seek medical expertise and feedback from peers. Technology has lowered the barrier for patients to become aggressive advocates on their own behalf. Empowered patients bring high expectations into healthcare relationships, expectations that can improve the way the system interacts with them and the way care is delivered (Brennan, 1996; Ferguson, 2000; Landro, 2000; Landro, 1999; Slack, 1998; Slack & Slack, 1972).

Our early work demonstrates that technologies designed to enhance patient participation in medical care can dramatically improve perceptions of care quality. The data further suggest that such systems can significantly impact hard outcomes measures like length of stay. Common sense would dictate that families who have been educated in the continuing care of their premature children, and who have additional reassurance in the form of a "tele-umbilical" cord, would likely take their children home earlier from the hospital. The systematization of this process provides some assurance that results can be duplicated.

Because our framework for patient empowerment reflects core processes for developing and maintaining healthcare relationships, we are optimistic that similar systems can work in many domains, including transplant medicine, diabetes, and heart failure management. Technology enables the empowerment framework by virtually extending the reach of the patient and creating efficiencies for care providers. If such systems are deployed on a wide scale, they will lose their domain specificity and become ubiquitous components of the healthcare system.

While the next generation of patient-centered systems is an idea with great appeal, we must establish who will pay for their development and deployment. Although new clinical systems may bring about significant cost reductions to third-party payers, the systems will likely achieve the greatest benefits within clinical settings, where patients and families can interact with their own care providers. Given the current healthcare funding dilemma, healthcare delivery enterprises themselves probably cannot fund the deployment and integration of additional information technology. Furthermore, while system costs may be amortized over large populations, the cost to provide appropriate security and confidentiality credentials to each participant—which may include an authentication token or smart card, a digital signature, and an encryption key—carries significant expense. Before we see deployment of comprehensive systems like the CareLink system, innovative partnerships must form among payers, providers, government, and the public.

These efforts will effect ample rewards: technology that empowers patients will alter healthcare relationships and supports the healthcare system as a whole. With the Internet's improvements in information access, we have already begun to witness positive change. Once partnerships are formed to fund and deploy patient-centered systems, technology will help reduce costs, facilitate data collection and quality initiatives that are currently impractical on a broad scale, and—most importantly—improve the quality of clinical care.

References

Brennan PF, Ripich S. 1994. Use of a Home Care Computer Network by Persons with AIDS. International Journal of Technology Assessment in Health Care 10(2):258–272.

Brennan PF. 1995. Characterizing the Use of Health Care Services Delivered Via Computer Networks. Journal of the American Medical Informatics Association 2(3):160–168.

Brennan PF, Moore SM, Smyth KA. 1995. The Effects of a Special Computer Network on Caregivers of Persons with Alzheimer's Disease. Nursing Research 44(3):166–172.

Brennan PF. 1996. The Future of Clinical Communication in an Electronic Environment. Holistic Nurse Practitioner 11(1):97–104.

Brennan PF. 1999. Health Informatics and Community Health: Support for the Patients as Collaborators in Care. Methods of Information in Medicine 38:274–278.

Ferguson T. 1995. Consumer Health Informatics. Health Care Forum Journal 38(1):28–33.

Ferguson T. 2000. Online Patient-Helpers and Physicians Working Together: A New Patient Collaboration for High Quality Health Care. British Medical Journal 321(7269):1129–1132.

Goldsmith DM, Chapman RH, Wandel J, Reiley PJ, Safran C. 1997. The Development of a Practice Based Nursing Home Page. Proceedings of the 6th International Congress of Nursing Informatics.

Goldsmith DM, Feldman ME, Cooney K, Costa MJ, Chapman R. 1998. Ambulatory Surgery Nurses Reaching Out to Patients from the Web. MedInfo 98. Proceedings of the Eighth World Conference on Medical Informatics.

Goldsmith D, Feldman ME, Cooney K, Safran C. 1998. The Development and Design of an Ambulatory Surgery Web Site. Proceedings of the American Medical Informatics Association Spring Congress.

Goldsmith DM, Safran C. 1999. Using the Web to Reduce Postoperative Pain Following Ambulatory Surgery. Journal of the American Medical Informatics Association (Suppl)6:780–784.

Gray J, Safran C, Weitzner GP, et al. 2000. Baby CareLink: Using the Internet and Telemedicine to Improve Care for High Risk Infants. Pediatrics 106(6):1318–1324.

Gustafson DH, McTavish F, Hawkins RP, Pingree S, Arora N, Mendenhall J, Simmons GE. 1998. Computer Support for Elderly Women with Breast Cancer. JAMA 280(15):1305.

Gustafson DH, McTavish F, Boberg E, Owens BH, Sherbeck C, Wise M, Pingree S, Hawkins RP. 1999. Empowering Patients Using Computer Based Health Support Systems. Quality Health Care 8(1):49–56.

Halamka JD, Osterland C, Safran C. 1999. CareWeb, a Web-based Medical Record for an Integrated Health Care Delivery System. International Journal of Medical Informatics 54(1):1–8.

Landro L. 1999. Patient-Physician Communication: An Emerging Partnership. Oncologist 4(1):55–58.

Landro L. 2000. Patient-Physician Communication: An Emerging Partnership. Annals of Oncology 11(Suppl 3):53–55.

Mandl KD, Kohan IS, Brandt AM. 1998. Electronic Patient-Physicians Communication Problems and Promise. Annals of International Medicine 129(6):495–500.

McTavish FM, Gustafson DH, Owen BH, Hawkins RP, Pingree S, Wise M, Taylor JO, Apantaku FM. 1995. CHESS (Comprehensive Health Enhancement Support System): An Interactive Computer System for Women with Breast Cancer Piloted with an Underserved Population. Journal of Ambulatory Care Management 18(3):35–41.

Pingree S, Hawkins RP, Gustafson DH, et al. 1996. Will the Disadvantaged Ride the Information Highway? Journal of Broadcasting and Electronic Media 40:331–353.

Safran C, Rind DM, Davis RB, Ives D, Sands DZ, Currier J, Caraballo E, Rippel K, Wang Q, Rury C, Slack WV, Makadon HJ, Cotton DJ. 1995. Guidelines for the Management of HIV Infection in a Computer-Based Medical Record. Lancet 346: 341–346.

Safran C, Jones PC, Rind D, Bush B, Cytryn KN, Patel VL. 1998. Electronic Communication and Collaboration in a Health Care Practice. Artificial Intelligence in Medicine 12(2):139–153.

Safran C, Rind DM, Sands DZ, Davis RB, Wald JS, Slack WV. 1996. Development of a Knowledge-Based Electronic Patient Record. MD Computing 13(1):46–54.

Shaw BR, McTavish F, Hawkins R, Gustafson DH, Pingree S. 2000. Experience of Women with Breast Cancer: Exchanging Social Support over the CHESS Computer Network. Journal of Health Communications 5(2):135–159.

Slack WV. 1977. The Patient's Right to Decide. Lancet 2(8031):240.

Slack WV. 1998. Cybermedicine: How Computing Empowers Patients for Better Healthcare. Medinfo 1:3–5.

Slack WV. 1999. The Patient Online. American Journal of Preventive Medicine 16(1):43–45.

Slack WV, Slack CW. 1972. Patient-Computer Dialogue. New England Journal of Medicine 286(24):1304–1309.

Vandenberg TA, Gustafson DH, Owen B, Gavin A, Cooke A, Anderson E, Markland S. 1997. Interaction Between the Breast Cancer Patient and the Health Care System: Demands, Constraints, and Options for the Future. Cancer Prevention and Control 1(2):152–153.

21 Increasing Clinical Trial Awareness and Accrual Via the Web

Joyce C. Niland and Douglas C. Stahl

The tremendous public and professional demand for online cancer information (Benjamin et al., 1996) is part of an emerging health care delivery paradigm in which information technology helps individuals access information about their medical conditions and potential treatment options (Widman & Tong, 1997). The Internet has had an impact on the evolving relationship between patients and physicians. There has been a growing movement advocating the view that patients are healthcare consumers with rights to information, interaction with health professionals, and participation in decision making (Sutherland et al., 1989). "Baby boomer" and post-baby boomer patient populations are found to be more autonomous, assertive, and demanding than patients of the past (Huber, 1993).

Because the public is increasingly well-educated, curious, and used to seeking healthcare information from printed media, it is natural for them to turn to electronic sources of information such as the Internet, which provides an expanding volume of information that previously was inaccessible (Widman & Tong, 1997; Jadad & Gagliardi, 1998). Cancer patients in particular possess an increasing level of medical sophistication, and are actively seeking the information they need to make rational decisions about treatment options (Huber, 1993; Mansour, 1994; Ho, 1994).

A significant factor limiting the availability of promising new therapies has been inadequate accrual of patients into clinical trials. The efficacy of any new treatment that is to be accepted as the standard of care by the medical community must be established by evaluating it against the "state of the art" treatment in a well-conducted, randomized clinical trial (Lawrence, 1990; Benson et al., 1991). Such trials are designed to evaluate new therapies in human subjects while minimizing investigator bias, design flaws, and subjective evaluation of treatment data, and are essential for understanding the effects of different treatment approaches (Mansour, 1994; Jenkins & Hubbard, 1991). Conclusions drawn solely from non-experimental data may lead to years of unnecessary costly treatment and immeasurable suffering (Farrar, 1991).

Although surveys of the general public have shown widespread support for the concept of clinical trials, and somewhere between 12% to 44% of patients with cancer are eligible for enrollment, it is widely reported that only 1% to 3% of over 1.2 million patients diagnosed with cancer in the United States each year are enrolled (Mansour, 1994; Lawrence, 1990; Farrar, 1991; Taylor et al., 1994; Morrow, Hickok & Burish, 1994; Fisher et al., 1991). In hospitals conducting clinical trials, on average less than 20% of eligible cancer patients are enrolled (Benson et al., 1991). It has been suggested that if only 10% of eligible patients routinely participated in oncology clinical trials, many trials could be completed in one year instead of the current 3 to 5 years that often are required (Farrar, 1991). This increased accrual would greatly expedite advances in cancer treatment and facilitate conclusions drawn from longer-term follow-up studies.

The barriers to clinical trial enrollment are numerous: Physicians are generally aware of the importance of trial participation, but frequently are unaware of trial availability at nearby centers (Mansour, 1994; Afrin et al., 1997). They also find it difficult to remember which clinical trials are active for a particular malignancy and their corresponding eligibility criteria (Mansour, 1994; Fisher et al., 1991). Although physicians may be willing to allow their patients to participate, they often do not have the resources to identify eligible participants (Mansour, 1994; Hunninghake, Darby, Probstfield, 1987). Many studies have relied primarily or exclusively on physicians, hospital records, or clinical laboratories for recruitment, and this approach generally has been unsuccessful if used alone (Hunninghake et al., 1987). Paper-based information distribution methods are known to be expensive, slow, and error-prone (Afrin et al., 1997). It has been unusual for patients to be the ones to initiate a discussion of clinical trials with physicians because their level of awareness about such trials also is generally low (Mansour, 1994).

A summary of the barriers to clinical trial enrollment and proposed strategies for eliminating them is shown in Table 21.1. Strategies for minimizing these barriers include heightening public awareness through improved information distribution methods and the dissemination of clinical trial synopses (Lawrence, 1990; Morrow et al., 1994; Afrin et al., 1997). An optimal medium for delivering timely, readily searchable data is the Internet. This chapter describes *Clinical Trials On-Line*, an interactive database system developed by the City of Hope National Medical Center to deliver clinical trials information via the Web. *ClinicalTrials.gov*, a government mandated system developed by the National Library of Medicine (NLM) is described by Alexa McCray in Chapter 22.

Clinical Trials On-Line

Located in Duarte, California, City of Hope National Medical Center is one of only 38 National Cancer Institute (NCI) designated Comprehensive Cancer Centers in the nation, and a founding member of the National

TABLE 21.1. Summary of barriers to the enrollment of patients into clinical trials and recommendations for removing them

Barriers to the enrollment of patients into clinical trials	Strategies for removing the barriers
• Physicians are often unaware of clinical trials available at nearby centers	• Increased public awareness of and access to clinical trials information
• Physicians find it difficult to remember eligibility criteria and which clinical trials are active for a particular malignancy	• Improved methods for disseminating clinical trial information to clinicians, patients, and the general public
• Paper-based distribution of clinical trials information	• Development and dissemination of synopses of active clinical trials
• Low patient awareness of the clinical trials process	
• Considerable time and effort required to explain complex clinical trials to patients	• Provision of a toll free number for clinical trial inquiries and information requests
• Lack of physician resources to identify eligible patients	• Increased patient education, complemented by discussions with clinical trial experts

Comprehensive Cancer Network (NCCN). Based on an analysis of the barriers to clinical trial enrollment and the emergence of the Internet as a new paradigm in healthcare information delivery, in 1998 City of Hope National Medical Center was motivated to develop a Web-enabled database of oncology clinical trials called *Clinical Trials On-Line*. Although several organizations have developed Internet-based information systems to distribute clinical trial information, many are limited by incomplete information, infrequent updates, and difficult user interfaces (Afrin et al., 1997), limitations that *Clinical Trials On-Line* overcomes.

System Features

Clinical Trials On-Line (found at clinicaltrials.coh.org) was designed to actively present City of Hope's research programs and ongoing cancer-related clinical trials to clinicians, patients, and the general public. The system contains descriptions of more than 100 ongoing trials at City of Hope at any given time, along with physician biographical information, research program descriptions, links to other Web sites, a glossary of terms maintained by the NCI, and a mechanism for the submission of user inquiries and feedback. The *Clinical Trials On-Line* home page is shown in Figure 21.1.

The Web interfaces for *Clinical Trials On-Line* were developed using Microsoft Active Server Page (ASP) technology and JavaScript, supported by Microsoft Internet Information Server (IIS) and SQL Server. The server hardware consists of two Dell PowerEdge 4300 Servers (400 MHz CPU,

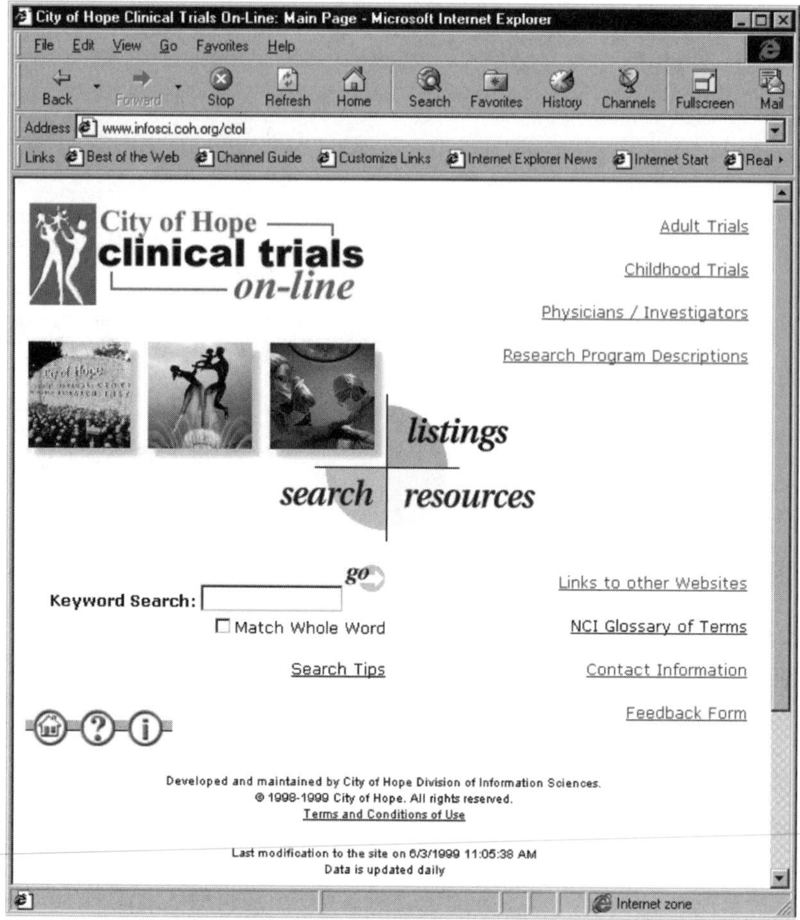

FIGURE 21.1. The home page for City of Hope's *Clinical Trials On-Line*. (Reprinted with permission from clinicaltrials.coh.org)

128 Mb RAM). IIS activity logs are routinely analyzed using WebTrends software (Portland, OR) to determine usage statistics for the Web site. The contents of the *Clinical Trials On-Line* database are updated daily using exports from the Biostatistics Information Tracking System (BITS), an inhouse relational database system created at City of Hope over 11 years ago to track data on all Cancer Center protocols and research participants.

Clinical Trials On-Line can be used to identify cancer clinical trials by patient age category (adult or child), the physician conducting the trial, or by keyword search (i.e., drug name, side effect, etc). If age categories are used, the information is then sub-categorized by cancer type. All of the clinical trial information is dynamically generated from database queries. When a specific disease category is selected, the user receives a list of clinical

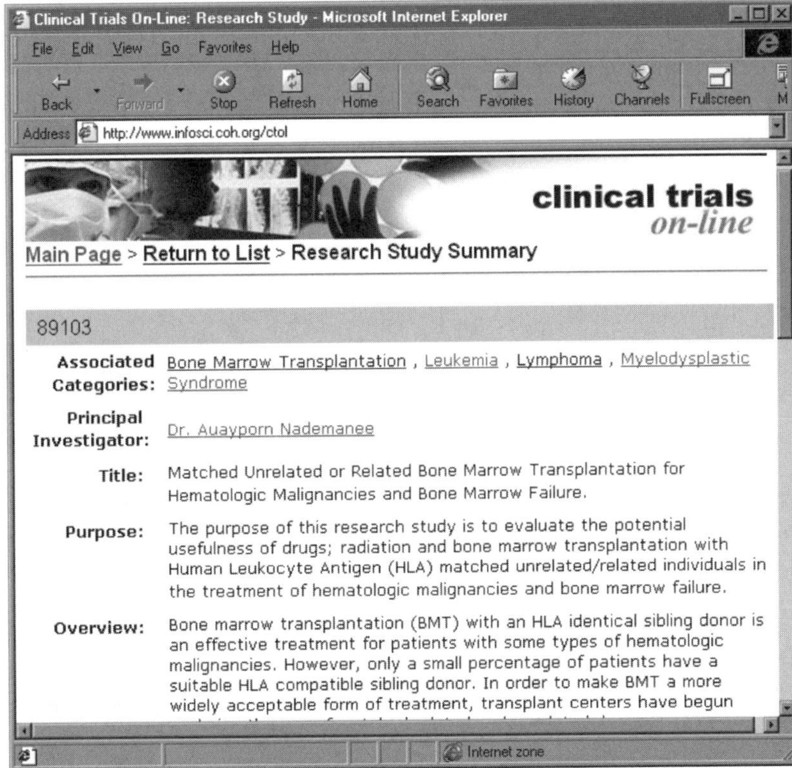

FIGURE 21.2. Lay summary of a specific clinical trial for childhood leukemia. (Reprinted with permission from clinicaltrials.coh.org)

trials that are open for accrual in that category. When the "summary" for a particular study is requested, *Clinical Trials On-Line* presents a synopsis of the study that has been specifically designed for the lay public, as shown in Figure 21.2. Each clinical trial summary provides a subset of the basic eligibility criteria, with a recommendation to contact City of Hope for more detailed information and to be considered for treatment. Because they are considered to be a form of "advertising" for the study, all clinical trial synopses must be reviewed and approved by the City of Hope Institutional Review Board (IRB). The IRB assures that all human subjects research, including clinical trials, conforms with current ethical standards and all regulatory mandates. The IRB's role in the *Clinical Trials On-Line* review is to ensure that there is no potential coersion to enter into the study in the phrasing of the text and that the summary information is accurate. This is an expedited review carried out by the IRB staff, administrator, and chair.

If an individual wishes to contact City of Hope, *Clinical Trials On-Line* supports inquiries via fax, regular mail, a toll-free 800 number unique to the *Clinical Trials On-Line* Web site, or via direct interaction with an online form linked to an inquiry database. All inquiries are transmitted to a trained oncology nurse, who triages the requests and responds via the desired mode specified, be that telephone, e-mail, or regular mail. Some of the inquiries are directed toward a particular clinical trial, while others are seeking more general cancer information or procedures for becoming a new patient. The unique toll-free number posted on the Web allows us to determine the number of call center inquiries generated by *Clinical Trials On-Line*, as recorded transparently by call detail reports, a less obtrusive information technology/telephony-based approach than interrogating potential new patients regarding whether or not they have seen a particular Web site.

Originally *Clinical Trials On-Line* supported both e-mail inquiries and direct submission to an inquiry database via an online information request form. However we subsequently discontinued the use of e-mail as a method of submitting information requests for the following reasons:

- The online form prompts users for specific contact information that is often not included in e-mail requests, while also providing comment fields for additional input.
- The online form places user inquiries directly into a database; in contrast, e-mail inquiries must be processed independently.
- Transactions with the online form are protected using the Secure Socket Layers (SSL) protocol supported by most Web browsers, allowing us to increase the security and confidentiality of sensitive patient information beyond that possible via e-mail.

Measuring Effectiveness

As with most information systems, the development and maintenance of a clinical trials Web site requires a substantial investment of resources. Although it may seem natural to assume that many "hits" on a clinical trials Web site will result in increased clinical trial enrollment, there is little direct evidence to support this premise. Tangible measures of effectiveness are required to justify and sustain the investment. When such evidence is not available, it may lead to the demise of potentially viable systems, as reported by one center at the 2000 Fall Conference of the American Medical Informatics Association (AMIA) (Afrin et al., 2000).

To track usage patterns of *Clinical Trials On-Line*, detailed logs of all user interactions are recorded by the Web server software and analyzed via WebTrends. The log contains Internet Protocol (IP) addresses, resources requested, and the time of the request. This log is a very important and powerful aspect of information publishing via the Internet because it provides feedback required to evaluate the site's impact (Benjamin et al., 1996). As an example, we determined that during the first 14-week period after *Clinical Trials On-Line* went live, there were 4,339 user sessions recorded by the *Clinical Trials On-Line* Web server. (A user session is synonymous with a "visit," and is defined as a session of activity [all hits] for

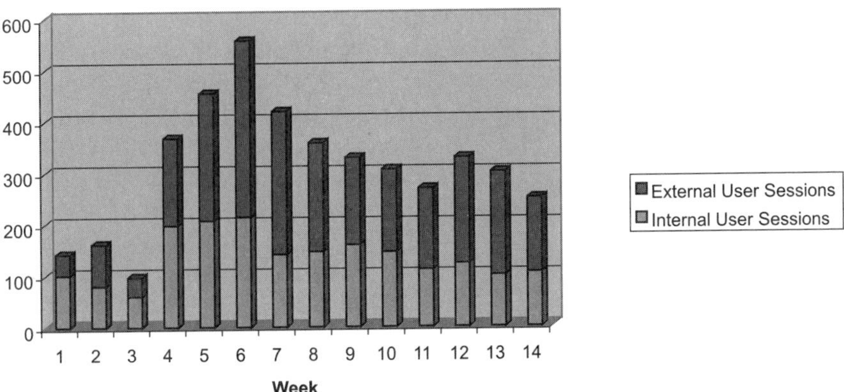

FIGURE 21.3. Graph of internal and external *Clinical Trials On-Line* user sessions for the first 14-week period. Weeks are identified on the X-axis, and number of user sessions per week is identified on the Y-axis.

one user for a specified period of time [WebTrends Corporation, 1998].) We quickly recognized that the system was useful not only to external visitors, but equally importantly serves as a critical resource for our internal physicians and research staff. The activity logs for this period revealed that 44% (1889 sessions) originated from the City of Hope intranet, with the remaining 56% (2450 sessions) originating from the Internet. A summary of internal and external user activity for the first 14-week period of operation is shown in Figure 21.3. The increase in internal activity seen in weeks four through six is believed to be the result of several articles about *Clinical Trials On-Line* that were published in City of Hope internal newsletters.

With regard to external visitors, through the IP addresses we have identified *Clinical Trials On-Line* information requests from the National Library of Medicine, National Institutes of Health, National Childhood Cancer Foundation, National Breast Cancer Coalition, and many of our fellow NCCN Cancer Centers. In the first 14-week period there also were many inquiries from North American universities, community hospitals, pharmaceutical companies, health maintenance organizations, insurance companies, and news organizations, as well as 168 international user sessions from over 20 different countries. The steady increase in external activity in weeks three through six (Figure 21.3) is believed to be the result of efforts to register *Clinical Trials On-Line* with major Internet search engines, and a message about *Clinical Trials On-Line* (including a hyperlink to the Web site) sent to several cancer-related USENET news groups.

Both the quantitative and qualitative data suggest that *Clinical Trials On-Line* is capable of making a positive contribution toward increased clinical trial awareness and accrual. The most credible evidence of the impact of *Clinical Trials On-Line* is the direct feedback we have received from cancer patients and their families. Over two thirds of our *Clinical Trials On-Line* information inquiries request specific treatment advice/information about clinical trials. The triage nurse also summarizes the nature of each inquiry, her mode of response, and the outcome when known.

Results suggest that *Clinical Trials On-Line* is providing valuable information and emotional support for its users. It has also been suggested, and our experience confirms, that Web sites like *Clinical Trials On-Line* can improve users' skills for self-help and reduce the financial burden of their care (Jaddad & Gagliardi, 1998).

Looking Ahead

The most perfectly designed Web-based system is of no use for information dissemination if users searching for relevant information cannot easily locate and access the site. Web site developers/owners need to make continual efforts to register their sites with search engines and Internet health information directories. The use of "push" technology can be used to provide automatic e-mail notification of clinicians and support groups about new clinical trials. Software such as WebTrends should be employed to analyze the usage of these new features as they are deployed.

Inter-connections between the more general *ClinicalTrials.gov* Web system (see Chapter 22) and those developed by individual organizations, like the City of Hope's *Clinical Trials On-Line*, will provide the optimal means for making a significant positive impact on clinical trial awareness and accrual. If centralized clinical trials repositories rely upon individual centers for content updates, the update frequency will vary among contributing organizations, and the quality of the repository as a whole will be compromised. An alternative approach used by *Clinicatrials.gov* is the creation of a "meta directory" with hyperlinks to *Clinical Trials On-Line* and other local clinical trial repositories. This approach allows the meta directory to be as up-to-date as the local systems it indexes, yet presents other challenges in terms of the inability to present users with a consistent interface. The most effective mode for integrating such centralized and individual organizational resources should be explored as directions for future research. This will further reduce enrollment barriers to clinical trials, and effectively exploit the Internet and its emerging role as a global medical information resource.

References

Afrin LB, et al. 1997. Electronic Clinical Trial Protocol Distribution via the World Wide Web: A Prototype for Reducing Costs and Errors, Improving Accrual, and Saving Trees. Journal of the American Medical Informatics Association 4:25–35.

Afrin LB, et al. 2000. How Useful Is the Web for Clinical Trial Accrual? Three Years of Experience with ACT: Proceedings of the American Medical Informatics Association, p 944.

Benjamin I, et al. 1996. OncoLink: A Cancer Information Resource for Gynecologic Oncologists and the Public on the Internet. Gynecologic Oncology 60:8–15.

Benson III, AB, et al. 1991. Oncologists' Reluctance to Accrue Patients onto Clinical Trials: An Illinois Cancer Center Study. Journal of Clinical Oncology 9(11):2067–2075.

Farrar WB. 1991, Clinical Trials: Access and Reimbursement. Cancer 67:1779–1782.

Fisher WB, et al. 1991. Clinical Trials in Cancer Therapy: Efforts to Improve Patient Enrollment by Community Oncologists. Medical and Pediatric Oncology 19:165–168.

Ho RCS. 1994. The Future Direction of Clinical Trials. Cancer 74:2739–2744.

Huber SL. 1993. Impact of Clinical Trial Protocols on Patient Care Systems at the University of Texas M.D. Anderson Cancer Center. Cancer 72:2824–2827.

Hunninghake DB, Darby CA, Probstfield JL. 1987. Recruitment Experience in Clinical Trials: Literature Summary and Annotated Bibliography. Controlled Clinical Trials 8(Suppl):6s–30s.

Jadad AR, Gagliardi A. 1998. Rating Health Information on the Internet. The Journal of the American Medical Association 279(8):611–614.

Jenkins J, Hubbard S. 1991. History of Clinical Trials. Seminars in Oncology Nursing 7:228–234.

Lawrence W. 1990. Improving Cancer Treatment by Expanding Clinical Trials. Cancer Journal for Clinicians 40(2):69–70.

Mansour EG. 1994. Barriers to Clinical Trials: Part III: Knowledge and Attitudes of Healthcare Providers. Cancer 74:2672–2675.

Morrow GR, Hickok JT, Burish TG. 1994. Behavioral Aspects of Clinical Trials: An Integrated Framework from Behavior Theory. Cancer 74:2676–2682.

Sutherland HJ, et al. 1989. Cancer Patients: Their Desire for Information and Participation in Treatment Decisions. The Royal Society of Medicine 82:260–263.

Taylor KM, et al. 1994. Fundamental Dilemmas of the Randomized Clinical Trial Process: Results of a Survey of the 1,737 Eastern Cooperative Oncology Group Investigators. Journal of Clinical Oncology 12(9):1796–1805.

WebTrends Corporation. 1998. User Manual. Portland, OR: WebTrends Corporation.

Widman LE, Tong DA. 1997. Requests for Medical Advice from Patients and Families to Health Care Providers Who Publish on the World Wide Web. Archives of Internal Medicine 157(2):151–152.

22
ClinicalTrials.gov: Linking Patients to Medical Research

Alexa T. McCray

ClinicalTrials.gov is a system designed to provide patients, families, and other members of the public with easy access to Web-based information about clinical research studies. The system owes its creation to a section of the Food and Drug Administration Modernization Act (1997), which charged the National Institutes of Health (NIH) with creating such a resource. The scope of this legislation is broad, requiring publicly available information on all clinical trials—whether federally or privately funded—for experimental treatments for serious or life-threatening diseases and conditions. On behalf of all NIH Institutes, the National Library of Medicine (NLM) developed *ClinicalTrials.gov* and made it available to the public in February 2000.

There are currently over 5,700 records in the database, representing primarily NIH-sponsored trials, though trials from other federal agencies and the private sector are increasingly being included. Each record in the database includes a summary of the purpose of the trial, its recruiting status, the criteria for patient participation, the location of the trial, and specific contact information. An important feature of the database is its "just-in-time" access to other online health resources, such as NLM's MEDLINE and MEDLINE*plus*. These resources help place clinical trials in the context of a patient's overall medical care. Figure 22.1 shows a sample search for "leukemia" and "bone marrow transplant."

Figure 22.2 shows the result of the search. Before clicking on any specific record, the user can easily see not only which trials are currently recruiting patients, but also which conditions those trials are studying. Once users choose a trial record, they may click on a link to related information available through NLM's consumer health site, MEDLINE*plus*. Figure 22.3 illustrates this capability. As illustrated in Figure 22.4, users can access additional information for the trial, including links to MEDLINE references, through NLM's PubMed system. Underlying the public Web site of *ClinicalTrials.gov* is a system designed to receive, process, validate, manage, and maintain data from a large number of sources (McCray & Ide, 2000; McCray, 2000). We use the knowledge represented in the NLM's

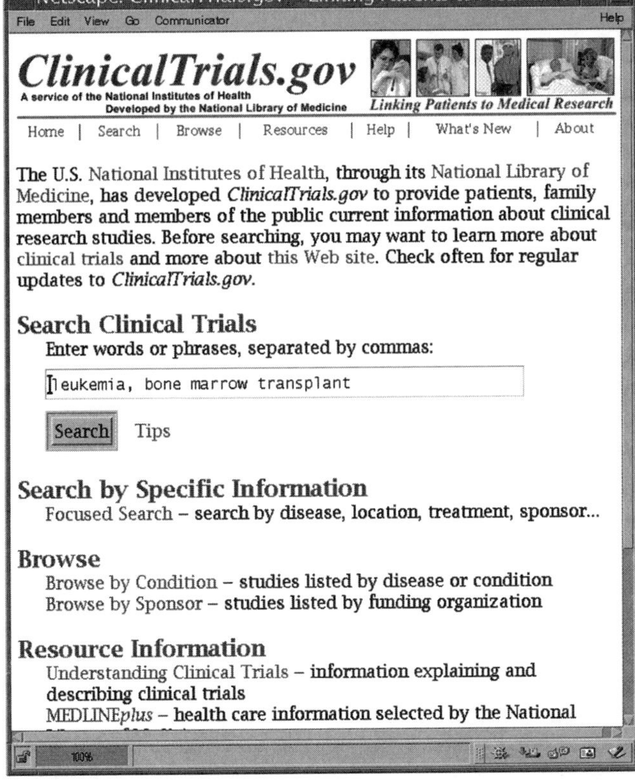

FIGURE 22.1. Simple search on *ClinicalTrials.gov* home page.

Unified Medical Language System (UMLS) Knowledge Sources (http://umlsinfo.nlm.nih.gov/) to ensure flexible access to the data. For example, we transform searches by adding UMLS synonyms to users' queries, and we create browsable condition name lists by mapping the disease terms found in our records to UMLS concepts.

For encoding the data, we have developed a standard set of data elements submitted to us according to an XML (eXtensible Markup Language) DTD (Document Type Definition). This standard set of data elements helps ensure that coverage and presentation are uniform, despite many different data providers. Deliberations about the optimal set of elements were informed by earlier work conducted at the NIH and elsewhere (Meinert, 1988; Spilker, 1996; International Collaborative Group on Clinical Trial Registries, 1993; International Conference on Harmonization of Technical Requirements for Registration of Pharmaceuticals for Human Use, 1996).

Table 22.1 shows a summary of the data elements.

ClinicalTrials.gov has been available to the public for approximately one and a half years. During that time, the number of visits to the site has

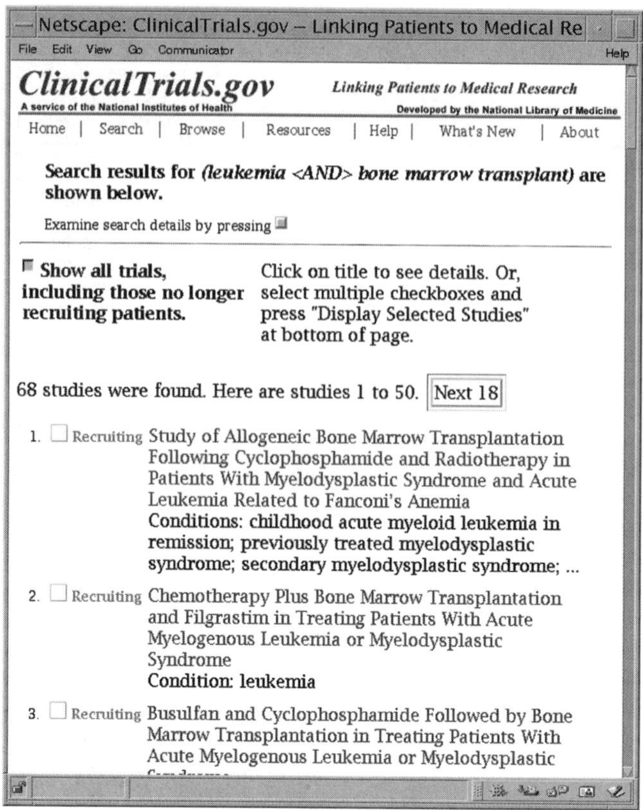

Figure 22.2. Search results for a simple search on *ClinicalTrials.gov*.

exceeded 33 million page hits, representing more than 5,000 individual users each day. As we add more trials from other federal agencies and the private sector, and as our broad base of users requests additional capabilities, the system will continue to grow in both coverage and functionality.

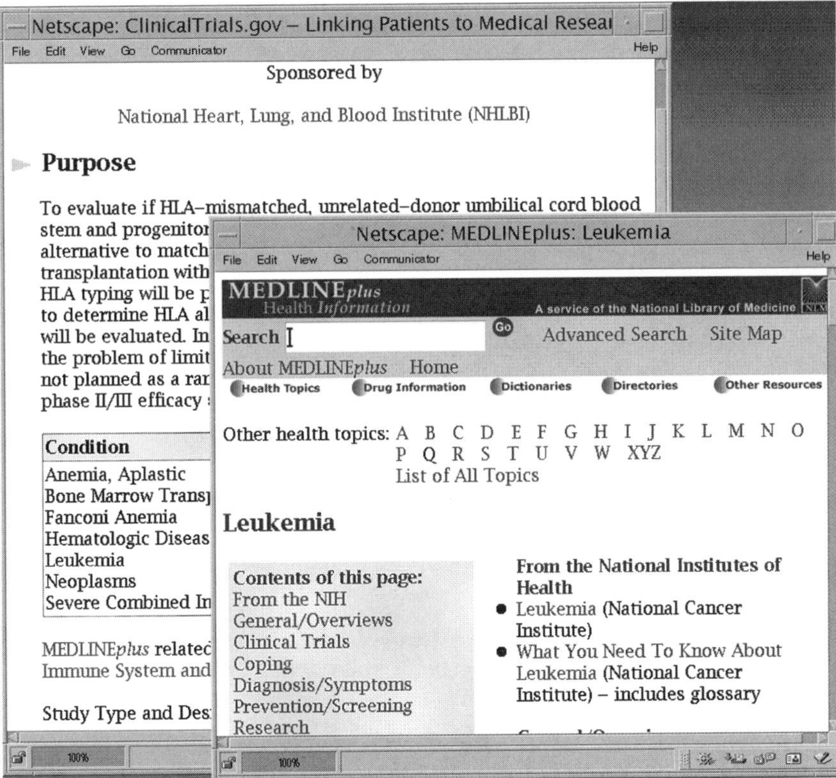

FIGURE 22.3. Portion of a *ClinicalTrials.gov* record with links to MEDLINE*plus*.

References

FDA Modernization Act of 1997, Public Law 105–115, Section 113. Information Program on Clinical Trials for Serious or Life-Threatening Diseases. http://www.fda.gov/cder/guidance/105-115.htm. Accessed 12/20/2000.

International Collaborative Group on Clinical Trial Registries. 1993. Position Paper and Consensus Recommendations on Clinical Trial Registries. Clinical Trials Metaanalysis 28:255–266.

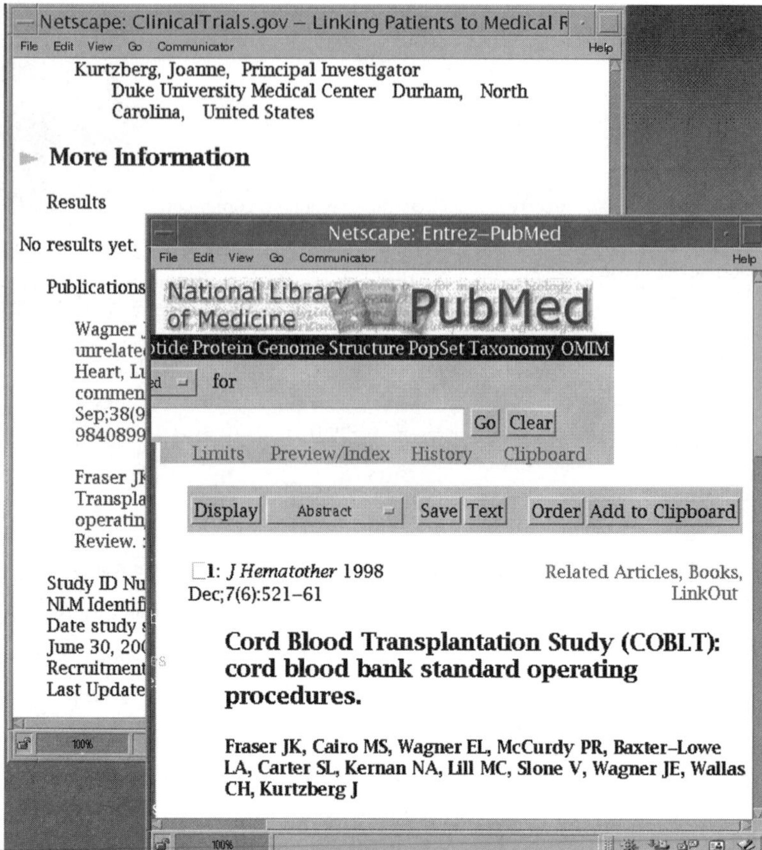

FIGURE 22.4. Portion of a *ClinicalTrials.gov* record with links to PubMed.

International Conference on Harmonization of Technical Requirements for Registration of Pharmaceuticals for Human Use. 1996. ICH Harmonized Tripartite Guideline. Guideline for Good Clinical Practice, 30–33. http://www.ifpma.org/pdfifpma/e6.pdf. Accessed 12/20/2000.

McCray AT, Ide NC. 2000. Design and Implementation of a National Clinical Trials Registry. Journal of the American Medical Informatics Association 7(3):313–323.

Table 22.1. Summary of data elements in *ClinicalTrials.gov*

Data Elements	Description
Unique identifier	Primary unique identifier assigned by the sponsoring organization; any secondary identifiers assigned by other groups
Title	Brief protocol title intended for the public; additional official title provided by the principal investigator, if desired
Sponsor information	Name of sponsoring organizations that initiate and take responsibility for the clinical investigation; information related to sponsor's Food and Drug Administration Investigational New Drug (IND) application
Study description	Brief summary describing the purpose of the trial intended for use by patients; detailed description, giving a technical summary for health professionals
Study status	Phase of the study investigation; type of investigation (e.g., interventional or observational); recruiting status (e.g., not yet recruiting, recruiting, completed); study start and stop dates
Study design	Primary investigative techniques used in the protocol, including reason for the protocol (e.g., treatment, prevention), allocation of subjects (e.g., randomization), masking (e.g., double blind), control (e.g., dose comparison), intervention assignments (e.g., cross-over), study endpoints.
Interventions	Intervention type (e.g., drug, vaccine, device); intervention name (using NLM's Medical Subject Headings if possible)
Conditions	Primary diseases or conditions being studied (using NLM's Medical Subject Headings)
Keywords	Additional important terms for search purposes (using NLM's Medical Subject Headings)
Eligibility criteria	Summary of specific criteria for subject selection, including age and gender
Location and contact information	Name and location of each facility where the trial is being conducted; name and phone number of a contact individual at each location; investigator information
Related information	Citations to published articles related to the protocol; pointers to Web sites that are relevant to the trial

McCray AT. 2000. Better Access to Information about Clinical Trials. Annals of Internal Medicine 133(8):609–614.

Meinert CL. 1988. Toward Prospective Registration of Clinical Trials. Controlled Clinical Trials 9:1–5.

Spilker B. 1996. Guide to Clinical Trials. Philadelphia: Lippincott-Raven. 816–819.

UMLS Information. http://umlsinfo.nlm.nih.gov/. Accessed 12/20/2000.

23
The National Cancer Institute's net-Trials™

Dianne M. Reeves and Douglas Hageman

In recent years, discussions of clinical research data management have shifted focus from manual to electronic processes. Although 95% of all clinical trials still used paper in 1996 (Vogel, 1997), more institutions have begun using electronic applications to enter, view, manage, and monitor clinical research data. Today, data can be collected in real time from study sites worldwide, and data quality can be verified at time of input or collection (Hageman & Reeves, 2001).

An automated approach offers many benefits over the paper-based approach. Electronic interchange of data can assist the human interface between clinical care data (the hospital/clinic systems) and clinical research data (the subset of clinical data dictated by protocol). Users can aggregate data for reports, search for patient-specific data, and quickly share information. Automation also enables front-end validation processes like range checking, simple edit checks, and cross-validation between variables measured on repeated occasions (Rotmensz, 1989; Day, Fayers, Harvey, 1998). Through new automated processes, organizations can streamline their workflow, introduce new data quality practices, and prepare for monitoring visits.

Simply put, information technology is the key to answering research questions and producing better information faster. Single and multi-center trials are realizing this, using Internet technology to collect data from multiple sites (Santoro et al., 1999; Lowe, 1999). Flexible, almost universally available, and unconstrained by geographic location, the Web-based approach supports the timely collection of complex medical information, displays it textually or graphically, and allows it to be stored and managed from a central database (Sippel & Ohmann, 1998; Vissers et al., 1998). Because it can operate from any site with an Internet connection and Web browser, it may be the best answer for fast and efficient data collection and administration in large randomized multi-center trials.

Lowe describes this as a paradigm shift in medicine toward Internet-based solutions for information management: "Perhaps the two most important applications to emerge in the next decade will be Internet-based clinical trials (in which patients and researchers, though geographically distributed, will be linked via secure Internet-based data collection, review, and reporting systems) and the Internet-based multimedia electronic medical record" (Lowe, 1999). The National Cancer Institute, through new applications like net-Trials™, has been part of this shift. In this chapter, we describe the evolution of net-Trials™, its characteristics and architecture, and the challenges and future considerations involved in its implementation and maintenance.

net-Trials™ at the National Cancer Institute

The Center for Cancer Research is the intramural component of the National Cancer Institute's clinical research program, located in Bethesda, Maryland. With more than 200 clinical trials in operation at any time, the Division's ten branches enroll approximately 2500 patients each year, primarily in phase I studies. The result of this research is clinical data, the center's most important asset.

By 1998, our center had over 20 systems collecting clinical trial information. Many of these had evolved slowly and addressed problems at the individual department level. Because these systems did not share a vocabulary to describe trials or the data collected, it was difficult to aggregate and report data across departments. Another ongoing challenge was supporting, maintaining, and modifying multiple systems. This resulted in uneven support across systems and a system not flexible enough to address changing protocol needs.

A major project initiative was unveiled in late 1998, supported by funding for a major system review and reengineering. The center's directive was to create a shared clinical data management solution that could be used intramurally and by NCI's collaborative sites.

Understanding Problems and Work Processes

Clinical trials in cancer are conducted in many different ways, depending on the phase of study, modality, institution policies, and other variables. In the NCI's intramural clinical program, there are department-specific ways of conducting business. Understanding all these processes and refining that understanding into system development requirements was a task that remains significant as we enter our first period of system operation.

Our initial goal was to support the entire protocol lifecycle: protocol development (authoring), patient recruitment, screening and registration, protocol implementation, and analysis and reporting. We gathered the requirements in two phases. In phase 1, we modeled the information flow and workflow as they currently existed in the protocol lifecycle stages, on a department-by-department basis (the "as-is" model). Phase 2 assembled groups of clinicians from multiple departments to walk through hypothetical information flows, again grouped by protocol lifecycle steps. This time, we questioned how processes should be done (the "to-be" model), not how they are already done.

This exercise produced process models, data models, and related conceptual representations of clinical trial operations. We also collected and analyzed examples of data collection forms, internal and external reports, sample protocols, and documentation (when available) from existing systems. With these intense, high profile exercises complete, we could begin developing the first iteration of the net-Trials™ system.

Although we could not have started technical development without the results of these activities, equally important was the feeling of ownership and input into the process by the clinical staff. The clinician community invested thousands of hours in the application during the first eight months of work. We believe our requirements gathering process allowed us to keep system ownership with the clinical staff using it.

The Buy Versus Build Decision

At first, we did not call this a development project; our idea was to implement a commercially available product, possibly with some customization. In the winter of 1998, we reviewed two consumer products designed predominantly for clinical trials implementation. Within six months, we evaluated a total of four commercially available products. Our evaluations focused on:

- **Technical functionality.** Would the product do what we needed it to do?
- **System compatibility.** Would the product work with our desktop hardware and security environment?
- **Ease of integration.** Was third-party integration viable, and would we be allowed into the source code?
- **Cost and schedule.** Could we integrate the product with available funding and in a reasonable timeframe?
- **Vendor performance and reliability.** Was the product from an established firm with a track record that would help us evaluate product risk?

Our analysis revealed that the commercially available products were not designed for enterprise-wide implementation, and none of them had multiplatform support or a browser interface. They offered no single underlying database and no direct support for the remote data entry highly desirable for multi-institutional trials. Furthermore, instead of offering a security approach, the products simply assumed we would deploy the software in a secure environment.

The two years since the initial product evaluation have introduced some interesting products that would have merited closer evaluation if we were near the beginning of the project. Fewer vendors tailor products to clinical research than to the broader clinical information system market, a fact that complicated the build versus buy decision. Given the products available at the time, we decided to pursue complete system development.

Basic Characteristics of net-Trials™

The net-Trials Clinical Trials Information System™ collects and reports clinical trials data sponsored by the NCI's Center for Cancer Research (CCR) and their collaborators. A Web-based application focusing solely on clinical trials, it frees the user from hardware constraints and the need for multiple approaches to creation, deployment, vocabulary, training, and maintenance. net-Trials™ was designed with the input of principal investigators, research nurses, data managers, and other staff involved in the day-to-day issues of clinical research.

Patient information management in the net-Trials™ system is based on the International Conference on Harmonisation's (ICH) Guideline for Good Clinical Practice, a set of standards-based processes developed for clinical research (ICH, 1997). This approach uses both case report forms and patient-centered views. When fully implemented, net-Trials™ will have the modules listed in Table 23.1 to simplify the clinical trials process and enhance the timeliness and usefulness of data. In the process, net-Trials™ will simplify administrative and regulatory reporting (including adverse

Table 23.1. Modules and descriptions

Module	Status	Description
Protocol development	Not currently implemented	Fulfills protocol authoring and document routing, mark-up, and electronic signature needs. Features tools for defining data requirements during protocol development
Patient recruitment	Not currently implemented	Assists with study categorization, patient-study matching, and information dissemination for patients and physicians
Patient screening and registration	Under development	Stores data beginning with the first patient encounter, including demographic information, patient history, eligibility assessment, and protocol enrollment and registration
Protocol implementation	Most functions completed	Includes protocol-specific data collection forms; reuse of information from the patient record, laboratory, and ancillary hospital services; automatic grading of laboratory data; and elements defined in the data dictionary, including international standards and organizationally defined terms
Analysis and publication	Under development	Includes predefined report fomats and allows users to define their own reports and perform ad hoc queries. This module also plots data and can export it to external statistical applications

event reporting) and incorporate automatic grading of such events by implementing the NCI's Common Toxicity Criteria.

In our clinical research program, we faced several problems stemming, in part, from our legacy information systems. Some basic goals of net-Trials™ evolved to address these issues; for example, it supports and enforces standardized clinical vocabulary, allows researchers to set up their protocols within the system, and allows unique representation of individual protocols. At the same time, each protocol is built on an enterprise data model shared by other protocols. It can display both protocol-specific views of information and patient-centered longitudinal views of data.

Data Challenges and Standards

In the area of clinical vocabulary, we aimed not to "solve" the complex issues, but to identify a consistent and repeatable way of identifying unique concepts in net-Trials™. We also planned to satisfy external mandates in several areas, particularly adverse event reporting. Our goals required a reasonable approach comprised of legacy system vocabulary, terminology useful to clinical research staff, creation of as few new vocabulary choices as possible, and adoption of as many nationally accepted vocabularies as possible. This would satisfy external requirements and create a framework we could use to evolve our approach to vocabulary as the science evolved. This framework is the net-Trials™ data dictionary.

After a complete inventory of our legacy systems, we catalogued over 8,000 non-unique data entities in areas like adverse events, investigational and concomitant agents, diagnosis, patient demographics, patient response, patient history, and procedures. Many hours of committee and workgroup activity produced a consensus dictionary based on legacy systems data and existing vocabularies. Our first consolidated data dictionary contained:

- ICD9-CM for diagnosis
- ICD-O for histology and body site
- Common Toxicity Criteria v. 2.0 for adverse event reporting
- First Data Bank (NDDF) for concomitant medications
- SNOMED for procedures
- CTEP (Cancer Therapy Evaluation Program) vocabulary for country, institution, group
- Office of Management and Budget codes for race/ethnicity
- Clinical Center Department of Clinical Pathology for Laboratory Tests
- other locally defined standards to provide consistent use.

The problems with our first data dictionary are obvious. ICD9-CM, for example, lacks depth in many areas necessary for clinical use and does not map easily into the MedDRA vocabulary required for adverse event reporting. Building a complete diagnostic picture by combining ICD9, ICD-O, and staging information from multiple sources allows reasonable depth and much flexibility, but as the variables increase, the goals of consistency and repeatability are severely tested. In addition, system logic to prevent nonsensical combinations was not yet in place.

Even with the limitations, our first approach was useful. It helped effect a culture shift in our organization, one that helped us acknowledge and understand the importance of standards. The data standards group became an important forum to engage clinicians in issues they valued and maintain their ownership of the developing new system.

Flexibility

The network environment in the National Institutes of Health's (NIH) Clinical Center is diverse, with many distinct physical networks in the building. In addition to the NIH Clinical Center network, the CCR's Medicine Branch has a significant clinical trials presence at the National Naval Medical Center, complete with its own network infrastructure. In this environment, security approaches like firewalls and private networks are difficult or impossible to apply across multiple networks. It also created a computing environment that the system architecture and security approach had to be designed to handle.

The system environment also includes multiple hardware platforms on the clinician desktops. Our users are almost evenly split between Macintosh and Windows-based personal computers. Given the dual platform environment and the physical network constraints on security, the system architecture leaned strongly toward a browser-based user interface. A browser application enables development of a single application for both Windows and Macintosh desktops, rather than a separate client version for each platform.

System Architecture

Because of the need to apply tight system security in an open network environment, as well as the diverse location and hardware of the users, net-Trials™ has a three-tier architecture.

- **Presentation.** The user interface is a Web browser (currently Netscape 4.7).
- **Application.** The business logic is codified and implemented by the application server (Silverstream v. 3.5).
- **Database.** Oracle database 8.16.

Security

There are several elements to consider here:

Physical Security

Communication between end-user computers and the servers is encrypted with certificate-based authentication of users, which is imposed via secure socket layer (SSL). All users will have IDs and passwords, and the system will enforce periodic password changes. Database and Web servers reside behind a firewall for protection.

Logical Security

With role-based security, system users are given access to specific groups of patients via protocol assignments and to specific functions like read, write, and report. Users see only patients being treated on the protocols on which they are working. Browsing through records is forbidden and detectable by a review of system audit files. Roles are divided generally by task area/ function; e.g., "system administration" or "write protocol data." Further, only two system administrators have access to all patients and protocols, so that risk is segmented across the user population.

Audit Trail

All access to the system, whether reading, writing, or reporting, is recorded in an audit trail. A complete record is maintained of what was viewed, what was written, and by whom.

Training and Usability Issues

By the time they attend formal training sessions for net-Trials™, most clinical staff are familiar with the electronic data collection forms, functions, and reports they helped design and develop. Through the involvement of the clinician community, net-Trials™ training has become primarily an opportunity to completely review the application's functionality. Training typically takes three to ten hours, based on the modules indicated for each user's role.

During training, information about user experience is collected for a profile of the Center for Cancer Research (CCR) user population. Attendees also complete a formal evaluation of the sessions. Their suggestions for enhancements, changes, and functionality are encouraged, collected, and added to the Requirements Database.

Building a major application useful for an intended audience also requires usability testing. Usability can be defined as the degree to which a piece of software helps users do their work. Through tools and structured methodological approaches, systems should be frequently assessed using several criteria:

- ease of learning the application
- ability to retain learning over time
- speed with which tasks are completed
- error rate associated with forms and functionality
- subjective level of user satisfaction with display and function.

Usability testing is observing, measuring, and evaluating the human-computer interaction characteristics of an application. Nearly any type of usability test can improve the product if the development group receives the results and incorporates them into the application appropriately. net-Trials™ users are participating in usability testing using the Software Usability Measurement Inventory (SUMI), developed in 1990 at the Human Factors Research Group at University College Cork (Ireland). It has undergone extensive development and research and rates high for reliability and validity. The tool has five scales to measure usability, is available in eleven languages, and is commercially available at a reasonable cost.

Looking Ahead

The net-Trials™ system promises numerous benefits to cancer researchers, physicians, and patients. It will unify systems, processes, and data to make participating in clinical trials easier than ever before. Users of net-Trials™ will collaborate by transmitting and receiving clinical trials data from a secure central database, eliminating complications that arise when researchers use multiple, and often incompatible, information systems.

As a key enabler of clinical research, net-Trials™ will replace standalone data management systems with a single system, accessible anytime and from anywhere. Developing and implementing net-Trials™ is an ongoing process. We expect that all the currently identified functions will be completed and implemented within the next two to three years.

Electronic processes like net-Trials™ not only require the same attention to coding conventions, workflow, and consistency as paper-based approaches; they also require an organizational commitment to reengineering work processes (Bartruff, 1999). Hammer and Champy (1993) note that most organizations view technology through the "lens of existing processes," asking how they can use technology to replicate processes, not how they can achieve entirely new goals (Vogel, 1997). Through redefined data management, personnel could enter clinical data directly from the source document into the computer, and auditors could review an activity log and aggregate data before a site visit. Internet-based technologies and multi-site, consistent work practices could enable geographically distanced sites, patients, and researchers to collaborate on clinical trial accrual (Lowe, 1999). When technology is used to transform, not merely replicate, these and other goals are possible.

References

Bartruff B. 1999. Issues in Clinical Trials Management: Part I. Clean Data: The Mark of Excellence. Research Nurse 5(2):12–15.

Day S, Fayers P, Harvey D. 1998. Double Data Entry: What Value, What Price? Controlled Clinical Trials 19:15–24.

Hageman D, Reeves DM. 2001. Research Data Management. In Cancer: Principles and Practice of Oncology, 6th ed. DeVita VT, Hellman S, Rosenberg SA. (eds.) Philadelphia: Lippincott Williams & Wilkins, pp. 539–545.

Hammer M, Champy J. 1993. Reengineering the Corporation. New York: Harper Collins Books.

International Conference on Harmonisation. 1997. Good Clinical Practice: Consolidated Guideline. Federal Register 9 May 62(90):1.24.

Lowe HJ. 1999. Transforming the Cancer Center in the 21st Century. MD Computing 16(3):40–42.

Rotmensz N (ed.). 1989. Data Management and Clinical Trials. EORTC Study Group on Data Management. Amsterdam: Elsevier Scientific Publishing.

Santoro E, Nicolis E, Franzosi MG, Tognoni G. 1999. Internet for Clinical Trials: Past, Present, and Future. Controlled Clinical Trials 19:194–201.

Silva JS. 1999. Fighting Cancer in the Information Age, an Architecture for National Scale Clinical Trials. MD Computing 16(3):43–44.

Sippel H, Ohmann C. 1998. A Web-Based Data Collection System for Clinical Studies Using Java. Medical Informatics 23(3):223–229.

Vissers MC, Hasman A, Stapert JW. 1998. Presenting Treatment Protocols with Web Technology. Medinfo 1:521–524.

Vogel R. 1997. Remote Data Capture. Applied Clinical Trials 6(5):36–40.

24
iN: A Community-Based Cancer Informatics and Clinical Trials Network

Donald W. Simborg

The first section of this book describes the principles of cancer informatics and clinical trials, the second examines their technical underpinnings, and the third explores standardization in cancer informatics. In this fourth and final section, we present examples of practical, implemented applications that use some of the infrastructure described in the preceding sections. These examples illustrate the issues involved in implementations, as well as potential successes. Focusing on one such implementation, the iKnowMed Network (iN), we examine a crucial aspect of cancer informatics: the relationship between clinical trials informatics and patient care informatics.

Rationale

Traditional attempts to meet the needs of patient care and clinical trials independently have produced parallel and redundant information systems. Most point-of-care electronic record products for clinicians do not satisfy the needs of clinical trials, and many young companies focus exclusively on clinical trial management functions like screening and case reporting. The idea behind iN, developed by the company iKnowMed, is to combine the needs of physicians and nurses at the point of care with the needs of organizations sponsoring clinical trials.

Clinical trial participants require the same medical record functions as any other patients. By combining patient care and clinical trial functions into a single operation where appropriate, organizations can reduce error, time delay, redundancy, and cost. Since most patient care in oncology and most clinical trials occur in the ambulatory environment, this combined solution applies to the physician office practice and the outpatient department of a medical center.

Benefits

Integrating clinical trial functions with patient care functions would yield significant benefits in two areas. The first is patient recruitment. Enrolling enough patients in clinical trials within the allotted time remains a challenge, particularly in oncology. According to 1999 data, only 2% to 3% of cancer patients enroll in clinical trials (Reuters, 1999). Additional data from the Southwest Oncology Group (SWOG) indicate that fewer than 10% of their patients eligible for a clinical trial actually get enrolled in one (Crowley J, personal communication, 2000). The gap between patients needed and patients enrolled has widened in recent years, and with the projected impact of genomics, proteinomics, and other areas of biotechnology, the need for clinical trials will increase dramatically.

The current patient recruitment process is inefficient. Either physicians must remember to consider trials during patient visits, or nurses and other staff members must scan patient records for candidates. Clinical research organizations and other trial managers have conducted direct-to-consumer advertising to supplement these methods. Although these techniques do yield patients, they suffer from insufficient sensitivity (have difficulty finding eligible patients) or specificity (refer patients who are not eligible).

If every patient encounter were documented electronically and key screening data were coded, the system could automatically alert the physician of a patient's potential eligibility during the encounter, which is the best time to consider trial participation. If this were a routine aspect of documentation, clinical trial screening would not only be a by-product of patient care, it would also increase the sensitivity and specificity of patient recruitment. As described later in this chapter, this is one feature of iN. Although iN does not alter other barriers to patient involvement in trials, such as resistance to experimental therapies, this technology addresses a major obstacle—inefficient patient recruitment.

Case reporting is the second area that would benefit from integrating the clinical trial and patient care process. The need to document patient care at an encounter overlaps with the need to report that encounter for clinical trials, although each purpose may require different documentation. The patient record must contain all clinically relevant information, even if it has no relevance to the clinical trial, but the trial imposes documentation requirements and diagnostic and therapeutic procedures that routine patient care may not have required.

With iN, a single point-of-care documentation process aims to meet both needs and eliminate redundancy. Since edits for errors and missing data can be moved to the point of care, the clinical trial monitor would save time and reduce errors on the case report form. The resulting ability to perform clinical trial analyses earlier could both speed the process and reduce the number of patients needed, freeing them for other clinical studies.

Requirements

Whether clinical trials are conducted or not, any point-of-care system must win clinician acceptance by enabling excellent patient care. Although this chapter does not review the broader issues regarding acceptance of electronic patient records (EPRs), we can identify fundamental requirements for a point-of-care system in both general practice and oncology.

In general, an EPR must save time and add value. More specifically, it must either save or not affect clinician time, and it must add clinical, financial, and workflow-related value in proportion to the added cost. Failure to fulfill all these requirements is still a barrier to widespread use of EPRs, which makes it a barrier to combining the needs of patient care and clinical trials. In oncology ambulatory settings, the complexity of treatment further complicates EPR use. In particular, chemotherapy administration requires a level of care in the ambulatory setting unlike that of almost any other specialty.

What, then, are the characteristics of a system that will integrate the clinical trial informatics components into a single point-of-care application? To embed clinical trial screening into the point-of-care process, the system must:

- electronically represent the eligibility requirements of a clinical trial
- electronically represent the encounter note
- include a standard coding system for representing both the eligibility requirements and the encounter note documentation
- include in the routine encounter note documentation of the high-level eligibility screening requirements for all clinical trials
- include software that quickly matches the encounter note data with the eligibility requirements.

Combining case reporting with encounter documentation carries several requirements.

- The point-of-care system must represent the clinical trial calendar and documentation requirements and integrate them with all other care plans for a single patient.
- The point-of-care system must incorporate and operationalize the special edits required for completeness and accuracy.
- The clinical care monitor must accept and the point-of-care system must send an electronic submission of the case report form.
- To ensure integrity, accuracy, and security of records, the point-of-care system must meet the 21 Case Report Form (CRF) 11 and other Food and Drug Administration (FDA) requirements for documentation. These are broad sets of requirements for system and user validation, auditability, and electronic signatures.

Elements of iN

Figure 24.1 illustrates the schematic of iN. The four major participants in the network are providers, patients, data users, and clinical trial sponsors, and the figure can represent an entity more than once. For example, providers are also data users and pharmaceutical companies are both clinical trial sponsors and data users. A set of software functions corresponds to each participant type. Data users access a Web-based reporting center, and the clinical trials module serves the clinical trial sponsors. The product for providers is called iKnowChart, and the one for patients is called iKnowMyChart. The following subsections describe each of these functions.

iKnowChart

Physicians, nurses, and all caregiver-related personnel use iKnowChart, a complete EPR that seamlessly integrates clinical trial functions. Here, we describe only the unique characteristics that will interest readers of this volume. The iKnowMed Web site (www.iknowmed.com) houses a more complete description of iKnowChart.

The iKnowChart user interface (patent # 5950168), a "single-screen" technology designed to speed the review and entry of patient information, is an essential component for patient care and clinician acceptance. During an encounter, clinicians view a summary screen of information specific to each

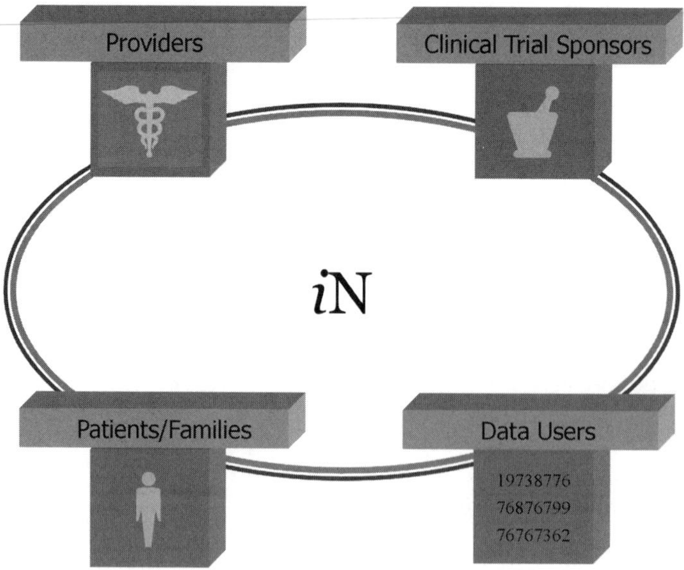

FIGURE 24.1. Schematic diagram of iN.

clinician/patient combination. The format and content of the data varies not only for each patient, but also for each clinician viewing that patient. If any information is not visible, clinicians can bring it into view without leaving the single screen. They can also enter all documentation, orders, and communications onto the same screen.

Data entry combines coded structured text dialogues and free text. Users enter free text by voice or keyboard, the voice converted to digital representation either through voice recognition or transcription. Free text is not coded, but it must exist to handle detailed patient care documentation. In iKnowChart, approximately 90% of data entry is performed with coded structured text, which is generally faster, avoids the cost and inconvenience of voice recognition technology or transcription, and is more valuable simply because it is coded.

Clinicians perform all encounter note documentation under the guidance of a Knowmed®, a form of protocol created with iKnowMed's proprietary tool set. This tool set, which integrates clinical trial functions with point-of-care documentation, includes the following components:

- vocabulary
- rules editor
- alerts editor
- Knowmed editor
- regimen editor.

Vocabulary

Structured text dialogues are created from coded vocabulary terms. Each term or phrase is a concept that can have "parents," "children," synonyms, and attributes, and each attribute can have values. For example, the concept "chest pain" may be a child of the general concept "pain" and the parent of a specific type of chest pain, "angina." It may have attributes like "location," "severity," and "duration," and an individual attribute like "severity" may have multiple values like "mild," "moderate," and "severe." By constructing a complete vocabulary and from it logical groupings of concepts, structured text input dialogues can be created for virtually any situation. The resulting records are coded and subject to use by the other tools.

Rules and Alerts

Rules are Boolean logic operations performed on the vocabulary. They can be as simple as "chest pain exists" or "chest pain exists and severity equals severe." Alternatively, they can be complex rules that string together many combinations of terms, operators, and conditions. Rules can be defined as inheritable or not inheritable to the children; for instance, a rule about "chest pain" can be applied to "angina" and all other children of "chest pain." Rules test as either true or false, and based on the findings, an alert can be created from a rule. For example: "if the rule 'Chest pain exists and severity equals severe' is true, then display the message 'Notify physician.'" Alerts can be simple, as in this example, or complex combinations of true and false rules.

Knowmeds

Sets of rules and alerts can string together to form a Knowmed, the most complex creation of the tool set. A Knowmed can represent cancer protocols for diagnosis and treatment decisions, such as those published by the National Comprehensive Cancer Network (NCCN). Any guideline or protocol from any organization may be represented by a Knowmed; the one that represents the MD Anderson Cancer Center Breast Cancer Treatment Guideline has over 10,000 lines of rules and alerts.

Knowmeds are modular and can be embedded in other Knowmeds. For example, eligibility criteria for a breast cancer clinical trial can be represented as a Knowmed, and the set of Knowmeds for all trials available for newly diagnosed breast cancer patients can be embedded in the Breast Cancer Guideline Knowmed used for initial encounters. In a transparent manner, the clinician can screen for all these clinical trials while documenting the initial visit of a breast cancer patient. The clinician does not have to remember all the trials; he or she simply enters an encounter note and the appropriate alerts and reminders of trial opportunities appear on the screen.

Figure 24.2 illustrates an example of a structured text dialogue session. This was the initial encounter of a test breast cancer patient whose history (as shown on the screen) included a segmental mastectomy for Stage IIB breast cancer. Recommendations at the bottom of the screen include four clinical trials for which this patient may be eligible.

In addition to the key benefit of alerting a physician to clinical trial options, the iN network enables streamlined, auditable management of clinical trials and guidelines. Those responsible for creating and altering the Knowmeds and deleting them from the network maintain them in a centralized location. A quality control process allows the Knowmed to be entered and altered in a test environment first, then "signed off" by authorized individuals and promoted to the live system. A complete audit trail of each step is maintained electronically.

Regimens

A regimen is a care plan with specific events (treatments, diagnostic tests, and documentation) that must occur according to a schedule. The regimen editor is the tool used to encode a chemotherapy or radiation therapy treatment regimen. Since a clinical trial is simply a form of regimen, the regimen editor is used to calendar a trial. At each encounter, the clinician

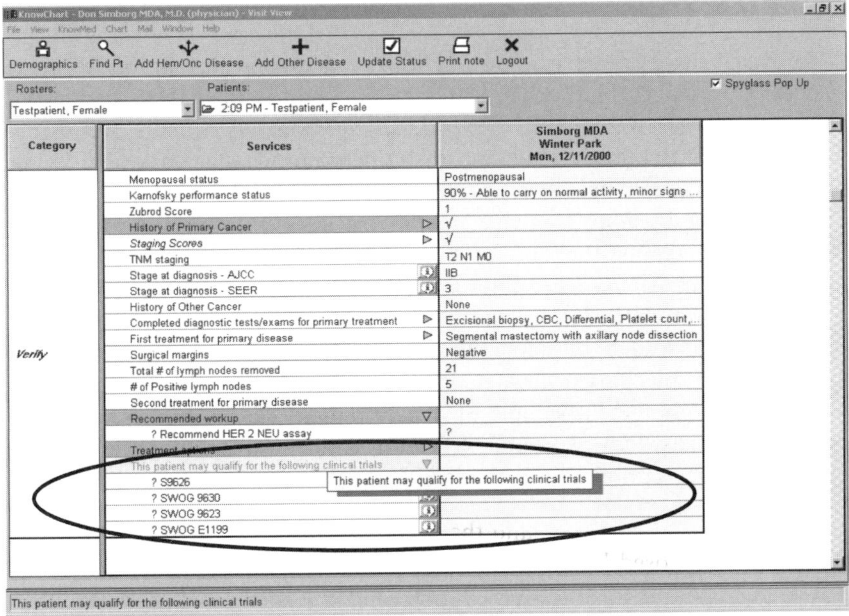

FIGURE 24.2. Screen shot showing screening for clinical trials.

enters an encounter note under the guidance of a Knowmed, and the events for all regimens that apply to that patient visit are displayed for documentation. Clinicians enter observations only once, even though multiple regimens or Knowmeds may use the data. In this way, clinical trial documentation and patient care documentation are integrated.

iKnowMyChart

Just as iKnowChart provides each clinician with a customized view of the patient record, iKnowMyChart creates a special view of the record for patients, including such key components as diagnosis, stage, test results, and treatments. Accessed through a secure Internet browser, iKnowMyChart allows the patient to respond to quality of life and other surveys and communicate with the physician practice about prescription refills, appointments, and e-mail. iKnowMyChart uses the data in each patient's record to link to online education about their problems, treatments, test results, and clinical trials.

iKnowMed has partnered with another company, CancerSource, to develop iKnowMyChart, and the first version of it was being tested as we were preparing this chapter. CancerSource is discussed in Chapter 25, coauthored by Deborah Meyer and Susan Hubbard.

Reporting Center

A browser-based reporting application is available to all data users, including providers, pharmaceutical companies, and others interested in the rich database iN participants generate. Data from all patients are aggregated into the database in a blind fashion, meaning that data identifying individual patients, providers, and provider organizations are removed. Provider organizations can view their own data with identification and benchmark it against the aggregate database; all other data users see only aggregate data. All access to data is HIPAA-compliant.

Since data are coded consistently across all providers and patients, the database is a source of detailed, longitudinal patient records available elsewhere only by chart review. As iN grows in volume and size, it provides a statistically competent sample of cancer patient characteristics, provider practice patterns, treatment and drug use, off-label drug usage, and other clinical and demographic information.

Clinical Trial Modules

Table 24.1 displays the informatics components needed for clinical trials and the functions that iKnowChart performs. The NCI has launched initiatives to standardize each of these components. The iN network participates in this effort and is collaborating with vendors chosen by the NCI to further develop standards. One experiment involves an interface with Protégé, an electronic authoring tool developed at Stanford under NCI sponsorship. (Protégé is described in Chapter 16.) An output of Protégé is an XML file of the eligibility criteria for clinical trials using the Common Data Elements described in Chapter 11 by Curtis Langlotz. In one project, SWOG is using Protégé to author clinical trials. The XML file is passed electronically to iKnowChart, and the rules for that clinical trial's Knowmed are created automatically so that screening can begin at the point of care for selected iKnowChart users. Evaluation will determine how effectively this shortens the time between clinical trial creation and approval and initiation of patient recruitment. The evaluation will also compare the effectiveness of iKnowChart with that of traditional techniques for patient accrual.

TABLE 24.1. Informatics components of clinical trials

- Authoring
- ***Recruiting and screening***
- ***Inclusion/exclusion criteria***
- ***Enrollment and randomization***
- ***Calendaring and execution of trial***
- ***Reporting***
- Analysis

Components in ***bold italics*** are iKnowChart functions.

The iN Value Proposition

The provider participants in iN benefit from the EPR features and functions of iKnowChart, as these compare favorably with other EPR products. In addition, because of its participation in a national network of similar providers, iN extends the benefits of an EPR. This dimension helps overcome traditional barriers to the use of point-of-care technology.

The main benefits of participating in iN are:

- The providers are part of a national network for clinical trials, which means they have access to a wider variety of trials from multiple sponsors.
- The providers can benchmark their practice characteristics, patterns, and performance against a national sample of oncologists.
- The providers have access to guidelines of care available through iN.
- Providers obtain additional revenue from increased participation in clinical trials.
- The cost of the technology is subsidized as providers allow their patient data to be aggregated in the national database.

Using iN, clinical trial sponsors can increase their potential patient pool and improve the timeliness of trials. A common informatics platform with standard terminology further speeds data collection, error correction, and analysis.

For such data users as pharmaceutical companies, iN provides a rich source of detailed and longitudinal data coded consistently across a large, geographically diverse population of patients and physicians. Data is returned within days rather than months or years, meaning that drug utilization patterns and other market analyses are performed nearly in real time. These data also interest payer organizations, providers, investment analysts, and researchers.

Looking Ahead

A project as ambitious as iN involves many complex issues. Below we summarize the most pressing ones and offer some speculation about future directions.

Physician Acceptance

The most overwhelming issue is one the industry has struggled with for decades: physician information technology adoption. As long as physicians prefer dictation devices and pens as their primary input devices, the industry will not achieve standardization, collaboration, and the other benefits described in the value proposition. The emphasis will remain on improving point-of-care applications to win physician acceptance. As this barrier gradually dissolves, other issues will become more prominent.

Privacy and Security

Privacy and security are the next most serious issues confronting a national network involved in patient care and clinical trials. HIPAA will be a significant factor, though there is widespread confusion and misunderstanding about its regulations and future expectations. (As of this writing, HIPAA regulations are still pending on most of these issues.) Since iN crosses many states, the applicable laws and policies vary.

Chapter 5 by Neuman and Chapter 15 by Braithwaite have discussed privacy and security, so we will not cover them. *For the Record: Protecting Electronic Health Information* (Computer Science and Telecommunications Board, 1997) also provides an excellent review of issues related to patient information on networks.

Patient Access

In most states, information in a patient's medical record belongs to the patient, who has the right to read it. Still, some physicians believe patients should not be allowed to view their records online. Because online records eliminate the inconvenience of paper-based systems, patients are more likely to view them. Some physicians feel this is a drawback, because they might want to document something the patient should not read or discuss a test result with a patient before he or she sees it.

These legitimate concerns must be addressed appropriately. For example, certain software requires clinician review before lab results or other data are made available for patient viewing. As consumers expect their access to information to increase, the policies and procedures for patient access to medical records will further evolve.

Use of Aggregate Data

Another issue facing a project like iN is the difference between aggregate data and patient identifiable data. Regulations prevent disclosure of individually identifiable patient information but not of aggregate information in which individual patients cannot be identified. Still, some believe that access to aggregate data violates patient confidentiality and may require patient consent. It does not. Used widely for public health, research, financial, statistical, and educational purposes, aggregate patient data is within the public domain.

Fed by anecdotes about broken security and confidentiality in computer systems in general and health care in particular, many physicians remain concerned that insurers and payers will use aggregate data to the physicians' financial disadvantage. Even after assurances that physician and organizational identifiers have been removed from the database, this general mistrust persists.

Standards

Standards in health care are still a source of conflict. Health Level 7 (HL7), an organization formed 15 years ago to define standards for sending healthcare-related messages between computer applications (Marietti, 2000) has produced the most widely used data interchange standard in health care. The "Level 7" refers to a widely referenced, seven-level model of data communication between computers. The seventh and highest level, the application level, is specific to a particular domain like health care, and the other six levels cross domains like TCP/IP, used in the Internet. Many other healthcare-specific standards are used for purposes HL7 does not cover.

The NCI faces a dilemma in developing another application-level healthcare standard specific to oncology clinical trials. HL7 and the other existing standards do not standardize screening, eligibility, and execution of oncology clinical trials. On the other hand, elements of those needs, like patient demographic descriptions and clinical terminology, are defined in other standards, and some aspects of oncology clinical trials overlap with clinical trial components for any disease. In addition, because the NCI is not a formal standards organization, it lacks formal procedures.

Aware of this dilemma, NCI members involved in this effort are embedding other applicable standards while limiting the creation of new standards to those specific to the task. To manage this balancing act, the NCI will maintain its ongoing efforts to communicate and collaborate with other standards organizations.

The multiplicity of clinical trials and sponsors creates a logistical problem at the point of care. Virtually all the investigators involved in NCI-sponsored clinical trials also take part in trials sponsored by pharmaceutical companies, academic centers, and other organizations. Site management organizations (SMOs) and contract research organizations (CROs) manage some of the industry-sponsored trials, and the NCI uses cooperative groups like Southwest Oncology Group (SWOG) and Eastern Collaborative Oncology Group (ECOG) to manage its trials. Each of these organizations has oversight from the local IRB and national organizations like the FDA, and each has different methods, reporting procedures, and levels of automation. All these competing sponsors should one day adopt a single standard.

Within the NCI, standardization efforts are beginning to level inter-organizational differences. Because this is not yet true across all sponsors, any point-of-care system must serve many standards and many masters. This is a major value proposition for both the provider and the sponsors: iN enforces standardization of processes and terminology. Standardization helps dismantle many of the barriers discussed above, at least from the provider's point of view. Security and confidentiality technology can be applied consistently across all users, and when communication with sponsor organizations and data users must occur, interface and data translation functions will accommodate different requirements. These issues will become easier to manage when standards are widely adopted. As iN usage grows rapidly and users learn lessons that will benefit all, iN is proving a major first step in simplifying the process.

References

Computer Science and Telecommunications Board. 1997. For The Record: Protecting Electronic Health Information. Washington, DC: National Academy Press.

Marietti C. 2000. Toward More Perfect Integration. Healthcare Informatics 17(7):36,38.

Reuters News Release. 1999. Internet Sites to Recruit Patients for Clinical Trials. http://www.cnn.com

25
Consumer Health Informatics

Deborah K. Mayer and Susan M. Hubbard

The convergence of information and informatics technologies has aided two vital developments: the emerging field of consumer health informatics (CHI) and interactive health communications (IHC) applications (Eng & Gustafson, 1999). Because of the rapid increase in the availability and adoption of technology in the healthcare community, well-planned and well-developed CHI infrastructures and IHC applications are greatly improving the quality of cancer care and research.

The modern National Cancer Act was passed in 1971, when cancer was still considered a fatal illness. Clinical trials were being implemented in a newly developing cooperative group structure, and patients were starting to receive chemotherapy as part of the treatment. In the early 1970s, virtually no cancer patient education materials were available. By the 1980s, both disease and treatment-specific materials were being developed, and Physician Data Query (PDQ™) was launched to provide health professionals and patients with online peer-reviewed cancer information (Hubbard, Henney, Devita, 1987). In the early 1990s, PDQ™ statements on cancer detection, prevention, and symptom control reflected progress in these areas (Hubbard, 2000). Approaches to cancer-related health information also expanded from print to audiovisual, online, and interactive delivery systems. As cancer-related health data grew exponentially, consumers found it increasingly difficult to find relevant, accurate, and current information.

Since the National Cancer Act passed, four major societal trends have affected CHI in general and cancer care in particular:

- a shift from the patient assuming a passive role in the patient-doctor relationship to becoming a more active partner in care
- the expanding complexity of cancer prevention, detection, treatment, and care
- shifts in the healthcare delivery system from predominantly hospital-based to ambulatory and home care settings with a concomitant increase in self-care or care provided by caregivers
- communication and informatics technology changes.

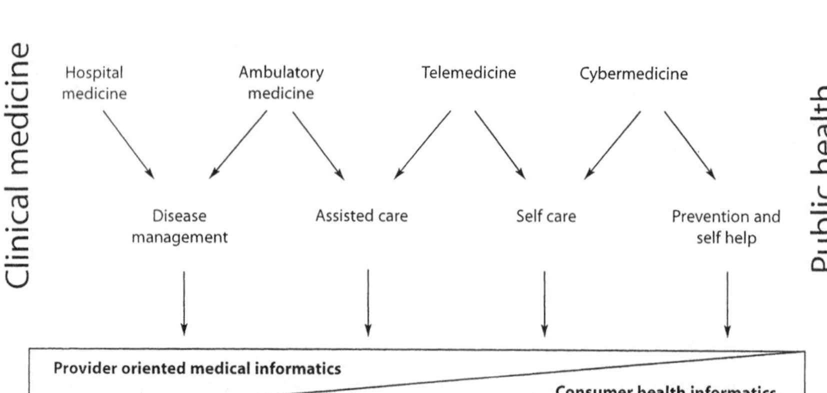

FIGURE 25.1. The focus of traditional medical informatics is shifting from health professionals to consumers.

These combined changes, shown in Figure 25.1, have irrevocably altered the information needs and options of people with cancer. They have significant implications for the CHI field.

CHI is a newly emerging branch of medical informatics that analyzes consumers' needs for information; studies and implements methods of making information accessible to consumers; and models and integrates consumer preferences into medical information systems (Eysenbach, 2000). Figure 25.2 provides a conceptual framework for the effects of informatics and variables affecting its usefulness in health-related behaviors and outcomes. An applied science, CHI combines health communication and education, behavioral medicine, and social network concepts and theories (Houston & Ehrenberger, 2001).

IHC, the application of CHI concepts and theories, has been defined as "the interaction of an individual—consumer, patient, caregiver, or professional—with or through an electronic device or communication technology to access or transmit health information, or to receive or provide guidance and support on a health-related issue" (Eng & Gustafson, 1999, p. 1). This chapter describes the functions and development of CHI, issues affecting adoption, outcomes, existing applications, and a research agenda for CHI in cancer care.

Functions of IHC

IHC has the potential to enhance health, minimize the burden of illness, and optimize relationships between consumers and their health providers

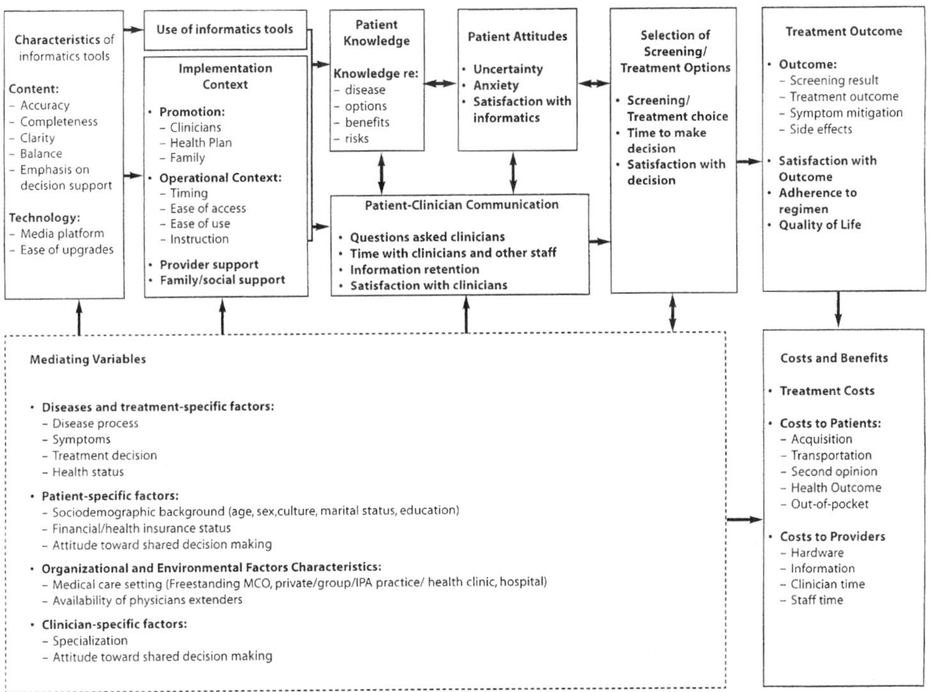

Figure 25.2. Conceptual frameworks for the effects of informatics on patient screening and treatment decision making.

(Ferguson, 2000; Jadad, 1999). These applications have been developed to expand and extend patient-provider interactions, provide opportunities for partnership in addressing healthcare issues, and empower consumers to care for themselves. Benefits of IHC include "just-in-time" learning, the ability to deliver and receive private, individualized, and self-paced learning, support, and help in decision making and self-care (Rolnick, Owens, Botta et al., 1999; Lewis, 1999; Tetzlaff, 1997). Other functions of IHC include relaying information, promoting healthy behaviors, encouraging peer information exchange and emotional support, and managing the demand for healthcare services (Eng & Gustafson, 1999). Many IHC applications address multiple functions.

The Comprehensive Health Enhancement Support System (CHESS), a well-studied and documented comprehensive IHC application, is a disease-specific computer system that provides information and support for those with HIV or breast cancer (Rolnick et al., 1999; Gustafson, McTavish, Hawkins et al., 1998; Gustafson, McTavish, Boberg et al., 1999). Several other CHI projects are achieving IHC's potential through the use of the Internet and other technologies. The Patient Education and Activation System (PEAS), developed at the University of Wisconsin, integrates education activities into an online medical history form to help individuals participate in and make decisions about their own care (McRoy, Liu-Perez, Ali, 1998). This prototype demonstrated the feasibility of developing and delivering patient-tailored Web-based interfaces to medical information. iKnowMyChart, a product of iKnowMed, takes a similar but broader approach in a cancer-specific population with tailored patient information based on all aspects of the individual's electronic medical record, the iKnowChart (see the Chapter 24 by Simborg).

CancerSource.com provides disease, treatment, and symptom management information and self-care guides, as well as a forum for online support through message boards and chats for consumers and health professionals. Patient education, an ongoing and evolving process throughout the cancer experience, is a way to transfer knowledge and skills to help patients cope with and manage their disease. The structure and functionality of CancerSource content does this by providing levels of content (introductory, basic, intermediate, and advanced) based on both reading level (sixth grade to graduate level) and depth of content (superficial overviews to detailed information) across the illness trajectory. The patient education wizard feature on the site allows health professionals to create, print or e-mail, and document tailored patient education from online content.

Telephone-linked care is another form of IHC. Here, clinical information is given and received to monitor patients with chronic diseases, provide counseling on health behaviors, and support caregivers by linking voice and database components (Friedman, Stollerman, Mahoney, Rozenblyum, 1997). Relevant printed reports are then shared with the patient and the caregiver. This methodology has been evaluated in the management of hypertension, medication adherence, diet, and exercise and has been associated with better disease control, improved health behaviors, and acceptance and satisfaction with their use.

Studies on electronic health communications have included computerized communication, telephone follow-up and counseling, telephone reminders, interactive telephone systems, and telephone access and screening in various patient populations (Balas, Jaffrey, Kuperman et al., 1997). These studies have demonstrated improved clinical outcomes in preventive care (immunizations); the management of diabetes, arthritis, cardiac rehabilitation; and emotional support for Alzheimer's caregivers as well as patient appointment keeping and medication adherence. Cancer-related findings included increased mammography use and decreased tobacco use with telephone follow-up and counseling.

The following sections underscore the importance of patient education by highlighting specific benefits.

Relay Information/Promote Learning

Patient education is designed to influence behaviors, knowledge levels, attitudes, and skills required for maintaining and improving health (Treacy

& Mayer, 2000). Specific needs identified across the illness trajectory include information related to diagnosis and treatment, side effect/symptom management, self-care needs, threat to personal well-being, and effects on work and relationships (Mayer, 1998). These needs vary in their timing, level of detail, and content based on individual factors (Tetzlaff, 1997; Mayer, 1998: Leydon, Boulton, Moynihan et al., 2000), including learning and coping styles, literacy level, anxiety or depression, poorly managed symptoms (e.g., pain or fatigue), and access to information (Mayer, 1999; Jones, Pearson, McGregor et al., 1999; Jones, Pearson, McGregor et al., 1999; McKinstry, 2000).

Lewis (1999) examined and compared computer-based approaches in patient education. Most programs were either interactive videos or CD-ROM programs for self-health promotion and disease self-management developed for adults with chronic diseases like diabetes. A significant change in outcomes in skill development or knowledge transfer was noted in 16 of 21 studies (14 were randomized trials, and 6 of the 21 studies were related to cancer education on topics like genetic susceptibility, pain, blood counts, and support groups). Other positive outcomes related to patient education include fewer symptoms, improved postoperative pain management, decreased length of hospital stay, and improved knowledge and patient satisfaction.

Enable Informed Decision Making

Including patients in decision making about their health care is an increasingly high priority, one that has raised new questions like which factors influence and facilitate decision making. The "empowered" cancer patient, a participating partner in his or her own care, is replacing the passive patient following physician orders (Mayer, 1999). Both patient and physician preferences influence the degree or amount of shared decision making that actually occurs, ranging from passive to active participation (McKinstry, 2000; Thompson, Pitts, Schwankovsky, 1993).

A 1997 report by the Agency for Healthcare Research and Quality (AHRQ) examined studies using several informatics tools, including interactive compact discs, videotapes, audiotapes, brochures, and computer-generated fact sheets to help patients make informed decisions about medical screening and treatment (AHCPR, 1997). Three of the studies reviewed were related to prostate cancer screening. Most of the studies examined the effects of the applications on knowledge and satisfaction rather than on interactions between healthcare providers and patients, healthcare behavior and outcomes, or healthcare costs. The report notes that most studies were small and exploratory and inconsistently employed rigorous controls, adequate samples, or standardized measurements. Although some studies report effects on treatment choices, the number of conditions and range of tools was limited, and there were no comparative studies examining differences between computerized and non-computerized tools or how people with low literacy or disabilities could use them.

Decision theory provides a framework for eliciting patient preferences for a given health state according to their values. Decision aids are tools that contain explicit components to help clarify the patient's personal values and elicit the utility or importance of the risks and benefits of each alternative treatment or test (Eysenbach, 2000). These preferences are assessed using visual analog scales, pair-wise comparisons, and standard gamble methods to measure patient utilities. Individual values and preferences are important in IHC applications that focus on decision making, since reliable assessment of individual preference and risk attitudes is often weak in clinical decision making (Jimison, Adler, Coye et al., 1999). Studies exploring the use of interactive applications to communicate about health outcomes, assess individual preferences, provide feedback in the learning process, and tailor messages have been performed, but more are needed to determine their effectiveness (Entwistle, Sheldon, Sowden, Watt, 1998; Skinner, Siegfried, Kegler, Strecher, 1993; Patrick, Robinson, Alemi, Eng, 1999).

Examples of IHC applications that have used tailoring include the shared decision-making program that helped individuals with breast, benign prostatic hyperplasia, and prostate cancer to make informed, complex decisions consistent with their individual values and preferences (DePalma, 2000; Barry, Cherkin, Chang et al., 1997; Volk, Cass, Spann, 1999). Computer-tailored messages have also had positive effects in smoking cessation programs (Brennan & Strombom, 1998; Brennan, 1999; Strecher, 1999). Patients preferred and were more satisfied with personalized information and were less anxious with the tailored information approach (Jones, Pearson, McGregor et al., 1999; Jones, Pearson, McGregor et al., 1999). Tailored or personalized information appears to have a greater and longer lasting impact (Rimer & Glassman, 1999).

O'Connor reviewed those decision aids in cancer screening, diagnosis, prevention, and treatment using a variety of media (O'Connor, Fiset, Degrasse et al., 1999). In her review, decision aids had a demonstrable effect on decisions made, improved determinants of the decision, improved comfort or satisfaction with the decision, and were acceptable to the patient. In another review of 17 studies, decision aids improved knowledge, increased patient participation in decision making, and lowered decisional conflict, but they had little effect on satisfaction or anxiety levels (O'Connor, Fiset, Degrasse et al., 1999; O'Connor, Rostom, Fiset et al., 1999). Six of the 17 studies were cancer-related, including BRCA1 gene testing, PSA screening, primary treatment for breast, and prostate cancer topics. Few of these studies, however, evaluated the impact of CHI on actual health behaviors or health outcomes. Most are still in development and in the research stage, not in wide clinical use.

Promote Healthy Behaviors

IHC, which has been used to promote adoption and maintenance of positive health behaviors, includes risk assessment and health promotion modules. In a meta-analysis of 16 randomized, controlled trials, computer-based reminders improved breast and colorectal cancer screening, vaccinations, and cardiovascular risk reduction, but not cervical cancer screenings, in ambulatory care settings (Shea, Dumouchel, Bahamonde, 1996).

Promote Peer Information Exchange and Emotional Support

IHC can provide a forum for social and emotional support and encouragement, personal empowerment, and information exchange through online support groups, message boards, and chats. In the CHESS program, women with breast cancer who accessed the message board left messages 42% of the time. Of those messages, 71% were related to social support and another 16% were related to treatment information (Gustafson, McTavish, Hawkins et al., 1998; Gustafson, McTavish, Boberg et al., 1999).

Promote Self-Care

Randomized trials of IHC in diabetes, asthma, hypertension, and rheumatoid arthritis and medication adherence in the elderly were reviewed. They demonstrated improved knowledge scores and self-care activities, two factors that also led to improved outcomes (Krishna, Balas, Spencer et al., 1997). Improvements in self-reported quality of life (QOL) in users of CHESS were also noted (Gustafson, McTavish, Boberg et al., 1999). IHC applications have also monitored and managed health problems between patient and provider.

Manage Demand for Health Services

IHC applications have been used to enhance effective use and reduce unnecessary use of health services. These applications include telephone advice systems, interactive voice response systems, e-mail, and other electronic consultations. The CHESS program demonstrated shorter ambulatory care visits, increased use of phone calls to providers, and fewer and shorter hospitalizations (Gustafson, McTavish, Boberg et al., 1999). These applications may also include requests regarding scheduling, refilling prescriptions, and other health-related transactions.

Although physicians have hesitated to embrace IHC, consumers are seeking and using these applications (Reents, 1999). Acceptance of IHC by both health professionals and consumers will evolve over time. IHC will become a widely accepted and used means to improve communication, satisfaction with care, and healthcare outcomes (Tang & Newcomb, 1998).

Development of IHC

Diverse organizations produce and disseminate IHC. These include government agencies, hospitals and clinics, employers, professional societies, voluntary health organizations, public libraries, the media, the pharmaceutical industry, and other components of the healthcare industry. Methods of dissemination include books, brochures, pamphlets, magazine articles and other printed materials, radio, TV and cable programs, videos, dial-in services like the NCI's Cancer Information Service, fax on demand services like CancerFax, interactive computer software, CD-ROM and DVD applications, health-oriented kiosks, and networked resources like bulletin boards, community health information networks, chat rooms, listservs, news groups, and Web sites providing health information and support.

Developing a usable and useful CHI application remains a challenge. Guidelines for designing usable systems that emphasize interactivity between users and the application are based on cognitive research on human computer interactions, often called usability engineering (Dumas & Redish, 1993; Neilson, http://www.usit.com; Spool, 1999). The guidelines call for an initial assessment of audience needs, development of core system objectives, and providing site and system structure design principles and tips on making systems intuitive and easy for the inexperienced to use. Given the anxiety related to diagnosis, this is particularly important for cancer patients and their families who may be trying to navigate an IHC application for the first time.

The guidelines also address interface issues like navigational elements and the look and feel of the system; consistency of layout and presentation; appropriate use of fonts, graphics, and terminology; tips on how to write for interactive systems and to structure search functions; and caveats on the typical technical constraints users face with hardware, software, access, and other platform issues. Other design considerations include the development of systematic mechanisms for maintaining accurate and current information; the selection of appropriate software tools if the system will "tailor" information for personalized health assessments, risk analyses, and decision support based on user input; and security and privacy issues.

The development of any consumer health application must start with clear articulation of the health issue, existing data, and gaps in knowledge; the rationale for the selection of a communication medium or media; and the strategy for communicating content and specific messages. Developers must also address the characteristics of the target audience(s) (e.g., age, race, gender, literacy, mode of learning, culture, socioeconomic status, and physical or cognitive disabilities). They must consider the level of personalization the system will provide and the short- and long-term process measures that will be used to evaluate the system (Edwards & Elwyn, 1999; Eng, Gustafson, Henderson et al., 1999; Jimison & Sher, 1995; Eng, Maxfield, Patrick et al., 1998; Jimison, Sher, Appleyard, Levernois, 1998; Noell & Glasgow, 1999; Robinson, Patrick, Eng, Gustafson, 1998).

Information delivered to the user must be accessible and meaningful. The current reading level of patient education material on the Web was measured to be tenth grade, on average, and twelfth grade for CancerNet. This makes the information difficult for many patients to access and comprehend (Graber, Roller, Kaeble, 1999; Wilson, Baker, Brown-Syet, Gollop, 2000). When planning better communication or health education strategies, developers must also understand the contextual factors that contribute to behavior change (National Cancer Institute, 1992). These include:

- predisposing factors, meaning the knowledge, attitudes, behavior, beliefs, and values that affect an individual's willingness to change
- enabling factors, meaning the situation, environment, and community that work to facilitate or inhibit change
- reinforcing factors, meaning the positive and negative effects of adopting a behavior that influence its continuation, including social support (Green, Kreuter, Deeds, Patridge, 1980).

Depending on the application, the needs of special populations must also be given careful consideration (e.g., education and literacy, ethnicity, and age-related considerations like a limited attention span or visual deficiencies). An iterative six-step process, developed by the National Cancer Institute and shown in Figure 25.3, provides a useful framework for development, implementation, and refinement of consumer health applications (National Cancer Institute, 1992).

When the NCI's CancerNet Web site was redesigned in 1998, usability guidelines were used to ensure that site development was user-driven (Iansiti & McCormick, 1997; Biermann, Golladay, Greenfield, Baker, 1999). At the outset, there was prospective gathering of data on the information needs of a spectrum of current and potential users. An online questionnaire provided input from more than 600 individuals on their needs and expectations (Hubbard, 2001). Following this, direct interviews were conducted with current and potential users to define their information requirements. Based on user feedback, the first prototypes were constructed and subjected to iterative evaluations with current and potential users to see if the prototypes were serving their needs. Volunteers from various backgrounds were recruited to search for information on the site in response to a series of specific questions. While attempting to find the required information, volunteers were prompted to "think out loud" so their thought processes could be captured and recorded on videotape. This would help identify flaws in the layout of information hierarchy, menu structure, and navigational elements.

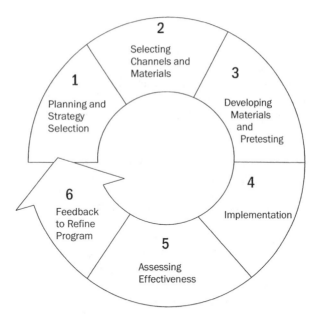

Figure 25.3. Stages in health communication.

The process effectively validated the information architecture and provided direction for developing the new site. Also addressed in this fashion was a broad spectrum of interface and system functionality issues, such as the organization, classification, and prioritization of information and navigational elements that provide multiple pathways to the same information to accommodate different learning and searching styles making it a more user-friendly site.

The NCI's usability guidelines are posted on the National Cancer Institute's usability Web site at http://usability.gov. These guidelines summarize research findings from the human computer interactions literature and provide citations from the literature that support the guidelines.

Quality

As Internet access and Web site development tools have become basic software for computer systems, anyone with a computer, an Internet connection, and the appropriate software can create a Web site. This fact has staggering implications for the amount and quality of medical information available to consumers. There are thousands of health-related Web sites and the number grows daily. A search on the term "cancer" via any of the popular Web search engines will retrieve thousands of sites offering cancer information.

For consumers, the plethora of health information on the Internet is often a mixed blessing. Because the Internet is still an unregulated, uncensored medium, many Web sites, e-mail services, and news and user groups contain anecdotal, unreviewed, and undated information. In an article on the accuracy of medical information on the Web, an oncologist searching for online information on Ewing's sarcoma found that half the material was irrelevant and 6% contained major errors (Biermann et al., 1999). Inaccurate information is not the only cause for concern. Some health-oriented sites promote healthcare products or refer users to e-commerce partners and then receive financial remuneration on those sales. Some also post information to advance unproven approaches to disease management that are not medically or scientifically sound.

The NCI has always had a formal review process for the inclusion of content in its databases and information services. All the information is reviewed by broadly based editorial boards composed of experts who ensure that the information is accurate, current, and of high quality. The NCI has also established a formal process for ensuring that CancerNet only provides hypertext links to accurate, useful, and current Web sites (http://cancernet.nci.nih.gov/wwwcritp.htm). Other cancer information providers, such as CancerSource.com, have recognized the need to ensure that patients are not exposed to false, outdated, or otherwise harmful cancer information; articulate the criteria used for selecting information to disseminate; and clarify any financial arrangements with other organizations that might pose a conflict of interest.

To help users determine which Web sites are credible, the Health on the Net (HON) foundation (http://www.hon.ch/honcode/conduct.html) has established criteria for evaluating Web sites. The principles embodied in these criteria have been widely adopted by credible health-related Web sites. Several other tools exist to help consumers evaluate the quality of health information on Web sites (Eysenbach, 2000; Jadad, 1999; Internet Health Coalition, 2000; Eysenbach & Diepgen, 1999; Charnock, Shepperd, Needham, Gann, 1999; Kim, Eng, Deering, Maxfield, 1999; Shepperd, Charnock, Gann, 1999; Sikorski & Peters, 1997).

Privacy and Security

The tension between the desire for privacy and for personalization is not unique to consumer health informatics (Patrick & Koss, http://nii.nist.gov/pubs/chi.html). In a recent Harris Interactive poll, 64% of respondents said that their biggest online worry was Web sites providing personal information to others without their knowledge (National Consumers League, http://www.nclnet.org/essentials/). Many do not know how they can change or update the information they have supplied. As the "profiling" of users becomes a more common feature of IHC, understanding how the application will maintain the confidentiality of personal information is increasingly important.

Users should understand what personally identifiable information the Web site collects from them; how the information will be used; with whom the information may be shared; what choices they have regarding the collection, use, and distribution of the information; what security procedures are in place to protect the loss, misuse, or alteration of information; and how they can correct any inaccuracies.

Developers should tell users if and how they protect the user's right to privacy. They should carefully determine that anonymity and privacy protection for users are stipulated in any partnerships that they establish (Krishna et al., 1997; Internet Health Coalition, 2000; Patrick & Koss, http://nii.nist.gov/pubs/chi.html; National Consumers League, http://www.nclnet.org/essentials/; National Research Council, 1997; Mabley, 2000). Current cookie tracking technology can track users across unrelated sites and permit partners to collect and link cookie profiles with third-party consumer databases containing demographic information on individual users. Specific technologies include strong data encryption tools for authentication and the protection of data integrity and confidentiality, uniform methods for authorization and access control, network firewall tools and virus protection software, rigorous management procedures, and effective use of system vulnerability monitoring tools (National Research Council, 1997). As IHC applications are linked with and integrated into health records to provide tailored information and services, these issues will become more important.

The European Union is already enforcing strict medical security standards, and the U.S. will demand improved standards for security and confidentiality under the provisions of the Health Insurance Portability and Accountability Act (HIPAA) (Mittman & Cain, 1990).

Although technologies are in place to safeguard electronic health information, the perception of insufficient security persists. Integrating features like e-mail consultations into standard medical practice will require an increased emphasis on security to ensure the privacy and confidentiality of sensitive health information (Patrick et al., 1999; Kane & Sands, 1998; Borowitz & Wyatt, 1998; Spielberg, 1998).

Message Framing

Increasingly, educated consumers are demanding convenience, choice, autonomy, and substantive involvement in the healthcare decision-making process. Research suggests that compliance with medical advice depends on access to basic information on the health problem. Consumers with this information understand the illness experience, are aware of viable alternatives, comprehend the potential benefits and risks associated with the alternatives, and understand how their own values affect these parameters. Once a consumer has a basic understanding of the problems and alternatives, it is easier to negotiate a mutually acceptable course of action and identify the priorities that must be addressed and the specific tasks that each must perform (Cunningham, Lockwood, Cunningham, 1991; Bopp,

2000). The capacity to elicit and provide feedback on factors that influence health behaviors can be used to tailor educational messages for individual patients (Volk et al., 1999; Strecher, 1999; Bopp, 2000; DeVries & Brug, 1999; Ruland, 1999).

The power of message framing is considerable. Several studies have shown that preferences for surgery depend on whether the outcomes are framed in terms of mortality or survival (Entwistle et al., 1998; Marteau, 1989; McNeil, Pauker, Sox, Tversky, 1982; Phillips & Bero, 1996).

Barriers

The rapid increase in technology use has important ramifications for CHI applications. It is occurring in most groups of Americans, regardless of income, education, race, ethnicity, location, age, or gender, suggesting that populations that were traditionally digital "have-nots" are making significant gains in closing the gap (McConnaughey, Lader, Chin, Everette, 2000). Despite this progress, a digital divide still exists between individuals of different income levels and education, different racial and ethnic populations, old and young, single and dual parent families, and those with and without disabilities. While less than 25% of people without a disability have never used a computer, close to 60% of people with a disability have never used one. Large gaps in Internet access remain among those with different racial and ethnic backgrounds. Asian Americans and Pacific Islanders have the highest level of home Internet access, at 56.8%. African Americans and Hispanics have the lowest levels, at 23.5 and 23.6% respectively.

Falling through the Net: Toward Digital Inclusion, the fourth report in a series of studies conducted by the National Telecommunications & Information Administration of the Department of Commerce, recently measured changes by looking at households and individuals with a computer and Internet access (National Telecommunications & Information Administration, 2000). The share of households with Internet access rose 58% in an 18-month period, and as of August 2000, more than 51% of U.S. households had computers. August 2000 data from the Digital Inclusion report show that schools, libraries, and public access ports continue to serve populations without home access (National Telecommunications & Information Administration, 2000). According to the report, the unemployed, African Americans, Asian Americans, and Pacific Islanders are far more likely than other underserved populations to access the Internet in public libraries.

Because underserved and minority populations often carry a particularly heavy burden of cancer incidence, morbidity, and mortality, developers must focus on addressing barriers to access. Studies have shown that when barriers to technology access are overcome and training is provided, underserved populations successfully use technology to address health concerns and rate these tools highly (Eng & Gustafson, 1999; Gustafson, Hawkins, Boberg et al., 1999; Eng, Gustafson, Henderson et al., 1999).

The cost associated with ensuring universal access to healthcare information and support is a significant barrier. As yet, third-party payers do not support reimbursement for the use of such tools. Infrastructure costs include the cost of hardware and software; content development and maintenance; user interface design, testing, and redesign; deployment and maintenance; and training for users and intermediaries.

As consumers assume greater responsibility for health-related decisions and care, health literacy programs that teach them to understand and interpret health science and scientific research will be increasingly important. A long-term strategy must include elementary, secondary, and community-based adult educational programs in areas like critical thinking, risk assessment, and understanding levels of evidence and bias (Gustafson, Hawkins, Boberg et al., 1999).

Another barrier to use of IHC applications is the failure of many IHC applications to address differences in the learning styles of consumers. Learning characteristics include literacy levels, age and aging issues, ethnicity and culture, gender, social support, knowledge, attitudes and beliefs, autonomy or empowerment, psychological profile, and readiness to learn (Walker, 1999). Leaffer and Gonda (2000) developed a successful train-the-trainer program for 100 senior citizens on accessing the Internet for healthcare information. In a 90-day follow-up, many participants continued to search the Internet and discuss the searches with their physicians.

Among physician concerns is the growing desire for e-mail consultation and communication. A study of free e-mail consultation in a pediatric gastrointestinal service at a metropolitan medical center reported that the service received an average of 38 e-mails each month from parents, relatives, or guardians (81%), physicians (10%) and other healthcare professionals (9%) (Borowitz & Wyatt, 1998). The central themes of the consultation related to a child's symptoms, appropriate diagnosis or treatment, a second opinion, or a request for general information about a disorder, treatment, or medication. Responses suggested treatment, gave general advice, and often contained references or directed the reader to educational materials on the Web. On average, reading and responding to each e-mail took less than four minutes, comparable to the time required to answer a patient-initiated telephone call. The authors concluded that e-mail was a viable way to provide patient- and disease-specific information from medical consultants. However, the authors emphasized the need for more studies examining workload, costs, outcomes, and legal and ethical ramifications.

Guidelines that address the key elements of a patient-provider agreement on the clinical use of e-mail also have been written and published (Kane & Sands, 1998). According to a recent survey conducted by Healtheon, many physicians have concluded that communicating with patients offers as many benefits to them as it does to patients. Of the physicians surveyed, 33% were communicating with patients by e-mail, up from 1 to 2% only two years earlier (Ferguson, 2000).

The American Association of Medical Colleges has emphasized the need for medical schools to update their curricula to address core competencies in information technology and medical informatics (Staggers, Gassert, Skiba, 1999). Similar mandates have been issued for nurses, health science librarians, and other health professionals.

Impact on Physician-Patient Relationships

Effective communication is central to effective, high-quality health care. Information can empower individuals to make informed decisions. Changes in the accessibility of medical information and the way the public can acquire it are altering health care and the relationship between healthcare professionals and patients. The use of the Internet as a channel for communicating health and medical information will continue to increase as interactive health communication applications become more sophisticated and the cost of electronic devices and Internet access decreases.

Although physicians and nurses have embraced information technology for routine administrative functions, many are reluctant to adopt technologies that could alter the physician-patient relationship (Ferguson, 2000; Entwistle et al., 1998; Mittman & Cain, 1990). They understand the value of having well-informed patients, but they remain concerned about and losing control of patient interactions and becoming overwhelmed with questions. While opportunities for online physician-patient communication are currently limited, the Internet is offering new opportunities for physicians and nurses to help patients access and manage the knowledge they need to participate in their health care.

Evaluation

The need for evaluation throughout the development of an IHC application has been emphasized in the literature (Eng & Gustafson, 1999; Entwistle et al., 1998; Patrick et al., 1999; Edwards & Elwyn, 1999; Eng et al., 1999; Eng et al., 1998; Robinson et al., 1998; Henderson, Noell, Reeves et al., 1999). The Science Panel on Interactive Communication and Health (SciPICH) has reported that reliable and valid evaluation guidelines are needed to evaluate and refine all types of interactive health communication applications. Current challenges include the rapidly evolving media and infrastructure that underlie these applications, the dynamic nature of the applications, the number of variables that influence health outcomes and the difficulty associated with assessing or controlling their impact, the lack of methodology sophistication of many developers, and the lack of systematic evaluation by developers (Robinson et al., 1998).

The Science Panel has also emphasized the need to integrate evaluation at the beginning of the IHC development cycle (Eng et al., 1999; Henderson et al., 1999; Patrick et al., 1999; Robinson, Patrick, Eng et al., 1998). Benefits of evaluation include improved quality, utility, and effectiveness; minimization of the likelihood of harm; promotion of innovation; conservation of resources; greater consumer participation in the development and implementation process; greater confidence among users; and a positive public image of the industry. The Science Panel has developed a detailed formal evaluation-reporting template for evidence-based evaluation of IHC applications (Eng & Gustafson, 1999; Entwistle et al., 1998; Robinson, Patrick, Eng et al., 1998) (Table 25.1). The reader is encouraged to visit the SciPICH Web site (http://www.scipich.org) and download the template, which has been widely published. Mullen (Mullen, Green, Persinger, 1985) has also proposed a coding scheme to evaluate the quality of research methods and the quality of educational interventions in a meta-analysis of educational programs for patients with chronic illness.

Consumer-oriented models for the evaluation of health informatics applications have also been developed (Eng & Gustafson, 1999; Gustafson, Hawkins, Boberg, Pingree et al., 1999; Jimison et al., 1999; Glenn, 1996). All of them emphasize the need for consumers to develop an evaluation framework that helps them make informed choices among applications, weighing factors like the quality of the information, guarantees of the confidentiality of personal information, performance measures, and the type, quality, and accessibility of evaluation data. Consumers also need to assess the features of the CHI to determine if the presentation of the information accommodates their learning style, social and personal characteristics, educational and computer skill levels, and any physical disabilities (Lewis, 1999; Tetzlaff, 1997). Evaluation components of interest to healthcare providers and purchasers have also been published (Eng & Gustafson, 1999; Entwistle et al., 1998).

Although cost is often cited as the reason for postponing evaluation, many IHC applications will not survive in a managed care environment without evidence of efficacy. Few cost-benefit and cost-effectiveness analyses have been performed, and few interventions have been adequately evaluated for potentially harmful effects, such as delaying the decision to seek medical attention or leading to the selection of an inappropriate treatment (Robinson et al., 1998).

As Patrick (1999) observes, knowledge about the evaluation of IHC applications is in its infancy. He suggests that a reasonable role for government is to help demonstrate the utility of these interventions in pilots, especially if effective IHC applications can help attain national health objectives. Demonstration projects that model how to improve healthcare practices with IHC applications may help demonstrate the potential return on investment for health plans and employers.

Table 25.1. Evaluation Reporting Template for Interactive Health Communication Applications, Version 1.0, Science Panel on Interactive Communication and Health

Description of Application

1 Title of product/application
2 Names(s) of developers(s)
3 Relevant qualifications of developer(s)
4 Contact(s) for additional information
5 Funding sources for development of the application (e.g., commercial company, government, foundation/nonprofit organization, individual)
6 Category of application (e.g., health information, clinical decision support, individual behavior change, peer support, risk assessment)
7 Specific goal(s)/objectives(s) of the application (What is the application intended to do? List multiple objectives if applicable)
8 Intended target audience(s) for application (e.g., age group, gender, educational level, types of organizations and settings, disease groups, cultural/ethnic population groups)
9 Available in languages other than English? No Yes (specify)
10 Technological/resource requirements of the applications (e.g., hardware, Internet, on-site support available)
11 Describe how confidentiality or anonymity of users is protected
12 Indicate who will potentially be able to get information about users

Formative and Process Evaluation*

1 Indicate the processes and information source(s) used to ensure the validity of the content (e.g., peer-reviewed scientific literature, in-house "experts," recognized outside "experts," consensus panel of independent "experts," updating and review processes and timing)
2 Are the specific original sources of information cited within the application? Yes No
3 Describe the methods of instruction and/or communication used (e.g., drill and practice, modeling, simulations, reading generic online documents, interactive presentations of tailored information, specifying methods used)
4 Describe the media formats used (e.g., text, voice/sound, still graphics, animation/video, color)
5 For each applicable evaluation question below indicate (1) the characteristics of the sample(s) used and how they were selected, (2) the methods(s) of assessment (e.g., specific measures used), and (3) the evaluation results:
6 If the text or voice is used, how was the reading level or understandability tested?
7 What is the extent of expected used of the application (e.g., average length and range of time, number of repeat uses)?
8 How long will it take to train a beginning user to use the application proficiently?
9 Describe how the application was beta tested and debugged (e.g., what users, in what settings)

Outcome Evaluation+

1 For each applicable evaluation question below, indicate (i) the type of evaluation design (I-III) (ii) the characteristics of the sample(s) used and how they were selected, (iii) the method(s) of assessment (e.g., specific measures used), and (iv) the evaluation results
2 How much do users like the application?
3 How helpful/useful do users find the application?
4 Do users increase their knowledge?
5 Do users change their beliefs or attitudes (e.g., self-efficacy, perceived importance, and intentions to change behavior, satisfaction)?
6 Do users change their behaviors (e.g., risk factor behaviors, interpersonal interactions, compliance, and use of resources)?
7 Are there changes in morbidity or mortality (e.g., symptoms, missed days of school/work, physiologic indicators)?

Table 25.1. (*Continued*)

8 Are there effects on cost/resource utilization (e.g., cost-effectiveness analysis)?
9 Do organizations or systems change (e.g., resource utilization, effects on "culture")?

Background of Evaluators

1 Names and contact information for evaluator(s)
2 Do any of the evaluators have a financial interest in the sale/dissemination of the application? No Yes (specify)
3 Funding sources for the evaluation(s) of the application (e.g., developer's funds, other commercial company, government, foundation/nonprofit organization)
4 Is a copy of the evaluation report(s) available for review on request? No Yes (specify)

This is an evaluation reporting template for developers and evaluators of interactive health communications (IHC) applications to help them report evaluation results to those who are considering purchasing or using their applications. Because the template is designed to apply to all types of applications and evaluations, some items may not apply to a particular application or evaluation. Users need only complete those items that apply. This and subsequent versions of the template and other resources on evaluation of IHC is available at http://www.scipich.org.

* *Formative evaluation* is used to assess the nature of the problem and the needs of the target audience with a focus on informing and improving program design before implementation. This is conducted prior to or during early application development and commonly consists of literature reviews and reviews of existing applications and interviews or focus groups of 'experts' or members of the target audience. Process evaluation is used to monitor the administrative, organizational, or other operational characteristics of an intervention. This helps developers successfully translate the design into a functional application and is performed during application development. This commonly includes testing the application for functionality and also may be known as alpha and beta testing.

\+ *Outcome evaluation* is used to examine an interventions's ability to achieve its intended results under ideal conditions (i.e., efficacy) or under real world circumstances (i.e., effectiveness), and also its ability to produce benefits in relation to its costs (i.e., efficiency or cost-effectiveness). This helps developers learn whether the application is successful at achieving its goals and objectives and is performed after the implementation of the application.

Design types are grouped according to level of quality of evidence as classified by the US Preventive Service Task and the Canadian Task Force on the Periodic Health Examination.

a Randomized controlled trials are experiments in which potential users are randomly assigned to use the application or to a control group. Randomization promotes comparability between groups. These designs can be (1) double-blinded–a study in which neither the participants nor the evaluators know which participants are in the intervention group or the control group, (2) single-blinded–a study in which the participants are not aware which experimental group they are in, or (3) nonblinded– a study in which both the participants and the evaluators are aware of who is in the intervention group and who is in the control group. The more a study is blinded, the less it is subject to bias.

b 1. Nonrandomized controlled trials are experiments that compare users and nonusers (or controls), but they are not randomly assigned to these groups. This type of design should specify how the participants were recruited, selected, and assigned to the groups and how the groups compare–similarities and differences between users and nonusers prior to the evaluation. 2. Cohort or observational studies evaluate users with no comparison or control group. 3. Multiple time series use observations of participants as they go through periods of use and nonuse of the application.

c These include such items as descriptive studies, case reports, testimonials, and "expert" committee opinions.

(*Source:* Science Panel on Interactive Communication and Health. Wired for Health and Well-being: the Emergence of Interactive Health Communication. Eng T.R., Gustafson D.H., editors. Washington, DC: US Department of Health and Human Services, US Government Printing Office, April 1999.)

Outcomes

Several factors make IHC applications an attractive addition to modern health care. One of the most important could be significant improvements in healthcare usage resulting from improved consumer understanding of health risks and disease management. If IHC applications can counsel patients effectively, the benefits may be greater than the development, deployment, training, and maintenance costs. Little is known about the operational factors that influence patient use of IHC tools, such as the need for repetitive exposure to them, or whether health professionals are required to optimize their use. Although these questions remain unanswered, evidence suggests potential for significant benefit.

Major gaps in knowledge exist about how consumers process and use health information, distinguish important from insignificant health risks, decide to modify risky behavior like smoking, deal with contradictory health messages, and make decisions about their healthcare options. We have not yet determined the long-term impact of IHC applications on healthcare, as measured by changes in knowledge and understanding, knowledge retention over time, adoption of healthy behaviors, skill development, shifts in decision preferences, healthcare utilization, and satisfaction with care and patient-professional relationships.

Almost all studies have focused on the retention of knowledge skills over short intervals (Lewis, 1999). Few assess whether knowledge and skill acquisition diminishes over time and whether they require ongoing remediation. Results of a randomized trial to evaluate the retention of benefits with three- or six-month implementation of CHESS in HIV-positive patients compared to controls demonstrated benefits in improved quality of life and more efficient use of health care (Gustafson, Hawkins, Boberg et al., 1999).

If tailored message framing of information is significantly more effective than standardized messages, we must develop innovative ways to integrate consumer values and preferences economically into IHC applications for use by diverse populations. For this integration to have value, we must determine if this information actually has an impact on the clinician's decision making (Ruland, 1999).

Future Research Priorities

Understanding how IHC works to promote and improve health will be critical in advancing the field of CHI. Major gaps in knowledge exist about how consumers process and use health information, distinguish important from insignificant health risks, decide to modify risky behavior such as smoking, deal with contradictory health messages, and make decisions about their healthcare options. Closing the gaps in our knowledge and understanding the impact of various technologies on these areas is also essential. How patients interact with computer-based informatics tools and how they digest and act on information must be explored further (Eng & Gustafson, 1999; Eysenbach, 2000; Agency For Health Care Policy and Research, 1997).

Future research priorities related to CHI and decision making include:

- identifying factors that promote the use of information tools
- assessing the effects of tools on the nature and content of patient/clinician communication and related clinician workload
- assessing the effects of tools on health outcomes and health behavior, including quality of life
- comparing and examining the cost effectiveness of different types of patient informatics tools for specified objectives, such as improved decision tools that focus on analysis compared with tools that focus on patient education.

Various authors have identified specific areas for research. We should study the use of video, audio, and graphics to improve comprehension of health information by functionally illiterate individuals or those with suboptimal reading skills (Jimison & Sher, 1995). Tools to help clinicians obtain and interpret patient health-related preference data could aid in complex decision making and should be developed, tested, and incorporated into informatics systems (Volk et al., 1999). These preferences may be related to the structure, process, and outcomes of health actions.

Lewis (1999) identified a research agenda to study how people learn best using technology. This agenda included the impact of CHI applications on long-term healthcare outcomes (as measured by knowledge transfer, knowledge retention, adoption of healthy behaviors, skill development, and decision support); the impact on patient-professional relationships; the interactions between age, race, culture, and learning style; the impact of low literacy and socioeconomic status on learning style; the impact of mode of knowledge acquisition on the ability to solve healthcare problems; and retention of knowledge over time.

Other issues include:

- cost-benefit analysis and cost effectiveness
- the consequences of providing health information without the opportunity to validate comprehension, understanding, and the ability to integrate information
- innovative ways of integrating consumer needs and preferences into information management systems in clinical practice, education, and research
- the impact of CHI applications on patient-professional relationships.

All of these topics are important and must be explored more fully. The real challenge will be encouraging, integrating, and supporting this type of research. Because many programs have commercial applications, evaluation and research efforts may be minimized or neglected to speed a product to market. Faster and more adequate funding and collaborations between researchers and IHC developers may help facilitate this type of evaluation.

Looking Ahead

Between 1990 and 1995, only one article identified in a MEDLINE search specifically addressed consumer health informatics. Between 1995 and 2000, there were six more. Because the number of IHC applications is growing exponentially, we can expect a rapid increase in related publications that address many of the topics covered in this chapter.

The SPICH identified four overarching strategies related to IHC:

- strengthen evaluation and quality of IHC
- improve basic knowledge and understanding of IHC
- enhance capacity of stakeholders to develop and use IHC
- improve access to IHC for all populations.

Specific recommendations are made for each strategy. For instance, policy issues relevant to IHC evaluations include issues like oversight, regulatory, and legal issues, privacy and confidentiality, liability, payment and reimbursement, and access. As this field grows, these must be addressed (Patrick et al., 1999; Patrick & Koss, http://nii.nist.gov/pubs/chi.html).

For most of this century, health care was isolated from many of the market forces that have driven other industries to become more efficient and provide excellent customer service. However, market forces like managed care, large employer purchasing coalitions, government regulations, and consumer organizations are at work, and these will affect the fate of many IHC applications (Patrick et al., 1999; Mittman & Cain, 1990). To help patients realize the potential impact of consumer health informatics in the twenty-first century, IHC applications must become much more tailored, interactive, and integrated into cancer care (McRoy et al., 1998; De Vries & Brug, 1999; Taylor, 1996). Studies suggest that the benefits of IHC applications are broad and within reach. As CHI develops and the number and type of IHC applications in oncology grows, we must address the issues identified in this chapter. It is "fraught with potential."

Acknowledgments. The authors would like to thank Don Simborg and Mike Campbell for their thoughtful critique of this chapter and Caroline Fitzpatrick and Philippe Heckly for their technical assistance.

References

Agency for Health Care Policy and Research (AHCPR). 1997. Consumer Health Informatics and Patient Decision-Making. Final Report. Rockville, MD: U.S. Department of Health and Human Services, Agency for Health Care and Policy Research. AHCPR Publication 98-N001.

Balas E, Jaffrey F, Kuperman G, Boren S, Brown G, Pincirioli F, Mitchell J. 1997. Electronic Communication with Patients: Evaluation of Distance Medicine Technology. JAMA 278(2):152–159.

Barry MJ, Cherkin DC, Chang Y, Fowler FJ, Skates S. 1997. A Randomized Trial of a Multimedia Shared Decision Making Program for Men Facing a Treatment Decision for Benign Prostatic Hyperplasia. Disease Management and Clinical Outcomes 1(1):7–11.

Biermann JS, Golladay GJ, Greenfield ML, Baker LH. 1999. Evaluation of Cancer Information on the Internet. Cancer 86(3):381–390.

Bopp KD. 2000. Information Services that Make Patients Co-Producers of Quality Health Care. Information Technology Strategies from the United States and the European Union. Amsterdam: IOS Press, 93–106.

Borowitz SM, Wyatt J. 1998. The Origin, Content, and Workload of E-Mail Consultations. JAMA 280:1321–1324.

Brennan P. 1999. Health Informatics and Community Health: Support for Patients as Collaborators in Care. Methods of Information in Medicine 38:274–278.

Brennan P, Strombom I. 1998. Improving Health Care by Understanding Patient Preferences: The Role of Computer Technology. Journal of the American Medical Informatics Association 5:257–262.

Charnock D, Shepperd S, Needham G, Gann R. 1999. DISCERN: An Instrument for Judging the Quality of Written Consumer Health Information on Treatment Choices. Journal of Epidemiology and Community Health 53:105–111.

Cunningham AJ, Lockwood GA, Cunningham AJ. 1991. A Relationship Between Perceived Self Efficacy and Quality of Life in Cancer Patients. Patient Educational and Counseling 17:71–78.

DePalma A. 2000. Prostate Cancer Shared Decision: A CD-ROM Educational and Decision-Assisting Tool for Men with Prostate Cancer. Seminars in Urologic Oncology 18(3):78–81.

De Vries H, Brug J. 1999. Computer-Tailored Interventions Motivating People to Adopt Health-Promoting Behaviours: Introduction to a New Approach. Patient Education and Counseling 36:99–105.

Dumas J, Redish J. 1993. A Practical Guide to Usability Testing. Norwood, MA: Ablex Publishing Company.

Edwards A, Elwyn G. 1999. How Should Effectiveness of Risk Communication to Aid Patients' Decisions Be Judged? Medical Decision Making 19:428–434.

Eng TR, Gustafson DH, (eds.). 1999. Wired For Health and Well-Being: The Emergence of Interactive Communication. Science Panel on Interactive Communication and Health. Washington, D.C.: U.S. Department of Health and Human Services, U.S. Government Printing Office.

Eng TR, Gustafson D, Henderson J, Jimison HB, Patrick K. 1999. Introduction to the Evaluation of Interactive Health Communication Applications. American Journal of Preventive Medicine 16(1):10–15.

Eng TR, Maxfield A, Patrick K, Deering M, Ratzan S, Gustafson D. 1998. Access to Health Information and Support: A Public Highway or a Private Road? JAMA 280:1371–1375.

Entwistle V, Sheldon T, Sowden A, Watt I. 1998. Evidence-Informed Patient Choice: Practical Issues of Involving Patients in Decisions about Health Care Technologies. International Journal of Technology in Health Care 14:212–225.

Eysenbach G. 2000. Recent Advances: Consumer Health Informatics. British Medical Journal 320:1713-1716.

Eysenbach G, Diepgen TL. 1999. Labeling and Filtering of Medical Information on the Internet. Methods of Information in Medicine 38:80–88.

Ferguson T. 2000. Online Patient-Helps and Physicians Working Together: A New Partnership for High Quality Health Care. British Medical Journal 321:1129–1132.

Friedman R, Stollerman J, Mahoney D, Rozenblyum L. 1997. The Virtual Visit: Using Telecommunications Technology to Take Care of Patients. Journal of the American Medical Informatics Association 4:413–425.

Glenn J. 1996. A Consumer-Oriented Model for Evaluating Computer-Assisted Instructional Materials for Medical Education. Academic Medicine 71:251–255.

Graber M, Roller C, Kaeble B. 1999. Readability Levels of Patient Education Material on the World Wide Web. Journal of Family Practice 48:58–61.

Green LW, Kreuter MW, Deeds SG, Patridge KB. 1980. Health Education Planning: A Diagnostic Approach. Palo Alto, CA: Mayfield Publishing Co.

Gustafson D, Hawkins, R, Boberg E, Pingree S, Graziano F, Chan C. 1999. Impact of a Patient-Centered, Computer-Based Health Information/Support System Amercian Hournal of Preventive Medicine 16(1):1–9.

Gustafson D, McTavish F, Boberg E, Owens B, Sherbeck C, Wise M, Pingree S, Hawkins R. 1999. Empowering Patients Using Computer Based Health Support Systems. Quality Health Care 8(1):49–56.

Gustafson D, McTavish F, Hawkins R, Pingree S, Arora N, Mendenhall J, Simmons G. 1998. Computer Support for Elderly Women With Breast Cancer. JAMA 280(15):1305.

Gustafson D, Robinson T, Ansley D, Adler L, Brennan P. 1999. Consumers and Evaluation of Interactive Health Communication Applications. American Journal of Preventive Medicine 16(1):23–29.

Henderson J, Noell J, Reeves T, Robinson T, Strecher V. 1999. Developers and Evaluation of Interactive Health Communication Applications. American Journal of Preventive Medicine 16:30–34.

Hubbard SM. 2001. Information Systems in Oncology. In Devita VT, Hellman S, Rosenberg S, eds. Principles and Practice of Oncology. 6th ed. Philadelphia: Lippincott Williams & Wilkins.

Hubbard SM, Henney JE, Devita VT. 1987. A Computer Data Base for Information on Cancer Treatment. New England Journal of Medicine 316:315–318.

Houston TK, Ehrenberger H. 2001. The Potential of Consumer Informatics. Seminars in Oncology Nursing, 3135–3147.

Iansiti M, McCormick A. 1997. Developing Products on Internet Time. Harvard Business Review 75(5):107–117.

Internet Health Coalition. 2000. Ethics and the Internet: Consumers vs. Webmasters. Conducted by Harris Interactive Inc. Executive Summary, http://www.ihealthcoalition.org/content/harris_report2000.pdf. Accessed 11-1-2000.

Jadad A. 1999. Promoting Partnerships: Challenges for the Internet Age. British Medical Journal 319:761–763.

Jimison HB, Adler LJ, Coye M, Mulley AG, Eng TR. 1999. Health Care Providers and Purchasers and Evaluation of Interactive Health Communication Applications. American Journal of Preventive Medicine 16(1):16–22.

Jimison HB, Sher PP. 1995. Consumer Health Informatics: Health Information Technology for Consumers. Journal of the American Medical Informatics Association 46(10):783–790.

Jimison HB, Sher P, Appleyard R, Levernois Y. 1998. The Use of Multimedia in the Informed Consent Process. Journal of the American Medical Informatics Association 5:245–256.

Jones R, Pearson J, McGregor S, Cawsey A, Barrett A, Craig N, Atkinson J, Gilmour W, McEwen J. 1999. Randomised Trial of Personalised Computer Based Information for Cancer Patients. British Medical Journal 319:124–127.

Jones R, Pearson J, McGregor S, Gilmour W, Atkinson J, Barrett A, Cawsey A, Mcewen J. 1999. Cross Sectional Survey of Patients; Satisfaction with Information about Cancer. British Medical Journal 319:1247–1248.

Kane B, Sands DZ. The AMIA Internet Working Group. 1998. Task Force on Guidelines for the Use of Clinic-Patient Electronic Mail. Guidelines for the Clinical Use of Electronic Mail With Patients. Journal of the American Medical Informatics Association 5:104–111.

Kim P, Eng TR, Deering MJ, Maxfield, A. 1999. Published Criteria for Evaluating Health Related Web Sites. British Medical Journal 318:647–649.

Krishna S, Balas E, Spencer D, Griffin J, Borem S. 1997. Clinical Trials of Interactive Computerized Patient Education: Implications for Family Practice. Journal of Family Practice 45:25–33.

Leaffer T, Gonda B. 2000. The Internet: An Underutilized Tool in Patient Education. Computers in Nursing 18(1):47–52.

Lewis D. 1999. Computer-Based Approaches to Patient Education: A Review of the Literature. Journal of the American Medical Informatics Association 6: 272–282.

Leydon G, Boulton M, Moynihan C, Jones A, Mossman J, Boudioni M, McPherson K. 2000. Cancer Patients' Information Needs and Information Seeking Behaviour: In Depth Interview Study. British Medical Journal 320:909–913.

Mabley K. 2000. Privacy Versus Personalization. Cyber Dialogue. http://www.cyberdialogue.com.

Marteau T. 1989. Framing of Information: Its Influence upon the Decisions of Doctors and Patients. British Journal of Sexual Psychology 28:89–94.

Mayer D. 1999. Cancer Patient Empowerment. Oncology Nursing Updates 6(4):1–9.

Mayer D. 1998. Information. In Johnson B, Gross, J. (eds.) Handbook of Cancer Nursing 3rd ed. Boston: Jones and Bartlett, 263–277.

McConnaughey JW, Lader W, Chin R, Everette D. Falling Through the Net II: New Data on the Digital Divide. National Telecommunications and Information Administration, http://www.ntia.doc.gov/ntiahome/

McKinstry B. 2000. Do Patients Wish to be Involved in Decision Making in the Consultation? A Cross Sectional Survey with Video Vignettes. British Medical Journal 321: 867–871.

McNeil BJ, Pauker SG, Sox HC, Tversky A. 1982. On the Elicitation of Preferences for Alternative Therapies. New England Journal Medicine 306:1259–1262.

Mcroy S, Liu-Perez A, Ali S. 1998. Interactive Computerized Health Care Education. Journal of the American Medical Informatics Association 5(4):347–356.

Mittman R, Cain M. 1990. The Future of the Internet in Health Care. Oakland: California Health Care Foundation.

Mullen P, Green L, Persinger G. 1985. Clinical Trials of Patient Education for Chronic Conditions: A Comparative Meta-Analysis of Intervention Types. Preventive Medicine 14:753–781.

National Cancer Institute. 1992. Making Health Communication Programs Work: A Planner's Guide. Washington, D.C.: U.S. Department of Health and Human Services. NIH, 92–1493.

National Consumers League. E-Consumer Confidence Study. Posted on the Consumer Guide to Internet Safety Security and Privacy. http://www.nclnet.org/essentials/. Accessed 11/1/2000.

National Research Council. Committee on Maintaining Privacy and Security in Health Care Applications of the National Information Infrastructure. 1997. For the Record: Protecting Electronic Health Information. Washington, D.C.: National Academy Press, 1–288.

National Telecommunications and Information Administration. 2000. Falling Through the Net: Toward Digital Inclusion. Washington, D.C.: U.S. Department of Commerce.

Neilson J. http://www.usit.com

net2/falling.html. Accessed 11/1/2000.

Noell J, Glasgow R. 1999. Interactive Technology Applications for Behavioral Counseling: Issues and Opportunities for Health Care Settings. American Journal of Preventive Medicine 17(4):269–274.

O'Connor A, Rostom A, Fiset V, Tetroe J, Entwistle V, Llewellyn-Thoma H, Holmes-Rovner M, Barry M, Jones J. 1999. Decision Aids for Patients Facing Health Treatment or Screening Decisions: Systematic Review. British Medical Journal 319:731–734.

O'Connor V, Fiset V, Degrasse C, Graham I, Evans W, Dawn S, Laupacis A, Tugwell P. 1999. Decision Aids for Patients Considering Options Affecting Cancer Outcomes: Evidence of Efficacy and Policy Implications. Journal of the National Cancer Institute Monographs 25:67–80.

Patrick K, Koss S. Consumer Health Information White Paper. http://nii.nist.gov/pubs/chi.html. Accessed 11/2/00

Patrick K, Robinson T, Alemi F, Eng T. 1999. Policy Issues Relevant to Evaluation of Interactive Health Communication Applications. American Journal of Preventive Medicine 16(1):35–42.

Phillips KA, Bero LA. 1996. Improving the Use of Information in Medical Effectiveness Research. International Journal for Quality in Health Care 8(1):21–30.

Reents S. 1999. Impacts of the Internet on the Doctor-Patient Relationship: The Rise of the Internet Health Consumer. Cyber Dialogue. Available on www.cyberdialogue.com

Rimer B, Glassman B. 1999. Is There a Use for Tailored Print Communication in Cancer Risk Communication? Journal of the National Cancer Institute Monographs 25:140–148.

Rolnick S, Owens B, Botta R, Sathe L, Hawkins R, Cooper L, Kelley M, Gustafson D. 1999. Computerized Information and Support for Patients with Breast Cancer or HIV Infection. Nursing Outlook 47(2):78–83.

Robinson T, Patrick K, Eng TR, Gustafson D. 1998. An Evidence-Based Approach to Interactive Health Communication: A Challenge to Medicine in the Information Age. JAMA 280:1264–1269.

Ruland C. 1999. Decision Support for Patient Preference-Based Care Planning: Effects on Nursing Care and Patient Outcomes. Journal of the American Medical Informatics Association 6:304–312.

Shea S, Dumouchel W, Bahamonde L. 1996. A Meta-Analysis of 16 Randomized Controlled Trials to Evaluate Computer-Based Clincial Reminder Systems for Preventive Care in the Ambulatory Setting. Journal of the American Medical Informatics Association 3:399–409.

Shepperd S, Charnock D, Gann B. 1999. Helping Patients Access High Quality Health Information. British Medical Journal 319:764–766.

Sikorski R, Peters R. 1997. Oncology ASAP: Where to Find Reliable Cancer Information on the Internet. JAMA 277(18):1431–1432.

Skinner C, Siegfried J, Kegler M, Strecher V. 1993. The Potential of Computers in Patient Education. Patient Education and Counseling 22:27–34.

Spielberg A. 1998. Sociohistorical, Legal, and Ethical Implications Of E-Mail For The Patient-Physician Relationship. JAMA 280:1353–1359.

Spool J. 1999. Web Site Usability: A Designer's Guide. San Francisco, CA: Morgan Kaufmann Publishers, Inc.

Staggers N, Gassert CA, Skiba DJ. 1999. Health Professionals' Views of Informatics Education: Findings from the AMIA 1999 Spring Conference. Journal of the American Medical Informatics Association 7:550–558.

Strecher VJ. 1999. Computer Tailored Smoking Cessation Materials: A Review and Discussion. Patient Education and Counseling 36:107–117.

Tang P, Newcomb C. 1998. Informing Patients: A Guide for Providing Patient Health Information. Journal of the American Medical Informatics Association 5:563–570.

Taylor P. 1996. Consumer Health Informatics: Emerging Issues. Washington, D.C.: U.S. General Accounting Office. GAO/AIMD-96-86.

Tetzlaff L. 1997. Consumer Informatics in Chronic Illness. Journal of the American Medical Informatics Association 4:285–300.

Thompson S, Pitts J, Schwankovsky L. 1993. Preferences for Involvement in Medical Decision-Making: Situational and Demographic Influences. Patient Education and Counseling 22:133–140.

Treacy J, Mayer DK. 2000. Perspectives on Patient Education. Seminars in Oncology Nursing 16(1):47–56.

Volk RJ, Cass AR, Spann SJ. 1999. A Randomized Controlled Trial of Shared Decision Making for Prostate Cancer Screening. Archives of Family Medicine 8(4):333–340.

Walker EA. 1999. Characteristics of the Adult Learner. The Diabetes Educator 25(Suppl 6):16–24.

Wilson F, Baker L, Brown-Syed C, Gollop C. 2000. An Analysis of the Readability and Cultural Sensitivity of Information on the National Cancer Institute's Web Site: CancerNet. Oncology Nursing Forum 27(9):1403–1409.

26
An Internet-Based Data System for Outcomes Research

Joyce C. Niland

As the Division of Cancer Control and Population Sciences (DCCPS) of the National Cancer Institute outlined in their 1999 report, *Surveillance Research Implementation Plan*, there is a paucity of resources available for collecting high-quality data focusing on the processes and outcomes of cancer care. A 1999 National Cancer Policy Board (NCPB) report also emphasized the significant deficiencies in the delivery system for cancer care, particularly related to the measurement of the appropriateness and outcomes of cancer care. Unfortunately there are no uniform standards in existence for measuring the quality of cancer care, and the scant evidence that is available suggests that the quality of care is very uneven at best. Further, an increasing number of people in the United States are receiving health care from managed care organizations that have a financial disincentive to provide expensive treatments, and subsequently many are concerned that they may be receiving cost-effective but suboptimal medical care (Widman & Tong, 1997).

With cancer ranking as the second leading cause of death in the United States, these issues have a substantial impact on our nation's health and healthcare expenditures. The NCPB report went on to describe an effective system for quality of cancer care as one that would capture information about individuals with cancer; their condition; their treatment, including significant outpatient treatments; their providers; site of care delivery; type of care delivery system; and the patients' outcomes. The assertion was made that it is unlikely that a single database can meet all of the various objectives of such systems, including cancer surveillance, research, and quality monitoring. However, over the past four years the City of Hope National Medical Center has created and maintained an Internet-based data system for the National Comprehensive Cancer Network (NCCN) Outcomes Research Project that we believe meets all of these objectives. The system described here is proving to yield extremely valuable data that can be used to improve the quality of cancer care across the nation.

The NCCN Outcomes Research Project

The NCCN is a coalition of 19 cancer centers from across the United States (located at City of Hope National Medical Center, Dana-Farber Cancer Institute, Duke Comprehensive Cancer Center, Fox Chase Cancer Center, Fred Hutchinson Cancer Research Center, H. Lee Moffit Cancer Center and Research Institute, University of Utah, Johns Hopkins, M.D. Anderson Cancer Center, Memorial Sloan Kettering Cancer Center, Northwestern University, Ohio State University, Roswell Park Cancer Institute, Stanford University Medical Center, St. Jude's Children's Research Hospital, University of California at San Francisco, University of Alabama at Birmingham, University of Michigan, University of Nebraska, and University of Utah). The NCCN's mission is to identify the most efficacious and cost-effective strategies for the management of common oncologic conditions. To this end 42 active disease panels made up of experts from these centers have developed and published evidence-based guidelines for the diagnosis, primary treatment, adjuvant treatment, and follow-up of the majority of cancer sites, based on clinical trials results whenever available. More than 90 guidelines have been developed, covering over 95% of all cancer sites, and these are updated annually to remain current.

The NCCN Outcomes Research Project, initiated in 1997, has as its goals the recording of the patterns of care and outcomes for patients treated in the NCCN institutions and their affiliates. The objectives are to assess the degree of concordance between actual treatment administered and the recommended treatment based on NCCN guidelines, and to provide a feedback loop to the disease panels to continually improve the guidelines in practice. Improving our knowledge about the quality of care requires the adoption of a common set of data elements to be collected, creation of a central database system and repository to store these elements, and a mechanism for querying and reporting the results. City of Hope was selected as the Data Coordinating Center of the Outcomes Research Project, and was charged with the design and implementation of a database system to support these goals.

In 1997 relatively few research studies were utilizing the Web for data collection/transmission, owing to the inherently public nature of the Internet and the complexity of the technological aspects of building such systems. However, we recognized the power and efficiencies that could be gained from deployment of a system via the Internet, particularly in such a widespread, nationally coordinated project. Therefore our database design specifications called for the implementation of a central repository that combined the familiarity of the Web environment with its cross-platform compatibility and real-time data access and submission capabilities via the Internet.

In describing this system we will organize the discussion around the mnemonic with which we began the introduction to Section 4, "HIT": the human, information, and technological aspects. We present these factors in reverse sequence, which we believe follows an increasing degree of difficulty when developing and deploying informatics applications.

The Technology

To provide nationwide access to the system in real time, the Internet seemed to be the natural choice for the database system interchange platform. The database system designed at City of Hope consists of a relational database system based on a client-server model. A Web browser interface is deployed on the client side, and the database utilizes Microsoft's MS SQL Server, Version 6.5, on the server side. Client-side tools include Active Server Pages (ASP), Java, and JavaScript. The application allows direct data entry via Web screens, incorporating pull-down menus, close-ended coding, and built-in error checking to preserve high data quality.

We also wanted to leverage existing forms of electronic data at the Cancer Centers and to avoid redundant effort and data entry. Therefore the system provides the alternative of transmitting electronic files to City of Hope using the File Transfer Protocol (FTP) as the mode of transmission. One consideration is that this option imposes programming overhead on the centers that choose FTP transmission. In contrast, data entry over the Web requires no local programming support, so this is a key factor that must be considered in setting up a new center to contribute to the database. The various options for data transmission and the high-level system architecture are represented in Figure 26.1.

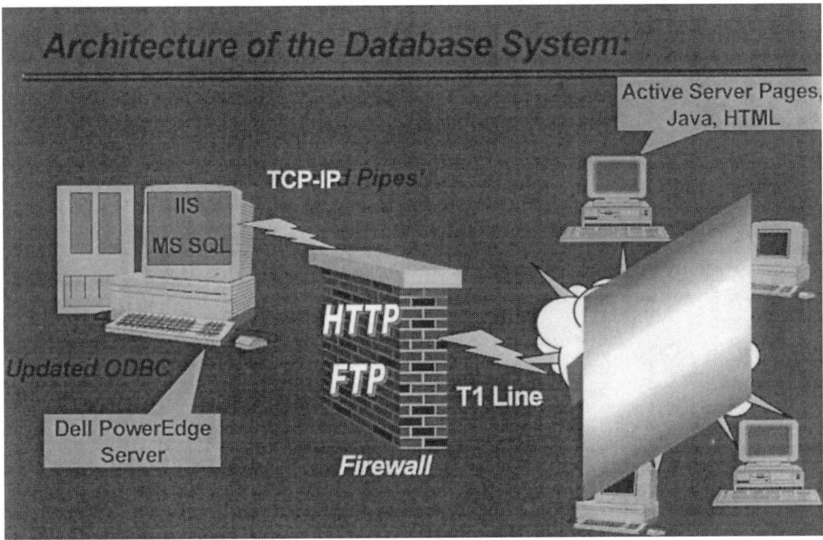

FIGURE 26.1. High-level architecture of the Internet-based outcomes research database system.

Fiberoptic cabling links the Internet through the City of Hope firewall, a security precaution to ensure that only valid users are allowed into City of Hope systems. A T1 line connects the system to the Internet "cloud," that in turn provides the connection to each of the work stations at the various centers located nationwide. The system is platform-independent such that it can be utilized on any type of workstation. The Web screens are browser-independent, and this interface is now very familiar to most people, minimizing the amount of training required and facilitating ease of use.

Since the system was first deployed in July 1997, improvements and enhancements have been made to the application architecture. Initially two separate servers were located at City of Hope, one on which the Internet Information Server (IIS) resided for Internet access, connecting to a separate server running MS SQL Server. However, after several months of deployment, user feedback indicated that this was not the optimal approach to ensure stable and efficient database connectivity. Therefore IIS and MS SQL were loaded onto a single server. This, along with an updated ODBC connection, greatly improved system performance factors.

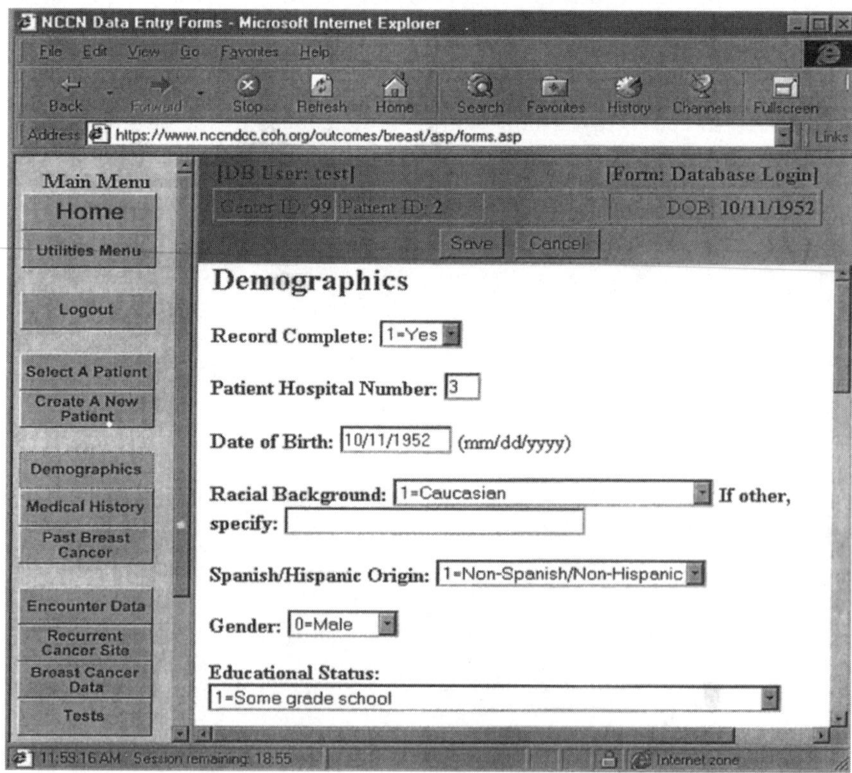

FIGURE 26.2. Web-based demographic data entry screen. (Reprinted with permission from nccndcc.coh.org)

An example of a Web-based data entry screen, showing fictitious demographic data, is provided in Figure 26.2. The menu bar on the left side of the screen displays the relational tables of the database into which data are entered. The user creates a new patient or selects an existing one to call up a form display for a particular table of the database for the patient. A convenient status bar at the top of the screen always indicates which patient has been selected. Date of birth is used as a secondary cross-check to ensure that the correct study number has been selected. For every field that involves a closed system of codes, drop-down menus of code selections are employed. The user clicks on the code desired and the corresponding value is automatically entered into the field.

A significant issue in Web application development is the ability to ensure that the database and the user interface are synchronized with respect to the application's current "state." When a user is progressing through a Web-enabled database application, pressing the "forward" and "back" buttons on the Web browser can result in a mismatch between the application state reflected in the user interface and the application state of the database. To maintain state synchronization, the application disables the ability to "cache" user interface pages in display memory. The Web browser is then forced to regenerate (synchronize) all pages from information maintained in application memory. When users press the "save" button in a data entry form, the information is committed to the database and immediately followed by a refresh to reflect the updated content on the screen. When users press the "cancel" button, an immediate refresh discards all input associated with the cancelled operation and prepares the data entry form for the next update.

While system security is of the utmost importance for any clinical research system, this is particularly crucial when transmitting data over the Internet. We have included two levels of ID/password authorization within the application, one at the document management page and another at the actual data entry/view level. This allows differing levels of access rights to be assigned to users, appropriate to their relationship to the study. For example, the data manager and investigator may have access to the data entry/view level, while the project secretary is given access to the document management page. New versions of the data dictionary, manual of operations, and system specifications are posted here for the centers to download and print the material at their sites. This eliminates the need for mailing paper, facsimile transmission, or sending attachments of electronic files by e-mail, which can often lead to incompatibility issues.

Data encryption is in place for both the Web entry (via Secure Socket Layers) and FTP transmission (via Pretty Good Privacy). User authentication is achieved via digital certificates issued by Verisign. View restriction has been built into the system to ensure that each center is allowed to view and edit only their own data. Daily and weekly backup tapes and disaster recovery are in place, and routine system assessments and audit trails are employed. These security procedures for the NCCN data system conform with all the recommendations of the National Research Council for protecting electronic health information (Frawley and Asmonga, 1997). A summary of the data security features of the outcomes research database system is given in Table 26.1.

The Information Structure

The initial cancer site chosen by the NCCN for this national outcomes study was breast cancer, due to its high incidence and significant impact on public health. One of the most challenging efforts to date in the NCCN project was the development of and agreement upon a standardized common data dictionary to support outcomes research for breast cancer. This process required monthly conference calls and regular meetings of the investigators throughout the first year of the project. Variables were iteratively proposed, aligned with the project objectives, and refined. Critical to the process was the use of standard coding schemas and vocabularies to ensure alignment with existing electronic data sources and other national studies. The result is a set of well-defined and documented process and outcome measures necessary to collect uniform accurate data on care patterns, treatment results, and concordance with treatment guidelines.

The data dictionary contains approximately 250 elements, considered to be the minimal set required to capture all necessary treatment fields and key outcomes. Major classes of data elements include:

- ***Demographics.*** Age, ethnicity, zip code, education, employer, insurer, employment status
- ***Clinical Data.*** Stage, histology, menopausal status, comorbidity, type and duration of all surgery, chemotherapy, and radiation, clinical trial participation
- ***Outcomes.*** Employment status, days lost from work, hospital days, performance status, tumor response, overall survival, disease-free survival.

Automated tools are being developed for creating and managing the metadata, "data about the data", and workflow analysis is on-going to optimize the processes associated with information collection, transmission, and management (Jimenez, Dicksen, Nob et al., 1996). This is particularly critical in a multi-center study of this nature, with the intention to scale up to additional cancer sites that will require extension of coding schema and addition of new disease-specific fields. The metadata repository is crucial to those centers that are transmitting data to the repository by creating export files from their legacy data systems. In this instance the local programmers need to map their existing data to the precise codes and terms specified by the NCCN common data dictionary. This process can be quite complex, and requires review and input from the Data Coordinating Center and Scientific

TABLE 26.1. Features of the Internet-based outcomes research data system

Security Features	Description
Data encryption (SSL)	The Secure Socket Layer (SSL) protocol is enabled on the NCCN Web server. Since data being transmitted over the Internet/intranet to the NCCN application include patient information and user passwords, SSL establishes a secure, encrypted channel between the Web server and each client browser, protecting all data in transit from eavesdroppers.
Web authentication	The Web application is password-protected, requiring users to submit a valid user name and unique password before access is granted. A limited number of application-level activities can be performed without access to the database (i.e., downloading release notes, data collection forms, and other documents). However, access to the database requires an additional unique password. Once established, all password-authenticated connections are maintained throughout the session duration.
User sensitive selection	Once the application and the database authenticate a user's identity, the user may choose to display only those options that are relevant to them. For example, each user can only enter information about patients at the center to which the user belongs. Information from patients at other participating institutions will not be available to the user through this application.
View restriction	Because the source code of HTML pages cannot be hidden from the users, technically oriented users may attempt to save a page locally, modify the selection list, and submit the data from their local machine. This action potentially compromises the restrictions set for the users in the HTML code. Therefore, a more rigid protection scheme is involved on the database server back end, by placing users in a database view where they can only access data that they are authorized to use. If users fabricated the selection list and tried to access unauthorized data, their action would be blocked by the view restriction. This scheme, combined with the User Sensitive Selection described above, makes the application operate within a very restricted realm of the database.
Side door access	When users are issued a database password, they are, in theory, entitled to access the database using any program that is capable of communicating with Microsoft SQL Server. Many such programs and utilities are readily available on the Internet and can be considered "unofficial side doors" for accessing the database, would explicitly bypass the data validation and integrity checks that have been added to the "official" Web application. To prevent unauthorized side door access, when users login to the database through the Web application via their regular account, the application automatically switches them to a "secret" account. All subsequent database requests are performed through this secret account, so that the user cannot inadvertently or deliberately utilize a side door access.

Table 26.1. (*Continued*)

Disaster Recovery	Description
Database backup	The database transaction log is copied to a 4-mm tape drive four times per day, and a full database backup is performed weekly. Each 4-mm tape is used to hold one week of backup data, and each tape is kept for three months before being overwritten.
Off-site tape storage	Monthly tapes are delivered to the Information Technology Services department for local storage in their fireproof vault. In addition a copy is transported to an off-site storage location in Phoenix, Arizona (well away from California earthquake fault lines!).
System Audit Trails	**Description**
Web level	Microsoft's Internet Information Server provides built-in functionality to record every request submitted to the Web server, including username, date, time, IP address, and a variety of additional usage statistics. This information is placed directly into an MS SQL Server table and is reviewed using WebTrends (Portland, OR) analysis software.
Database level	Although MS SQL Server does not include a built-in auditing system, a simple yet effective alternative was implemented in the Web application by recording every SQL command, the submitting user, and the time it was captured in separate database table hidden from users. Data in this audit log can easily be retrieved, analyzed, and cross-checked with Web level audit reports to resolve any inconsistencies and database errors.

Office staff before implementation, to ensure that the mapping is correct and that common definitions are being applied correctly.

The data in the central repository are "de-identified" and a unique study number is assigned to each patient for transmission to City of Hope; no other primary identifiers such as name or medical record number are included in the central repository. The patient's medical record number and name are retained at the individual NCCN member institution, along with the linkage to the unique study number. Still the data cannot be considered fully "anonymous," in that certain data elements are included that might allow ultimate identification of a case if intentional efforts were made to match the study data against some other source of information. An example might be matching the combination of date of birth, specific histology, and zip code. Yet these fields are considered essential elements for the type of research that is being conducted and must be captured for analysis purposes. Therefore additional precautions are being taken in case an intruder should attempt to intercept the data as they are being transmitted over the Internet. A secure, encrypted channel is established between the Web server and each client browser, protecting the data in transit from "eavesdroppers." The data are also protected behind the City of Hope firewall, as noted previously.

Data quality and completeness are critical features of the information structure. Strict quality control procedures are in place for the project, similar to the conduct of a multi-centered national clinical trial. These measures include standardized operating procedures, initial on-site staff training, online data entry editing, computerized quality assurance checks of the centralized data, annual audits of a randomly chosen subset of the medical records at each institution, Web posting of responses to FAQs (Frequently Asked Questions), and on-going staff training annually. Quality assurance mechanisms are built into the system through error checking at the time of data entry. For example, if a user makes an error in format when entering a date field, the system will flash a warning message and will not allow further data entry until the error has been corrected. Logic checks are also run on the tables of the central pooled database after the data have been transmitted to City of Hope.

Quarterly reports of the data are run and centrally distributed to all participating centers, including averages and ranges of treatment modalities for all centers in the database combined. In addition, the principal investigators at each Cancer Center receive the results for their particular institution. Individual center results are not revealed to the other NCCN members. Each center also receives a list of those patients who were treated in some manner that was inconsistent with the guidelines, so they can examine these cases individually. Reasons for non-concordance may include patient preference, local practice patterns, individual treatment choice of a given physician, or a reflection that the guidelines need further enhancement or revision. In this last instance this information is transmitted to the disease committee for consideration for possible revision or updating of the guidelines as needed, thus closing the feedback loop.

In addition to the adherence and patterns of care analyses that can be performed using the NCCN database, hypothesis-driven analyses to examine relationships between treatment patterns and outcomes are underway as well. The analytic and reporting tools paired with the database system are on the leading edge of recent advancements of the SAS statistical software package. The SAS system connects directly with Microsoft's SQL Server, providing a seamless interface to the database. This provides an extremely efficient and powerful tool for data analysis of the central repository. Another new feature of SAS includes Web tools that will direct the results generated by SAS procedures to an HTML-formatted file that can be directly viewed and printed from a Web browser.

The initial data model was for a single disease site while we established proof of concept that common outcomes data could be collected from multiple centers via the Internet. Once this had been successfully confirmed, we needed to ensure that the database design was sufficiently scalable as the project grows to include a number of different cancer sites. In 1999 the data dictionary was extended to capture outcomes data on the second major cancer diagnosis to be studied, non-Hodgkins lymphoma (NHL). An integrated database model was developed to support the incorporation of additional oncologic disease sites with relative ease, and with minimal future reprogramming of the file structure for those sites using the FTP transmission mode. In this new model, common data tables are utilized for all data that are shared across disease sites, and a minimal set of disease-specific tables are added to capture elements that are unique to the new oncologic condition. Data from the breast cancer project have now been migrated into this integrated data model, and the NHL-specific data tables have been added. Data collection for NHL began in December 2000, and the first transmissions of NHL data from the FTP sites took place in 2001. The application is now poised to scale up readily to study several additional major forms of cancer care and outcomes over the next few years.

The Human Factor

Probably the most important and complex issue to deal with in the deployment of a database application is the *human-computer interface* (HCI). A primary goal in the system design must be to ensure a high level of user acceptance of the application. Therefore we elicited frequent user feedback during the design and testing phase, and piloted early prototypes of the Web screens with our local data management staff, to raise the likelihood of user acceptance when the system was deployed nationwide.

One of our main objectives was to ensure that the Web data-entry process was efficient and simple. Therefore the system was designed to be natural and consistent with respect to navigation. The tool bars and menus always appear in the same location on the screen, allowing the user to move around the system easily. Drop-down coding boxes provide the capability to "point and click" on the correct code to enter a coded value. "Save" and "cancel" buttons are located at both the top and bottom of each screen for ease of use. Changes to the data can be made easily by calling up an existing patient's record, correcting the information, and clicking on the "save" button. Wherever possible the data dictionary coding conforms with other coding systems already commonly in place, such as that for the American College of Surgeons, so that terms and definitions are familiar to the users. This allows future comparisons with other major databases that utilize these coding schemes as well.

A key feature designed to enhance user acceptance is the ease with which the individual centers can obtain access to their own data stored in the central repository. Centers using the Web site for data entry are capturing very valuable information, but then immediately send it off to the central repository at City of Hope by a click on the "save" button. It was recognized that investigators at these centers would want to have local access to their own data. This was incorporated through a download feature that can be invoked by the user at any time, retrieving their most recent data directly from the central database and downloading the file to their own hard disk. For centers with minimal programming support, a "seed" Access database shell also is maintained on the Web site. The database shell can be downloaded and merged with the exported data files for subsequent analysis and reporting at the center. (As with data entry, the system allows retrieval of only the individual center's data and not the pooled aggregate data.)

When we began this project in 1997 there were many challenges associated with adopting such relatively new technology for critical entry and transmission of medical research data. To determine the success of this medium in the users' eyes, we conducted a survey of the 35 system users performing data entry via the NCCN Web application after several months of experience with the system. The majority of respondents rated the system as "good" to "excellent" with respect to layout and flow of the Web site, ease of downloading documents, ease of use as a database entry system, usefulness of online logic checks, and ease of use as a database reporting system.

The training that was provided was found to be very satisfactory in orienting the users to the system. However, some less experienced users indicated that on-going advice would be helpful with this new technology. Therefore our lead programmer was added as a participant on the monthly data management conference calls to field questions and discuss new system features as they are introduced. It was also determined that computer training would be an integral component of the annual training program held for the research staff.

The survey made us aware of a simple yet important logistical problem. While the technical support provided by the Data Coordinating Center generally was found to be very helpful to users, some users cited the lack of technical support in the early morning hours for centers on the East Coast, due to the different time zone at City of Hope, located 20 miles from downtown Los Angeles. Once recognized, this issue was resolved readily by providing our lead developer with a cell phone that is manned during all working hours for the spectrum of time zones encompassed by the study. If simple matters like this remain undetected and are not addressed, they can lead to dissatisfaction and "revolt" among the system users.

The survey queried the users regarding the speed and consistency of access to the Web-based system. Compared to other Web sites the users rated the connection speed as "about the same" in most cases, but as being "a little slower" for some users. This led to the most surprising and critical finding of the survey, that many users had been encountering connectivity problems over the past few months. The frequency of interruptions ranged from less than once per month to close to daily problems for two users. Diagnostics run at City of Hope showed that most of these interruptions were occurring at the database connection level, making data entry slower than necessary. This result led to system architecture re-design and database connectivity upgrades, which greatly improved system performance and stability, as determined by central testing and a follow-up user survey.

Continued user feedback over the years has led to several application enhancements over time, including: user-specified record completion flags to indicate when a record has been completely researched and data entered; posting of quality assurance checks on the Web for rectification by the data manager; the ability to conditionally link main menus with the appropriate sub-item menu based on the entered choice; the capability of the user to change and maintain their own passwords online; an automated patient scheduling function to facilitate data collection on returning patients; and a technique to allow the FTP sites to run diagnostics on their data file prior to submission to City of Hope, ensuring that the files will load correctly into the central database.

After 4 years of data collection the NCCN database now contains more than 240,000 records of longitudinal data on over 7000 women with breast cancer, and we have begun accumulating data on NHL patients. Analyses of the accumulating data have been presented at the annual NCCN Outcomes Conferences held in Fort Lauderdale in March of 1999 and 2000 (Weeks & Niland, 1999; Niland, 2000).

Looking Ahead

A recent "request for proposal" was issued by the DCCPS of the NCI, with the goals of determining organizational and structural changes necessary to improve the cost efficiency, accuracy, completeness, and standardization of data collection beyond the Cancer Center setting. City of Hope was awarded a one-year grant to extend the Internet-based outcomes research application to five community-based facilities distributed across Southern California. We are developing a graphical decision support interface that will be contrasted with the standard Web data entry process to determine the most effective mode of capturing data while simultaneously promoting guideline usage in the community oncology setting.

This community study will help determine the quality and completeness of data collected in this setting, and increase our understanding of the time and effort required to extend collection of medical, treatment, and outcomes data to practicing oncologists and community hospitals. Efforts to determine how the assembled population compares to the population-at-risk will be important in developing later studies designed to include additional settings and targeting patients from those populations, especially within underserved and minority communities. We will also study the impact of providing decision support at the point of care on concordance levels with nationally developed treatment guidelines.

Our observation to date in the NCCN setting is that the mere fact of measuring and reporting on patterns of care has already improved awareness, surveillance, and treatment patterns in the participating centers. Extending such data collection efforts to the community could well result in improved quality of care in this setting as well, through the feedback loop provided and the heightened awareness that access to such valuable information will bring. The potential impact of such an Internet-based outcomes data application on generating uniform standards and data for measuring and improving the quality of cancer care throughout the nation is tremendous.

References

Frawley KA, Asmonga D. 1997. For the Record: Protecting Electronic Health Information, Committee on Maintaining Privacy and Security in Health Care Applications of the National Information Infrastructure, National Research Council. Washington, D.C.: National Academy Press 68(5):12–14.

Jimenez A, Dicksen K, Noble W, Butler S, Gunther K, Niland JC. 1996. Data Dictionary: A Tool to Expedite Information Systems Integration. Journal of the American Medical Informatics Association, Symposium Supplement, 83.

Niland JC. 2000. NCCN Outcomes Research Database: Data Collection Via the Internet. Oncology 14:11A.

Weeks JC, Niland JC. 1999. NCCN Oncology Outcomes Database: An Update. A Report from NCCN's 1999 4th Annual Conference. Managed Care and Cancer 32–35.

Widman LE, Tong DA. 1997. Requests for Medical Advice from Patients and Families to Health Care Providers Who Publish on the World Wide Web. Archives of Internal Medicine, 157(2):151–152.

Index

O

P

Health Informatics Series
(formerly Computers in Health Care)

Computerizing Large Integrated Health Networks
The VA Success
R.M. Kolodner

Organizational Aspects of Health Informatics
Managing Technological Change
N.M. Lorenzi and R.T. Riley

Transforming Health Care Through Information
Case Studies
N.M. Lorenzi, R.T. Riley, M.J. Ball, and J.V. Douglas

Trauma Informatics
K.I. Maull and J.S. Augenstein

Advancing Federal Sector Health Care
A Model for Technology Transfer
P. Ramsaroop, M.J. Ball, D. Beaulieu and J.V. Douglas

Medical Informatics
Computer Applications in Health Care and Biomedicine, Second Edition
E.H. Shortliffe and L.E. Perreault

Filmless Radiology
E.L. Siegel and R.M. Kolodner

Cancer Informatics
Essential Technologies for Clinical Trials
J.S. Silva, M.J. Ball, C.G. Chute, J.V. Douglas, C.P. Langlotz, J.C. Niland, and W.L. Scherlis

Knowledge Coupling
New Premises and New Tools for Medical Care and Education
L.L. Weed